Client Management
and Leadership **Success**

A Course Review Applying Critical Thinking Skills to Test Taking

Client Management and Leadership Success

A Course Review Applying Critical Thinking Skills to Test Taking

Ray Hargrove-Huttel, RN, PhD
Trinity Valley Community College
Kaufman, Texas

Kathryn Cadenhead Colgrove, RN, MS, CNS, OCN
Trinity Valley Community College
Kaufman, Texas

F. A. DAVIS COMPANY • Philadelphia

F. A. Davis Company
1915 Arch Street
Philadelphia, PA 19103
www.fadavis.com

Printed in the United States of America

Last digit indicates print number: 10 9 8 7 6 5

Publisher, Nursing: Robert G. Martone
Director of Content Development: Darlene D. Pedersen
Senior Project Editor: Padraic J. Maroney
Design and Illustrations Manager: Carolyn O'Brien

As new scientific information becomes available through basic and clinical research, recommended treatments and drug therapies undergo changes. The author(s) and publisher have done everything possible to make this book accurate, up to date, and in accord with accepted standards at the time of publication. The author(s), editors, and publisher are not responsible for errors or omissions or for consequences from application of the book, and make no warranty, expressed or implied, in regard to the contents of the book. Any practice described in this book should be applied by the reader in accordance with professional standards of care used in regard to the unique circumstances that may apply in each situation. The reader is advised always to check product information (package inserts) for changes and new information regarding dose and contraindications before administering any drug. Caution is especially urged when using new or infrequently ordered drugs.

ISBN 10: 0-8036-2043-8
ISBN 13: 978-0-8036-2043-8

Reviewers

Valerie Allen, RN, MSN
Professor
Somerset Community College
Somerset, Kentucky

Patrica Balkcom, RN, MSN
Director of Nursing
Central Georgia Technical College
Milledgeville, Georgia

Doreen Biondolillo, RN, MSN
Nurse Educator
West Suffolk BOCES
Suffolk County Community College
East Northport, New York

Wonda L. Brown, RN, MSN
Nursing Instructor
Connors State College
Muskogee, Oklahoma

Lindsey L. Carlson, MSN, RN
Adjunct Instructor
William Jewell College
Liberty, Missouri

Carmela Theresa de Leon, BSN, RN, MAN
Active Medical Surgical RN
Banner Gateway Medical Center
Mesa, Arizona

Donna M. Garbacz Bader, MA, MSN, RN,
BC D-ABMDI
Assistant Professor
BryanLGH College of Health Sciences
Lincoln, Nebraska

Jan Hartig, MSN, RN
Assistant Professor
BryanLGH College of Health Sciences
Lincoln, Nebraska

Karla R. Jones, RN, MS
Associate Professor
University of Alaska
Anchorage, Alaska

Tami J. Rogers, DVM, MSN, BSN
Professor
Valencia Community College
Orlando, Florida

Patricia Rondaris, RN, MSN, MBA
Director, Risk/Quality/Education
METRO HEALTH
Old Brooklyn Campus
Case Western Reserve University
Cleveland, Ohio

Karen Moore Schaefer, PhD, RN
Associate Chair
Temple University
Philadelphia, Pennsylvania

Karla Scholl, MSN, RN
Assistant Professor
BryanLGH College of Health Sciences
Lincoln, Nebraska

Cynthia Small, RN, MSN, APRN-BC
Instructor
Lake Michigan College
Benton Harbor, Michigan

Lisa Streeter, MS, RN
Instructor
St. Elizabeth College of Nursing
Utica, New York

Sharon J. Thompson, PhD, RN, MPH
Assistant Professor
Gannon University
Erie, Pennsylvania

Marjorie Vogt, PhD, CNP
Associate Professor
Otterbein College
Westerville, Ohio

Acknowledgment

We would like to thank the sophomore students of Trinity Valley Community College Associate Degree Nursing program for their support in this endeavor. They unselfishly spent time piloting the questions and providing feedback for this book. Without Robert Martone's vision and continuous support, this book would not have been possible. Barbara Tchbovsky is the best editor with whom anyone could have the honor of working. With her editorial abilities and expertise, this dream has become a book of which we are very proud. Thanks go to Glada Norris for her phenomenal computer skills; she always makes it look pretty.

Ray A. Hargrove-Huttel

This is my fourth book since I started my nursing career over 30 years ago. Without the support of my nursing colleagues, my college chums, my bowling buddies, and my wonderful friends, none of this would have been possible. To all of you, and you know who you are, thank you. My family has always been my rock: my sisters Gail and Debbie, my nephew Benjamin and Paula, my grandparents, my aunts, uncles, and cousins have always been there for me. My children, Teresa and Aaron, always keep my life interesting, and without them life would be so boring. As always, I dedicate this book to my father and mother, TSgt. Leo R. and Nancy Hargrove, and to my husband, who will always be with me, Hans Jorgen "Bill" Huttel.

Kathryn Cadenhead Colgrove

I would like to acknowledge my friend Sandra Chilcoat and the people who have formed my nursing experiences; my nursing school colleagues; the staff of 4 North, IV Team, IV Clinic, and the administration of Doctors Hospital from 1974 to 1995; and the faculty, staff, and students of Trinity Valley Community College from 1995 to now. I truly have learned and grown and been blessed to have been associated with you. My family has always been the most important aspect of my life. Thank you for your love and patience. Special thanks go to my husband, Larry, daughter, Laurie, and son-in-law, Todd, son, Larry Jr., and daughter-in-law, Mai, and the most wonderful group of young people in the world, my grandchildren Christopher, Ashley, Justin C., Justin A., Connor, and Sawyer.

Table of Contents

Critical Thinking Strategies Related to Nursing and Client Management

"Each problem that I solved became a rule which served afterwards to solve other problems."

—René Descartes

This book is part of a series of books, published by F.A. Davis Company, designed to assist the student nurse in nursing school and in taking examinations, particularly the NCLEX-RN exam for licensure as a registered nurse (RN).

Client Management and Leadership Success: A Course Review Applying Critical Thinking Skills to Test Taking focuses on three aspects of management: setting priorities for client care, delegating and assigning nursing tasks, and managing clients and staff. It contains practice questions on these topics in a wide variety of nursing arenas, including medical, surgical, critical care, pediatric, geriatric, rehabilitation, home health, and mental health nursing. Answers—and why each possible response is correct or incorrect—are given for all questions.

Management, prioritizing, and delegation questions are some of the most difficult questions for the student and new graduate to answer because there is no reference book in which to find the correct answers. Answers to these types of questions require knowledge of basic scientific principles, leadership, standards of care, pathophysiology, and psychosocial behaviors, as well as the ability to think critically. The test taker should not read the rationale for the incorrect answers. During an examination, the test taker will remember reading the information but not if it is correct or incorrect data. The test taker should go back to the textbooks and try to understand why the correct answer is correct.

Many of the answers in this book include tips to help the test taker. Termed "Making Nursing Decisions," these tips provide help for the student in identifying exactly what the question is asking, in analyzing the question, and in determining the correct response. A Comprehensive Examination with answers and rationales is also included for each field of nursing.

Practice questions and answers and practice examinations are valuable in preparing for an examination, but the test taker should remember that there is no substitute for studying the material. For general information on how to prepare for an examination and on the types of questions used in nursing examinations, refer to *Fundamentals Success: A Course Review Applying Critical Thinking to Test Taking* by Patricia Nugent, RN, MA, MS, EdD, and Barbara Vitale, RN, MA.

NCSBN BLUEPRINT FOR QUESTIONS

The National Council of State Boards of Nursing (NCSBN) provides a blueprint that assists nursing faculty in developing test questions for the NCLEX-RN. Content included in management of care provides and directs nursing care that enhances the care delivery setting to protect clients, family/significant others, and health-care personnel. Related content includes, but is not limited to, advance directives, advocacy, case management, client rights, collaboration with the interdisciplinary team, delegation, establishing priorities, ethical practice, informed consent, information technology, and performance improvement. Other topics also include legal rights and responsibilities, referrals, resource management, staff education, supervision, confidentiality/information security, and continuity of care. The questions in this book follow this blueprint.

GUIDELINES FOR MAKING A DECISION

Nurses* base their decisions on many different bodies of information in order to arrive at a course of action. Among the basic guidelines to apply in nursing practice—and in answering test questions—are the nursing process and Maslow's Hierarchy of Needs.

The Nursing Process

One of the basic guidelines to apply in nursing practice is the nursing process, which consists of five steps—assessment, nursing diagnosis, planning, intervention, and evaluation—usually completed in a systematic order.

Many questions can be answered based on "assessment." If a priority-setting question asks the test taker to choose which step to implement first, the test taker should look for an answer that would assess for the problem discussed in the stem of the question.

EXAMPLE

The nurse is caring for a client diagnosed with congestive heart failure who is currently complaining of dyspnea. Which intervention should the nurse implement first?
1. Administer furosemide (Lasix), a loop diuretic, IVP.
2. Check the client for adventitious lung sounds.
3. Ask the respiratory therapist to administer a treatment.
4. Notify the health-care provider of the problem.

Answer: 2. Checking for adventitious lung sounds is assessing the client to determine the extent of the client's breathing difficulties causing the dyspnea. There are numerous words, such as "check," that can be used to indicate assessment. The test taker should not discard an option because the word "assess" or "assessment" is not used. Alternatively, the test taker should not assume that an option is correct merely because the word "assess" is used.

The test taker must also be aware that the assessment data must match the problem stated in the stem, regardless of terminology. The nurse must assess for the correct information. If option 2 in this example said to assess urinary output, it would not be a correct option even though it includes the word "assess," because urinary output is not directly related to heart failure and breathing difficulties.

In addition, the test taker should be aware that assessment is not always the correct answer when the question asks which should be done first. Suppose, for example, that the earlier question had listed option 3 as follows:

3. Apply oxygen via nasal cannula at 2 LPM.

In that case, assessment does not come first. The nurse would first attempt to relieve the client's distress and then assess.

When a question asks what a nurse should do next, the test taker should determine from the information given in the question which steps in the nursing process have been completed and then should choose an option that matches the next step in the nursing process.

---

*In this book, the term "nurse," unless otherwise specified, refers to a licensed RN. An RN can assign tasks to a licensed practical nurse (LPN) or delegate to unlicensed assistive personnel (UAP), which may be known under other terms such as medical assistant or nurse's aides. An LPN can delegate tasks to a UAP. Each state has specific regulations that govern what duties/tasks can be delegated/assigned to each of these types of personnel.

The term "health-care provider," used in this book, refers to a client's primary provider of medical care. It includes physicians (including osteopathic physicians), nurse practitioners (NPs), and physician assistants (PAs). Depending on state regulations, many NPs and some PAs have prescriptive authority at least for some categories of prescribed drugs.

EXAMPLE

The client diagnosed with peptic ulcer disease has a blood pressure of 88/42 and an apical pulse of 132, and respirations are 28. The nurse writes the nursing diagnosis "altered tissue perfusion related to decreased circulatory volume." Which intervention should the nurse implement first?
1. Notify the laboratory to draw a type and crossmatch.
2. Assess the client's abdomen for tenderness.
3. Insert an 18-gauge catheter and infuse lactated Ringer's.
4. Check the client's pulse oximeter reading.

Because the client has assessment data and the nursing diagnosis has been formulated, the next step is to implement a nursing intervention appropriate to the situation.

Answers
1. This would be an appropriate intervention because the client is showing signs of hypovolemia, but it is not the first intervention because it would not directly support the client's circulatory volume.
2. The stem of the question has provided enough assessment data to indicate the client's problem of hypovolemia. Further assessment data are not needed.
3. The vital signs indicate hypovolemia, which is a life-threatening emergency that requires the nurse to intervene to support the client's circulatory volume.
4. A pulse oximeter reading would not support the client's circulatory volume.

These types of questions are designed to determine whether the test taker can set priorities in client care.

Maslow's Hierarchy of Needs

If the test taker has looked at the question and the nursing process cannot help in determining the correct option, then using a tool such as Maslow's Hierarchy of Needs can assist in choosing the correct answer.

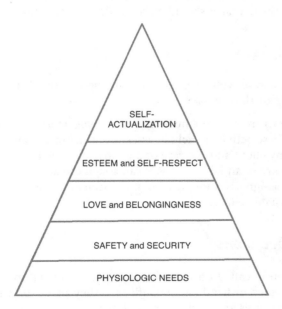

Remember that the bottom of the pyramid—physiologic needs—represents the top priority in instituting nursing interventions. If a question asks the test taker to determine which is the priority intervention and a physiologic need is not listed, then safety and security take priority, and so on up the pyramid.

TYPES OF QUESTIONS

Although most of the questions on the NCLEX-RN are multiple-choice questions, a few are what is known as alternate format questions. These include choosing more than one option that correctly answers a question, ranking procedures or actions in correct order, as well as drop and drag and fill in the blank questions. As stated earlier, the questions involving leadership/management involve prioritizing, delegation/assignment, and management of clients and staff.

Prioritizing Questions/Setting Priorities

In test questions that ask the nurse which action to take first, two or more of the options will be appropriate nursing interventions for the situation described. When choosing the correct answer, the test taker must decide which intervention should occur *first* in a sequence of events or which intervention directly affects the situation.

With a question that asks which client should the nurse assess first, the test taker should first look at each option and determine whether the signs/symptoms the client is exhibiting are normal or expected for the disease process; if so, the nurse does not need to assess that particular client first. Second, if two or more of the options state signs/symptoms that are not normal or expected for the disease process, then the test taker should select the option that has the greatest potential for a poor outcome. Each option should be examined carefully to determine the priority by asking these questions:

- Is the situation life threatening or life altering? *If yes, this client is the highest priority.*
- Is the situation unexpected for the disease process? *If yes, then this client may be priority.*
- Are the lab data abnormal? *If yes, then this client may be priority.*
- Is the situation expected for the disease process? *If yes, then this client may be—but probably is not—priority.*
- Is the situation or is the data normal? *If yes, this client can be seen last.*

The test taker should try to make a decision pertaining to each option. On pencil-and-paper examinations, it may be helpful to note the decision near the option. On a computerized test, the test taker should make the decision and move on to the next question.

Delegating and Assigning Care

Although each state and province has its own Nursing Practice Act, there are some general guidelines that apply to all professional nurses.

- When delegating to an UAP, the nurse may not delegate any activity that requires nursing judgment. These activities include assessing, teaching, evaluating, or administering medications to any client and the care of any unstable client.
- When assigning care to an LPN, the RN can assign the administration of some medications but cannot assign assessing, teaching, or evaluating any client and cannot delegate the care of an unstable client.

Management Decisions

The nurse is frequently called on to make decisions about staffing, movement of clients from one unit to another, or handling of conflicts as they arise. Some general guidelines for answering questions in this area include the following:

- The most experienced nurse gets the most critical client.
- A graduate nurse can take care of any client who is receiving care from a student with supervision.
- The most stable client can move or be discharged, whereas the most unstable client must move to the intensive care unit (ICU) or stay in the ICU.

When the nurse must make a decision regarding a conflict in the nursing station, a good rule to follow is to use the chain of command. The primary nurse should confront a peer (another primary nurse) or a subordinate unless the situation is illegal (such as stealing drugs). The primary nurse should use the chain of command in situations that address superiors (a manager or director of nursing); then the nurse should discuss the situation with the next in command above the superior.

PUTTING THE PIECES TOGETHER

The nurse is required to acquire information, analyze the data, and make inferences based on the available information. Sometimes this process is relatively easy, and at other times the pieces of information do not seem to fit. This is precisely where critical thinking and nursing judgment must guide in making the decision.

Medical Nursing

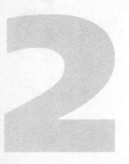

"When you do the common things in life in an uncommon way, you will command the attention of the world."

—George Washington Carver

ABBREVIATION LIST

ABG	Arterial Blood Gas	**IV**	Intravenous
ACE	Angiotensin-Converting Enzyme	**IVPB**	Intravenous Piggy Back
		K+	Potassium
AP	Apical Pulse	**LPN**	Licensed Practical Nurse
BP	Blood Pressure	**MAR**	Medication Administration Record
CNO	Chief Nursing Officer		
COPD	Chronic Obstructive Pulmonary Disease	**MRSA**	Methicillin-Resistant *Staphylococcus aureus*
DKA	Diabetic Ketoacidosis	**NCSBN**	National Council of State Boards of Nursing
DVT	Deep Vein Thrombosis		
ED	Emergency Department	**NPO**	Nothing per (by) Os (Mouth)
GI	Gastrointestinal	**PTT**	Partial Thromboplastin Time
H&H	Hemoglobin and Hematocrit	**R**	Respiration
HCP	Health-care Provider	**RBC**	Red Blood Cell
HHNC	Hyperglycemic Hyperosmolar Nonketotic Coma	**RN**	Registered Nurse
		UAP	Unlicensed Assistive Personnel
HIPPA	Health Information Privacy and Portability Act	**WBC**	White Blood Cell
HTN	Hypertension		

PRACTICE QUESTIONS

Setting Priorities When Caring for Clients

1. The 7:00 P.M. to 7:00 A.M. nurse has received the shift report from the outgoing nurse. Which client should the nurse assess first?
   1. The male client who has just been brought to the floor from the emergency department (ED) with no report of complaints.
   2. The female client who received pain medication 30 minutes ago for pain that was a level "8" on a 1-to-10 pain scale.
   3. The male client who had a cardiac catheterization in the morning and has been allowed to use the bathroom one time.
   4. The female client who has been turning on the call light frequently and stating that her care has been neglected.

2. The client diagnosed with breast cancer who is positive for the *BRCA* gene is requesting advice from the nurse about treatment options. Which statement is the nurse's best response?
   1. "If it were me in this situation, I would consider having a bilateral mastectomy."
   2. "What treatment options has your health-care provider (HCP) discussed with you?"
   3. "You should discuss your treatment options with your HCP."
   4. "Have you talked with your significant other about the treatment options available to you?"

3. The nurse has finished receiving the morning change-of-shift report. Which client should the nurse assess first?
   1. The client diagnosed with pneumonia who has bilateral crackles.
   2. The client on strict bed rest who is complaining of calf pain.
   3. The client who complains of low back pain when sitting in a chair.
   4. The client who is upset because the food is cold all the time.

4. The nurse is preparing to administer medications after receiving the morning change-of-shift report. Which medication should the nurse administer first?
   1. The intravenous (IV) proton-pump inhibitor medication to a client who is to be given nothing by mouth (NPO).
   2. The loop diuretic to a client with a serum K+ level of 3.2 mEq/L.
   3. The rapid-acting insulin Humalog to a client who has the breakfast tray in the room.
   4. The stimulant laxative to a client who has not had a bowel movement in 3 days.

5. The charge nurse has received laboratory data for clients in the medical department. Which client would require intervention by the charge nurse?
   1. The client diagnosed with a myocardial infarction who has an elevated troponin level.
   2. The client receiving the IV anticoagulant heparin who has a partial thromboplastin time (PTT) of 68 seconds.
   3. The client diagnosed with end-stage liver failure who has an elevated ammonia level.
   4. The client receiving the anticonvulsant phenytoin (Dilantin) who has levels of 24 mg/dL.

6. The nurse is caring for clients on a medical unit. Which intervention should the nurse implement first?
   1. Change the leg wound dressing for a client who has ambulated in the hall.
   2. Discuss the correct method of obtaining a blood glucose level with the unlicensed assistive personnel (UAP).
   3. Check on the male client who called the desk to say he has just vomited.
   4. Place a call to the extended care facility to give the report on a discharged client.

7. The nurse is preparing a client diagnosed with peptic ulcer disease for a barium study of the stomach and esophagus (upper gastrointestinal [GI] system). Which intervention is the priority for this client?
   1. Obtain informed consent from the client for the diagnostic procedure.
   2. Discuss the need to increase oral fluid intake after the procedure.
   3. Explain that the client will have to drink a white, chalky substance.
   4. Tell the client not to eat or drink anything prior to the procedure.

8. After receiving the shift report, the 7:00 P.M. to 7:00 A.M. nurse is reviewing the medication administration record (MAR) of the client diagnosed with type 2 diabetes. Which intervention should the nurse implement?

Client's Name:		Account Number: 123456		Allergies: NKDA
Height: 70 inches	Weight: 265 pounds			
Date	Medication	2301–0700	0701–1500	1501–2300
	Regular Insulin by bedside glucose subcu ac & hs			
	<60 notify HCP 150 0 units 151–200 2 units		0730 DN BG 42 0 units	
	201–250 4 units 251–300 6 units		1130 DN BG 245 4 units	
	301–350 8 units 351–400 10 units >400 notify HCP			1630 DN BG 398 10 units
	Humulin N 48 units BID subcu ac		0730 DN	1630 DN
Signature/Initials		Day Nurse RN DN	Night Nurse RN NN	

   1. Make sure the client receives a snack at bedtime.
   2. Check the client's blood glucose level immediately.
   3. Have the UAP give the client some orange juice.
   4. Teach the client about the symptoms of diabetic ketoacidosis.

9. The nurse is administering medications for clients on a medical unit. Which medication should the nurse administer first?
   1. The narcotic pain medication to a client complaining that his pain is an "8."
   2. A loop diuretic to a client diagnosed with heart failure who has 3+ pitting edema.
   3. An anticholinesterase medication to a client diagnosed with myasthenia gravis.
   4. An antacid to a client with pyrosis who has called several times over the intercom.

10. The nurse is caring for clients on a medical unit. Which laboratory data warrants immediate intervention by the nurse?
   1. The PTT of 98 seconds with a control of 36 on a client diagnosed with deep vein thrombosis (DVT).
   2. The hemoglobin and hematocrit (H&H) of 10.4/31 for a client diagnosed with a bleeding gastric ulcer.
   3. The white blood cell (WBC) count of 4800 for a client diagnosed with leukemia.
   4. The triglyceride level of 312 mmol/L in a client diagnosed with hypertension (HTN).

Delegating and Assigning Nursing Tasks

11. The nurse and a UAP are caring for a client with right-sided paralysis. Which action by the UAP requires the nurse to intervene?
    1. The assistant places the gait belt around the client's waist prior to ambulating.
    2. The assistant places the client on the abdomen with the client's head to the side.
    3. The assistant places her hand under the client's right axilla to help the client move up in bed.
    4. The assistant praises the client for attempting to perform activities of daily living independently.

12. The charge nurse is making client assignments for a neuro-medical floor. Which client should be assigned to the most experienced nurse?
    1. The elderly client who is experiencing a stroke in evolution.
    2. The client diagnosed with a transient ischemic attack 48 hours ago.
    3. The client diagnosed with Guillain-Barré syndrome who complains of leg pain.
    4. The client with Alzheimer's disease who is wandering in the halls.

13. The nurse and the UAP are caring for clients on a medical-surgical unit. Which task should not be assigned to the UAP?
    1. Instruct the UAP to feed the 69-year-old client who is experiencing dysphagia.
    2. Request the UAP turn and position the 89-year-old client with a pressure ulcer.
    3. Tell the UAP to assist the 54-year-old client with toilet training activities.
    4. Ask the UAP to obtain vital signs on a 72-year-old client diagnosed with pneumonia.

14. The charge nurse is making assignments for clients on a cardiac unit. Which client should the charge nurse assign to a new graduate nurse?
    1. The 44-year-old client diagnosed with a myocardial infarction.
    2. The 65-year-old client admitted with unstable angina.
    3. The 75-year-old client scheduled for a cardiac catheterization.
    4. The 50-year-old client complaining of chest pain.

15. The charge nurse is making assignments for a 30-bed medical unit that is staffed with three registered nurses (RNs), three licensed practical nurses (LPNs), and three UAPs. Which assignment is most appropriate?
    1. Assign the RN to perform all sterile procedures.
    2. Assign the LPN to give all IV medications.
    3. Assign the UAP to complete the A.M. care.
    4. Assign the LPN to write the care plans.

16. The UAP tells the nurse that the client has a blood pressure (BP) of 78/46 and a pulse of 116 using a vital signs machine. Which intervention should the nurse implement first?
    1. Notify the HCP immediately.
    2. Have the UAP recheck the vital signs manually.
    3. Place the client in reverse Trendelenburg's position.
    4. Assess the client's cardiovascular status.

17. The charge nurse on a medical unit is working with a new unit secretary. Which statement concerning laboratory data is most important for the charge nurse to tell the secretary?
    1. "Be sure to show me any lab information that is called in to the unit."
    2. "Make sure to file the reports on the correct client's chart."
    3. "Do not take any laboratory reports over the telephone."
    4. "Verify all telephone reports by calling back to the lab."

18. The physical therapist has notified the unit secretary that the client will be ambulated in 45 minutes. After receiving notification from the unit secretary, which task should the charge nurse delegate to the UAP?
    1. Administer a pain medication 30 minutes before therapy.
    2. Give the client a washcloth to wash his or her face before walking.
    3. Check to make sure the client has been offered the use of the bathroom.
    4. Find a walker that is the correct height for the client to use.

19. The nurse on a medical unit has a client with adventitious breath sounds, but the nurse is unable to determine the exact nature of the situation. Which multidisciplinary team member should the nurse consult first?
    1. The HCP.
    2. The unit manager.
    3. The respiratory therapist.
    4. The case manager.

20. An RN is working with an LPN and a UAP to care for a group of clients. Which nursing task should not be delegated or assigned?
    1. The routine oral medications for the clients.
    2. The bed baths and oral care.
    3. Evaluating the client's progress.
    4. Transporting a client to dialysis.

Managing Clients and Nursing Staff

21. The female volunteer on a medical unit tells the nurse that one of the clients on the unit is her neighbor and asks about the client's condition. Which information should the nurse discuss with the volunteer?
    1. Determine how well she knows the client before talking with the volunteer.
    2. Tell the volunteer the client's condition in layman's terms.
    3. Ask the client if it is all right to talk with the volunteer.
    4. Explain that client information is on a need-to-know basis only.

22. The nurse on a medical unit is discussing a client with the case manager. Which information should the nurse share with the case manager?
    1. Discuss personal information that the client shared with the nurse in confidence.
    2. Provide the case manager with any information that is required for continuity of care.
    3. Explain that client confidentiality prevents the nurse from disclosing information.
    4. Ask the case manager to get the client's permission before sharing information.

23. The staff nurse is concerned about the documentation form for blood administration. The nurse thinks it is unclear and time consuming. The nurse has discussed this with the charge nurse and other staff members who agree the documentation is cumbersome and needs to be revised. Which action would be most appropriate for the staff nurse to implement first?
    1. Discuss the blood administration flow sheet with the chief nursing officer.
    2. Contact an individual to help design a new blood transfusion flow sheet.
    3. Learn to adapt to the present form and do not take any further action.
    4. Volunteer to be on an ad hoc committee to research alternate flow sheets.

24. The charge nurse is transcribing HCP orders for a client scheduled for a barium enema. In addition to the radiology department, which department of the hospital should be notified of the procedure?
    1. The cardiac catheterization department.
    2. The dietary department.
    3. The nuclear medicine department.
    4. The hospital laboratory department.

25. The medical unit is governed by a system of shared governance. Which statement best describes an advantage of this system?
    1. It guarantees that unions will not be able to come into the hospital.
    2. It makes the manager responsible for sharing information with the staff.
    3. It involves staff nurses in the decision-making process of the unit.
    4. It is a system used to represent the nurses in labor disputes.

26. The staff nurse answers the telephone on a medical unit and the caller tells the nurse that he has planted a bomb in the facility. Which actions should the nurse implement? Select all that apply.
    1. Do not touch any suspicious object.
    2. Call 911, the emergency response system.
    3. Try to get the caller to provide additional information.
    4. Immediately pull the red emergency wall lever.
    5. Write down exactly what the caller says.

27. The male visitor on a medical unit is shouting and making threats about harming the staff because of perceived poor care his loved one has received. Which statement is the nurse's best initial response?
    1. "If you don't stop shouting, I will have to call security."
    2. "I hear that you are frustrated. Can we discuss the issues calmly?"
    3. "Sir, you are disrupting the unit. Calm down or leave the hospital."
    4. "This type of behavior is uncalled for and will not resolve anything."

28. The new graduate working on a medical unit night shift is concerned that the charge nurse is drinking alcohol on duty. On more than one occasion, the new graduate has smelled alcohol when the charge nurse returns from a break. Which action should the new graduate nurse implement first?
    1. Confront the charge nurse with the suspicions.
    2. Talk with the night supervisor about the concerns.
    3. Ignore the situation unless the nurse cannot do her job.
    4. Ask to speak to the nurse educator about the problem.

29. The experienced male nurse has recently taken a position on a medical unit in a community hospital, but after 1 week on the job, he finds that the staffing is not what was discussed during his employment interview. Which approach would be most appropriate for the nurse to take when attempting to resolve the issue?
    1. Immediately give a 2-week notice and find a different job.
    2. Discuss the situation with the manager who interviewed him.
    3. Talk with the other employees about the staffing situation.
    4. Tell the charge nurse the staffing is not what was explained to him.

30. The charge nurse is making assignments on a medical unit. Which client should the nurse assign to the new graduate nurse?
    1. The client who has received 3 units of packed red blood cells (RBCs).
    2. The client going for an esophagogastroduodenoscopy in the morning.
    3. The client diagnosed with hyperosmolar hyperglycemic nonketotic syndrome.
    4. The client who has just returned from a cardiac catheterization.

Setting Priorities When Caring for Clients

1. 1. This client may or may not be stable. He may have "no complaints" at this time, but the nurse must assess this client first to determine that whatever the complaint was that brought him to the ED has stabilized. This client should be seen first.
   2. It is important for the nurse to assess for pain relief in a timely manner, but this client has been medicated, and the nurse can evaluate the amount of pain relief after making sure that the ED admission is stable.
   3. This client has been back from the procedure long enough to be allowed bathroom privileges; therefore, this client does need to be seen first.
   4. Psychological issues are important, but not more so than a physiologic issue, and the client admitted from the ED may have a physiologic problem.

   MAKING NURSING DECISIONS: The test taker should use some tool as a reference to guide in the decision-making process. In this situation, Maslow's Hierarchy of Needs should be applied. Physiologic needs have priority over psychosocial ones.

2. 1. This is boundary crossing because the nurse does not have breast cancer. The nurse should assess what information the client is really seeking and then explain the treatment or refer the client, as appropriate.
   2. The nurse must assess what information the client actually needs. To do this, the nurse must know what treatment options have been suggested to the client. Assessment is the first step in the nursing process.
   3. This may be needed after the nurse further assesses the situation, but this is not the first intervention.
   4. The client needs information about treatment options from a designated HCP; the significant other would not have such information/suggestions.

3. 1. A typical sign of pneumonia is bilateral crackles; therefore, this client would not need to be seen first.
   2. The client with calf pain could be experiencing deep vein thrombosis (DVT), a complication of immobility, which may be fatal if a pulmonary embolus occurs; therefore, this client should be assessed first.
   3. The client experiencing low back pain when sitting in a chair should be assessed but not prior to the client with suspected DVT.
   4. The nurse should address the client's concern about the food, but it is not priority over a physiologic problem.

   MAKING NURSING DECISIONS: When deciding which client to assess first, the test taker should determine whether the signs/symptoms the client is exhibiting are normal or expected for the client situation. After eliminating the expected options, the test taker should determine which situation is more life threatening.

4. 1. An IV proton-pump inhibitor would not be priority over a client receiving insulin.
   2. Because the client's serum K+ level is already low, the nurse should question administering a loop diuretic.
   3. Rapid-acting insulin, such as Humalog, peaks in 15 to 20 minutes and should be administered when or immediately before the client eats the food on the tray; therefore, this medication should be administered first.
   4. A laxative is not a priority medication over insulin.

5. 1. The nurse would expect the client diagnosed with a myocardial infarction to have an elevated troponin level; thus the nurse would not assess this client first.
   2. Because the client's PTT of 68 seconds is 1.5 to 2 times the normal range, it is considered therapeutic and would not warrant the nurse's assessing this client first.
   3. The nurse would expect a client with end-stage liver failure to have an elevated ammonia level.
   4. The therapeutic range for Dilantin is 10-20 mg/dL. This client's higher level warrants intervention because the serum level is above therapeutic range.

   MAKING NURSING DECISIONS: The test taker must know normal laboratory data. See Appendix A for normal laboratory data.

6. 1. This client should be seen in a timely manner but not before the client who is vomiting.
   2. This can take some time and should not be hastily completed because the nurse must know the task is being done correctly before delegating it to a UAP. This should be done at a time arranged between the UAP and the nurse.
   3. **This client has experienced a physiologic problem, and the nurse must assess the client and the emesis to decide on possible interventions.**
   4. The nurse could call the extended care facility after assessing the client who has vomited and after dressing the client's leg.

7. 1. A barium study of the upper GI system is an x-ray procedure and does not require the client to sign an informed consent.
   2. The barium can cause constipation after the procedure; therefore, the client should increase fluid intake, but this is not the priority intervention.
   3. The client will have to drink a white, chalky substance, but the priority intervention is to make sure the client is NPO.
   4. **The test is a barium study of the upper GI system and requires the client's upper GI system to be empty. This client should be made NPO at least 8 to 10 hours before the test.**

8. 1. **The client received an intermediate-acting insulin at 1630 plus the sliding scale insulin dose to lower the client's blood glucose level. This client should receive a bedtime snack to make sure the client does not experience a hypoglycemic reaction during the night. Intermediate insulin generally peaks 6 to 8 hours after administration, 2230 to 0030 for this client.**
   2. The nurse should check the client's blood glucose at 2100 hours, not at the current time.
   3. Nothing indicates the client needs an intervention for hypoglycemia at this time.
   4. The client with type 2 diabetes would experience hyperglycemic hyperosmolar nonketotic coma (HHNC) syndrome, not DKA.

9. 1. A pain medication is important to administer in a timely manner, but its administration is not priority over a medication that must be administered on time to prevent respiratory complications.
   2. For a client experiencing expected symptoms of a disease, such as pitting edema, administration of a loop diuretic has a

30-minute leeway—that is, it can be administered 30 minutes before to 30 minutes after the scheduled dosing time.
   3. **Anticholinesterase medications administered for myasthenia gravis must be administered on time to preserve muscle functioning, especially the functioning of the muscles of the upper respiratory tract. This is the priority medication.**
   4. Clients who have called for medications should be attended to, but this client would not receive an antacid for heartburn before the client diagnosed with myasthenia gravis or the client in pain.

10. 1. **Therapeutic levels for PTT should be 1-1/2 to 2 times the control—that is, 54 to 72 seconds when the control is 36; therefore, this client is at risk for bleeding. The prolonged PTT indicates the client is receiving heparin (drug of choice to treat DVT). The nurse should stop the infusion and follow the facility protocol.**
   2. Although this H&H is low (but not critically), it would be expected in a client diagnosed with a bleeding gastric ulcer.
   3. This WBC count is low (normal is 5000 to 10,000), but it would be considered good in a client diagnosed with leukemia.
   4. The nurse should notify the HCP on rounds of laboratory data that is abnormal but not immediately life threatening. The triglyceride level is high, but it will take weeks to months of a healthy heart diet and exercise and possibly medications to lower this level.

MAKING NURSING DECISIONS: When a question asks for immediate intervention, the test taker must decide whether there is an intervention the nurse can implement immediately or whether the HCP must be notified. If the data are abnormal—but not life threatening—then the option can be eliminated as a possible correct answer.

Delegating and Assigning Nursing Tasks

11. 1. Placing a gait belt prior to ambulating is an appropriate action for safety and would not require the nurse to intervene.
    2. Placing the client in a prone position helps promote hyperextension of the hip joints, which is essential for normal gait and helps prevent knee and hip flexion contractures; therefore, this would not require the nurse to intervene.

3. This action is inappropriate and would require intervention by the nurse because pulling on a flaccid shoulder joint could cause shoulder dislocation; the client should be pulled up by placing the arm underneath the client's back or using a lift sheet.
4. The client should be encouraged and praised for attempting to perform any activities independently, such as combing hair or brushing teeth.

12. 1. Because the client is having an evolving stroke, the client is experiencing a worsening of signs and symptoms over several minutes to hours; thus, the client is at risk for dying and should be cared for by the most experienced nurse.
2. A transient ischemic attack by definition lasts less than 24 hours; thus, this client should be stable at this time.
3. Pain is expected in clients with Guillain-Barré, and symptoms typically are on the lower half of the body, which wouldn't affect the airway. Therefore, a less experienced nurse could care for this client.
4. The charge nurse could assign this client to an unlicensed assistive personnel.

MAKE NURSING DECISIONS: When the test taker is deciding which client should be assigned to the most experienced nurse, the most critical and unstable client should be assigned to the most experienced nurse.

13. 1. The nurse should not delegate to the UAP feeding a client who is at risk for complications during feeding as a result of dysphagia. This requires judgment that the assistant is not expected to possess.
2. UAPs can turn and position clients with pressure ulcers. However, the nurse should assist with this process at least once during the shift to assess the wound area.
3. The UAP can assist the client to the bathroom every 2 hours and document the results of the attempt.
4. The assistant can obtain the vital signs on a stable client.

14. 1. This client is at high risk for complications related to necrotic myocardial tissue and will need extensive teaching; therefore, this client should not be assigned to a new graduate.
2. Unstable angina means this client is at risk for life-threatening complications and should not be assigned to a new graduate.

3. A new graduate should be able to complete a pre-procedural checklist and get this client to the catheterization lab.
4. Chest pain means this client could be having a myocardial infarction and should not be assigned to a new graduate.

MAKE NURSING DECISIONS: When the test taker is deciding which client should be assigned to a new graduate, the most stable client should be assigned to the least experienced nurse.

15. 1. The LPN can perform sterile procedures such as inserting indwelling catheters and IV catheters. The RN should perform the functions that require nursing judgment, such as planning and evaluating the care of the clients.
2. Although the LPN could administer most intravenous piggy back (IVPB) medications, only qualified RNs may administer intravenous push (IVP) medications and chemotherapy.
3. The UAP is capable of performing the morning care. This is an appropriate nursing task to delegate.
4. Writing a care plan for a client requires nursing judgment; therefore, the RN should be assigned this function.

MAKING NURSING DECISIONS: Tasks that cannot be delegated are nursing interventions that require nursing judgment. Remember that in most instances, options that include the word "all" (options 1 and 2) can be eliminated because if the test taker can think of one time when some other level of licensure could safely perform the task, then the option automatically becomes wrong.

16. 1. The nurse should first assess the client to determine the status prior to notifying the HCP.
2. The UAP has notified the nurse of a potentially serious situation. The nurse should personally assess the client.
3. The nurse might place the client in reverse Trendelenburg's position once cardiovascular shock is determined.
4. The nurse should immediately go to the client's room to assess the client.

MAKING NURSING DECISIONS: Anytime the nurse receives information about a client (who may be experiencing a complication) from another staff member, the nurse must assess the client. The nurse should not make decisions about

the client's needs based on another staff member's information.

17. 1. Because laboratory values called into a unit usually include critical values, the charge nurse should tell the unit secretary "to show me any lab information that is called in immediately." The charge nurse must evaluate this information immediately.
2. Posting laboratory results is the responsibility of the laboratory staff, not the nursing staff.
3. This is unrealistic because laboratory data are important information that must be called in to a unit when there is a critical value so that immediate action can be taken for the client's welfare. The secretary must know how to process the information.
4. The unit secretary should verify the information by repeating back the information at the time of the call, not by making a second telephone call to the lab.

18. 1. Administering pain medication is the nurse's responsibility, not that of the UAP.
2. A washcloth should be provided to the client before a meal, but not before ambulating with the physical therapist.
3. The client should be ready to work on therapy when the physical therapist arrives. The UAP should make sure that the client has used the bathroom or has not been incontinent before the therapist arrives, thus making the most efficient use of the therapist's time.
4. Obtaining a walker that is the correct height for the client is the physical therapist's responsibility, not that of the UAP.

19. 1. The client's HCP should be consulted if the nurse determines a need, but at this time, the nurse should discuss the client with the respiratory therapist.
2. The unit manager may or may not be capable of helping the nurse assess a client with adventitious breath sounds; therefore, this is not the first person the nurse should consult.
3. Respiratory therapists listen to and treat clients with lung problems multiple times every day. Therefore, this is the best person to consult when the nurse needs help identifying a respiratory problem.
4. The case manager is usually capable of maneuvering through the maze of health-care referrals but is not necessarily an expert in lung sounds.

20. 1. The LPN may be assigned to administer the routine oral medications to the clients.

2. Bed baths and oral care can be performed by the UAP.
3. The nurse cannot delegate or assign tasks that require nursing judgment, such as evaluating a client's progress.
4. The UAP can transport a client to dialysis.

MAKING NURSING DECISIONS: The nurse cannot delegate assessment, evaluation, teaching, or administration of medications to any client or the care of an unstable client to a UAP. Also, the nurse cannot assign assessment, evaluation, teaching, or tasks that require nursing judgment to an LPN.

Managing Clients and Nursing Staff

21. 1. The fact that the patient is a neighbor of the volunteer has no bearing on whether or not the nurse can discuss a client's condition with the volunteer. The nurse should inform the volunteer that information obtained inadvertently is still confidential.
2. The nurse cannot release the client's information in layman's or medical terms; this is a violation of the Health Insurance Portability and Accountability Act (HIPAA). In many facilities, the client can give a "password" to individuals who can receive information about the client's condition.
3. The nurse should not discuss the situation with the client. This would alert the client to potential breeches in confidentiality.
4. The nurse should remind the volunteer of the HIPAA and confidentiality rules that govern any information concerning clients in a health-care setting.

22. 1. Unless the information shared is directly connected to health-care issues, the nurse should not share confidential information with anyone else. The nurse should inform clients that information directly affecting the client's health care will be shared on a need-to-know basis only.
2. The case manager's job is to ensure continuity and adequacy of care for the client. This individual has a "need to know."
3. The case manager is part of the health-care team; therefore, information should be shared.
4. The client gave permission when being admitted to the hospital for information to be shared among those providing care. The case manager does not need to obtain further consent.

23. 1. The staff nurse should go through the chain of command when attempting to make a change.
    2. This may be an appropriate action at some point, but this would not be implemented until after assessing the old form and identifying areas to be changed.
    3. The nurse should be a change agent.
    4. **The staff nurse should be a part of the solution to a problem; volunteering to be on a committee of peers is the best action to effect a change.**

24. 1. Because this procedure is performed in the radiology department and is testing the gastrointestinal system, the cardiac catheter lab does not need to be informed of the procedure.
    2. **The client must be NPO for 8 to 10 hours before the procedure. Therefore, the dietary department should be notified to hold the meal trays.**
    3. The procedure is performed using barium or Gastrografin, neither of which contains any nuclear material. The nuclear medicine department does not need to be informed of the procedure.
    4. The procedure does not involve the clinical laboratory; this department does not need to be notified.

25. 1. Under shared governance, some nurses become so involved with the management of facilities that they are no longer eligible for representation by a bargaining agent (union), but there are no guarantees.
    2. The manager is responsible for disseminating information under a centralized system of organization.
    3. **Shared governance is an organizational framework in which the nurse has autonomy over his or her own practice. The nurse is given direct input into the working of the unit.**
    4. Shared governance is a system in which the nurse represents himself or herself.

26. 1, 3, and 5 are correct.
    1. **The nurse should begin a systematic search of the unit after activating the bomb scare emergency plan, and if any suspicious objects are found the nurse should not touch and should notify the bomb squad.**
    2. The nurse should notify the house supervisor and administration because they are responsible for notifying the police department.

3. **The nurse should stay calm and try to keep the caller on the telephone. The nurse should attempt to get as much information from the caller as possible. The nurse can jot a note to someone nearby to initiate the bomb scare procedure.**
4. The red emergency levers in hospitals are to notify the fire departments of a fire, not a bomb scare.
5. **The nurse should try to transcribe exactly what the caller says; this may help identify who is calling and where a bomb might be placed.**

MAKING NURSING DECISIONS: The nurse must be knowledgeable of hospital emergency preparedness. Students as well as new employees receive this information in hospital orientations and are responsible for implementing procedures correctly. The NCSBN NCLEX-RN blueprint includes questions on safe and effective care environment.

27. 1. This might be the second statement for the nurse to make if the client does not calm down and discuss the problems with the nurse. Because it could escalate the anger, it should not be the first statement.
    2. **The nurse should remain calm and try to allow the client to vent his frustrations in a more acceptable manner. The nurse should repeat calmly in a low voice any instructions given to the client.**
    3. This statement will escalate the situation and could cause the visitor to lash out at the nurse.
    4. This statement will escalate the situation and could cause the visitor to lash out at the nurse.

28. 1. The new graduate must work under this charge nurse; confronting the nurse would not resolve the issue because the nurse can choose to ignore the new graduate. Someone in authority over the charge nurse must address this situation with the nurse.
    2. **The night supervisor or the unit manager has the authority to require the charge nurse to submit to drug screening. In this case, the supervisor on duty should handle the situation.**
    3. The new graduate is bound by the nursing practice acts to report potentially unsafe behavior regardless of the position the nurse holds.
    4. The nurse educator would not be in a position of authority over the charge nurse.

MAKING NURSING DECISIONS: When the nurse is deciding on a course of action involving other staff members, a rule of thumb is this: If the individual the nurse is concerned about is superior in job title to the nurse, then go through the chain of command to the next level of superior. If the individual is subordinate in job title to the nurse, then the nurse should confront the individual.

29. 1. The nurse should leave if he determines that the staffing is not now or ever will be as it was relayed to him in the interview; however, there may be a temporary situation that can be resolved.
    2. The nurse should give the manager a chance to discuss the situation before quitting. A temporary problem, such as illness, may be affecting staffing.
    3. This action could cause the manager to think of the new nurse as a troublemaker.
    4. The nurse should not discuss this with the charge nurse because this may cause a rift between the charge nurse and the new nurse. The nurse should clarify the staffing situation with the unit manager.

30. 1. This client is unstable and should not be assigned to a new graduate nurse.
    2. This client is being prepared for a test in the morning and is the least acute of the clients listed. The new graduate should be assigned to this client.
    3. This client has a complication of diabetes mellitus type 2; a more experienced nurse should be assigned to this client.
    4. A client returning from a cardiac catheterization has potential for life-threatening complications such as hemorrhaging and should be assigned to a more experienced nurse.

MAKING NURSING DECISIONS: The test taker must determine which client is the most stable, which makes this an "except" question. Three clients are either unstable or have potentially life-threatening conditions.

COMPREHENSIVE EXAMINATION

1. At 0830, the day shift nurse is preparing to administer medications to the client. Which action should the nurse take first?

Client's Name:	Account Number: 123456		Allergies: NKDA	
Height: 62 inches	**Weight:** 105 pounds			
Date	**Medication**	**2301–0700**	**0701–1500**	**1501–2300**
	Lanoxin (digoxin) 0.125 mg PO every day		0900	
	Lasix (furosemide) 40 mg PO BID		0900	1600
	Zantac (ranitidine) 150 mg in 250 mL NS IV continuous infusion every 24 hours	0300 NN @11 mL/hr		
	Vancomycin 850 mg IVPB every 24 hours		1200	1800
Signature/Initials	**Day Nurse RN DN**		**Night Nurse RN NN**	

   1. Check the client's arm band against the medication administration record (MAR).
   2. Assess the client's IV site for redness and patency.
   3. Ask for the client's date of birth.
   4. Determine the client's last K$^+$ level.

2. Which client should the medical unit nurse assess first after receiving the shift report?
   1. The 84-year-old client diagnosed with pneumonia who is afebrile but getting restless.
   2. The 25-year-old client diagnosed with cellulitis of the left arm who has 2$^+$ edema.
   3. The 56-year-old client diagnosed with diverticulitis who has crampy left lower quadrant pain.
   4. The 38-year-old client diagnosed with a sinus infection who has green drainage from the nose.

3. The nurse on the telemetry unit notes the client's telemetry reading while the client is talking to the nurse on the intercom system.

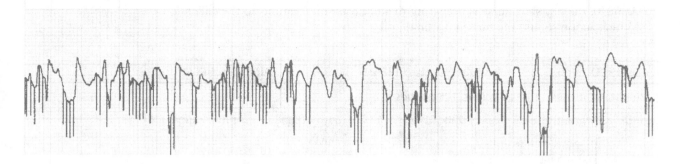

   Which task should the nurse instruct the UAP to implement?
   1. Call a Code Blue immediately.
   2. Check the client's telemetry leads.
   3. Find the nurse to check the client.
   4. Remove the telemetry monitor.

4. The nurse is planning the care of a client diagnosed with acute gastroenteritis. Which nursing problem is priority?
   1. Altered nutrition.
   2. Self-care deficit.
   3. Impaired body image.
   4. Fluid and electrolyte imbalance.

5. The nurse is preparing to administer morning medications to clients on a medical unit. Which medication should the nurse administer first?
   1. Methylprednisolone (Solu-Medrol), a steroid, to a client diagnosed with chronic obstructive pulmonary disease (COPD).
   2. Donepezil (Aricept), an acetylcholinesterase inhibitor, to a client with dementia.
   3. Sucralfate (Carafate), a mucosal barrier agent, to a client diagnosed with ulcer disease.
   4. Enoxaparin (Lovenox), an anticoagulant, to a client on bed rest after hip surgery.

6. The nurse is completing a head-to-toe assessment on a client diagnosed with breast cancer and notes a systolic murmur that the nurse was not informed of during report. Which action should the nurse implement first?
   1. Notify the HCP about the new cardiac complication.
   2. Document the finding in the client's chart and tell the charge nurse.
   3. Check the chart to determine whether this is the first time a murmur has been identified.
   4. Ask the client whether she has ever been told she has an abnormal heartbeat.

7. A major disaster has been called, and the charge nurse on a medical unit must recommend clients to discharge to the medical discharge officer on rounds. Which client should not be discharged?
   1. The client diagnosed with chronic angina pectoris who has been on new medication for 2 days.
   2. The client diagnosed with DVT who has had heparin discontinued and has been on warfarin (Coumadin) for 4 days.
   3. The client with an infected leg wound who is receiving vancomycin IVPB every 24 hours for methicillin-resistant *Staphylococcus aureus* (MRSA) infection.
   4. The client diagnosed with COPD who has the following arterial blood gas (ABG) levels: pH, 7.34; PCO_2, 55; HCO_3, 28; PaO_2, 89.

8. The client diagnosed with a cerebrovascular accident (CVA) has residual right-sided hemiparesis and difficulty swallowing, but is scheduled for discharge. Which referral is most appropriate for the case manager to make at this time?
   1. Inpatient rehabilitation unit.
   2. Home health-care agency.
   3. Long-term care facility.
   4. Outpatient therapy center.

9. The nurse and LPN are caring for a client diagnosed with a stroke. Which intervention should the nurse assign to the LPN?
   1. Feed the client who is being allowed to eat for the first time.
   2. Administer the client's anticoagulant subcutaneously.
   3. Check the client's neurologic signs and limb movement.
   4. Teach the client to turn the head and tuck the chin to swallow.

10. The nurse is caring for a client diagnosed with Alzheimer's disease. Which nursing tasks should not be delegated to the UAP? Select all that apply.
    1. Check the client's skin under the restraints.
    2. Administer the client's antipsychotic medication.
    3. Perform the client's morning hygiene care.
    4. Ambulate the client to the bathroom.
    5. Take the client's routine vital signs.

11. The client diagnosed with lung cancer has a hemoglobin and hematocrit (H&H) of 13.4 mg/dL and 40.1, a WBC count of 7800, and a neutrophil count of 62%. Which action should the nurse implement?
    1. Place the client in reverse isolation.
    2. Notify the HCP.
    3. Make sure no flowers are taken into the room.
    4. Continue to monitor the client.

12. The nurse has been named in a lawsuit concerning the care provided. Which action should the nurse take first?
    1. Consult with the hospital's attorney.
    2. Review the client's chart.
    3. Purchase personal liability insurance.
    4. Discuss the case with the supervisor.

13. The nurse has accepted the position of clinical manager for a medical-surgical unit. Which role is an important aspect of this management position?
    1. Evaluate the job performance of the staff.
    2. Be the sole decision-maker for the unit.
    3. Take responsibility for the staff nurse's actions.
    4. Attend the medical staff meetings.

14. The charge nurse notices that one of the staff takes frequent breaks, has unpredictable mood swings, and often volunteers to care for clients who require narcotics. Which priority action should the charge nurse implement regarding this employee?
    1. Discuss the nurse's actions with the unit manager.
    2. Confront the nurse about the behavior.
    3. Do not allow the nurse to take breaks alone.
    4. Prepare an occurrence report on the employee.

15. The charge nurse observes two UAPs arguing in the hallway. Which action should the nurse implement first in this situation?
    1. Tell the manager to check on the UAPs.
    2. Instruct the UAPs to stop arguing in the hallway.
    3. Have the UAPs go to a private room to talk.
    4. Mediate the dispute between the UAPs.

16. The graduate nurse is working with a UAP who has been an employee of the hospital for 12 years. However, tasks delegated to the UAP by the graduate nurse are frequently not completed. Which action should the graduate nurse take first?
    1. Tell the charge nurse the UAP will not do tasks as delegated by the nurse.
    2. Write up a counseling record with objective data and give it to the manager.
    3. Complete the delegated tasks and do nothing about the insubordination.
    4. Address the UAP to discuss why the tasks are not being done as requested.

17. A male HCP frequently tells jokes with sexual undertones at the nursing station. Which action should the female charge nurse implement?
    1. Tell the HCP that the jokes are inappropriate and offensive.
    2. Report the behavior to the medical staff committee.
    3. Discuss the problem with the chief nursing officer.
    4. Call a Code Purple and have the nurses surround the HCP.

18. The new graduate nurse is having difficulty in completing the workload in a timely manner. Which suggestion could the preceptor make to help the new graduate become more organized?
    1. Take a break whenever the nurse feels overwhelmed with the tasks.
    2. Start the shift with a work organization sheet for assigned clients.
    3. Take five deep breaths at the beginning of the shift and then begin.
    4. Review each day's assignments and organize the work for the new nurse.

19. The nurse is preparing to administer medications to clients on a medical unit. Which medication should the nurse question administering?
    1. Levothyroxine (Synthroid), a thyroid hormone, to a client diagnosed with hypothyroidism.
    2. Propranolol (Inderal), a beta-adrenergic, to a client diagnosed with hyperthyroidism.
    3. Nifedipine (Procardia), a calcium channel blocker, to a client with hypotension.
    4. Enalapril (Vasotec), an angiotensin-converting enzyme (ACE) inhibitor, to a client with diabetes.

20. The nurse has received the shift report. Which client should the nurse assess first?
    1. The client diagnosed with a DVT who is complaining of dyspnea and coughing.
    2. The client diagnosed with gallbladder ulcer disease who refuses to eat the food served.
    3. The client diagnosed with pancreatitis who wants the nasogastric tube removed.
    4. The client diagnosed with osteoarthritis who is complaining of stiff joints.

1. 1. Checking the client's arm band is done prior to actually administering the medications, but it is not the first action for the nurse to take.
   2. The nurse should have assessed the client's IV site on first rounds. At this time, all medications to be administered are oral.
   3. This is part of the two-identifier system of medication administration implemented to prevent medication errors, but it is not the first action for the nurse to take.
   4. **The nurse should assess the client's last potassium (K^+) level because hypokalemia (abnormally low K^+ level) is the most common cause of dysrhythmias in clients receiving digoxin secondary to clients concurrently taking diuretics. Furosemide (Lasix) is a loop diuretic. The nurse should check for digoxin and K^+ levels and apical pulse (AP) prior to administering digoxin.**

2. 1. **Elderly clients diagnosed with pneumonia may not present with the "normal" symptoms, such as fever. The client's becoming restless may indicate a decrease in oxygen to the brain. This client should be seen first.**
   2. Two-plus edema is expected in a client diagnosed with cellulitis.
   3. One of the typical main symptoms of diverticulitis is crampy left lower quadrant pain; therefore, this client does not require intervention.
   4. Sinus drainage is to be expected in a client diagnosed with a sinus infection.

3. 1. The telemetry strip indicates artifact, so there is no need for the UAP or any staff member to call a Code Blue, which is used when someone has arrested.
   2. **The UAP should be instructed to check the telemetry lead placement; this reading is artifact because the client is talking to the unit secretary over the intercom system.**
   3. The UAP can take care of this problem; there is no need for the primary nurse to check the client.
   4. The strip indicates artifact, but there is no indication that the client should be removed from telemetry.

4. 1. Altered nutrition is a concern, but a client can live for several weeks on minimal intake.
   2. Self-care deficit is a psychosocial problem; physiologic problems have priority.
   3. Impaired body image is a psychosocial problem; physiologic problems have priority.
   4. **Fluid and electrolyte imbalance can cause cardiac dysrhythmias. This is the priority problem.**

5. 1. This is a routine medication that has a time frame of 30 minutes before and after the scheduled time to be administered. This medication does not need to be the first medication administered.
   2. Aricept can be administered within the 30-minute time frame. This medication does not need to be the first medication administered.
   3. **A mucosal barrier agent must be administered before the client eats in order for the medication to coat the gastric mucosa. This medication should be administered first.**
   4. Lovenox can be administered within the 30-minute time frame. This medication does not need to be the first medication administered.

6. 1. This should be done if the murmur is a new finding; however, the nurse should investigate the finding further before notifying the HCP.
   2. This should be done, but assessing the client's situation is the nurse's priority.
   3. **Although the client was not admitted for a cardiac problem, she may have had a murmur for a while, and the previous nurse did not pick it up or did not mention it in the report because it was a long-standing physiologic finding in this client. The nurse should research the chart for a current history and physical to determine whether the HCP is aware of the condition.**
   4. The nurse should not ask the client because this could scare or alarm the client needlessly.

7. 1. This client has been on a medication to control the angina for 2 days and could be discharged.
   2. This client is currently completing the amount of care that would be provided in the hospital setting. The client can be taught to continue the Coumadin at home and return to the HCP's office for blood work, or a home health nurse can be assigned to go to the client's home and draw blood for the lab work.

3. Because resistant infections are very difficult to treat, this client should remain in the hospital for the required IVPB medication.
4. These blood gases are expected for a client diagnosed with COPD. This client could go home with oxygen and home health follow-up care.

8. 1. This client should be referred to an inpatient rehabilitation facility for intensive therapy before deciding on long-term placement (home with home health care or a long-term care facility). The initial rehabilitation a client receives can set the tone for all further recuperation. This is the appropriate referral at this time.
2. A home health-care agency may be needed when the client returns home, but the most appropriate referral is to a rehabilitation center where intensive therapy can take place.
3. A long-term care facility may be needed at some point, but the client should be given the opportunity of regaining as much lost ability as possible at this time.
4. The outpatient center would be utilized when the client is ready for discharge from the inpatient center.

9. 1. The nurse should be the first one to feed the client, in order for the nurse to evaluate the client's ability to swallow and not aspirate.
2. The LPN could administer routine parenteral medications. This is the best task to assign to the LPN.
3. This involves assessing the client; therefore, the nurse should not delegate this assignment to the LPN.
4. Teaching is the responsibility of the RN.

10. 1 and 2 are correct.
1. Checking the client's skin involves assessment; therefore, the nurse cannot delegate this assignment to the UAP.
2. The nurse cannot delegate medication administration to a UAP.
3. The UAP can perform routine hygiene care. The nurse must then make the time to assess the client's skin.
4. The UAP can ambulate a client to the bathroom.
5. The UAP can take routine vital signs.

11. 1. The client's lab work does not indicate an increased risk for infection. The client does not need to be placed in reverse isolation.

2. The lab work is within normal limits. The nurse does not need to notify the HCP.
3. The client is not at an increased risk for infection; therefore, the client may have flowers in the room.
4. This client's lab work is within normal limits. The nurse should continue to monitor the client.

12. 1. The nurse may wish to consult the hospital's attorneys or retain an attorney of his or her own, but this is not the first action for the nurse.
2. The nurse should be familiar with the chart and the situation so that details can be remembered. This should be the nurse's first action.
3. It is too late to purchase liability insurance to cover the current situation. The nurse may wish to purchase insurance for any future litigation.
4. The nurse should refrain from discussing the case with anyone who could be called as a witness or be named in the suit.

13. 1. One of the many jobs of a manager is to see that performance evaluations are completed on the staff.
2. The manager should receive input from many sources to make decisions. Some decisions are made for the manager by administration based on costs or any number of other reasons.
3. The nurses retain responsibility for their own actions because they practice under the state's nursing practice act. The manager retains responsibility for the functioning of the unit.
4. The nurse manager attends many meetings pertaining to nursing but attends medical committee meetings only when a nursing issue is being discussed.

14. 1. Usually, the charge nurse should attempt to settle a conflict at the lowest level possible, in this case, confronting the nurse. However, the charge nurse does not have the authority to require a drug screen, which is the intervention needed in this situation. The nurse should notify the unit manager.
2. The charge nurse does not have the authority to force the nurse to submit to a drug screening, which is what this behavior suggests. Therefore, the charge nurse should not confront the staff nurse. The nurse should notify the supervisor.

3. Nurses have the right to take breaks with or without their peers. The charge nurse cannot enforce this option.
4. An occurrence report is not used for this type of situation. This is a management or a peer review issue. The nurse can go through the manager or a peer review committee.

15. 1. The nurse should stop the behavior occurring in a public place. The charge nurse can discuss the issue with the UAPs and determine whether the manager should be notified.
2. **The first action is to stop the argument from occurring in a public place. The charge nurse should not discuss the UAPs' behavior in public.**
3. The second action is to have the UAPs go to a private area before resuming the conversation.
4. The charge nurse may need to mediate the disagreement; this would be the third step.

16. 1. The graduate nurse should handle the situation directly with the UAP first before notifying the charge nurse.
2. This may need to be completed, but not prior to directly discussing the behavior with the UAP.
3. The graduate nurse must address the insubordination with the UAP, not just complete the tasks that are the responsibility of the UAP.
4. **The graduate nurse must discuss the insubordination directly with the UAP first. The nurse must give objective data as to when and where the UAP did not follow through with the completion of assigned tasks.**

17. 1. **Telling jokes with sexual innuendos creates a "hostile work environment" and should be addressed with the HCP. This is a courtesy to the HCP to allow him to correct the behavior without being embarrassed.**
2. If the behavior is not corrected, then the nurse should report the HCP to the manager or chief nursing officer (CNO). The manager or CNO may find it necessary to report the behavior to the medical staff committee or president.
3. The charge nurse should first report the behavior to the manager and the, if the problem is not resolved, to the CNO, or, in other words, follow the chain of command.
4. Some facilities have a code for staff to use when an HCP is acting out, but it is rarely, if ever, used.

18. 1. The new graduate cannot take a break whenever he or she becomes overwhelmed because the work may never get done. The new graduate should schedule breaks throughout the shift, not when he or she wants to take them.
2. **The preceptor should recommend that the new graduate use some tool to organize the work so that important tasks, such as medication administration and taking vital signs, are not missed.**
3. Encouraging the new graduate to calm himself or herself down (five deep breaths) before beginning work is good, but it will not help the new graduate with time management.
4. The new graduate must find the best way to organize himself or herself. Doing the organizing for the new graduate will not help him or her.

19. 1. Synthroid is a medication used to treat hypothyroidism; therefore, the nurse would not question administering this medication.
2. Inderal is administered to decrease the heart rate in clients diagnosed with hyperthyroidism; therefore, the nurse would not question administering this medication.
3. **Procardia decreases blood pressure; therefore, the nurse should question administering this medication to a client with hypotension.**
4. Vasotec, an ACE inhibitor, is administered to clients with diabetes to help prevent diabetic nephropathy. The nurse would not question administering this medication.

20. 1. **This client is exhibiting signs and symptoms of a potentially fatal complication of DVT—pulmonary embolism. The nurse should assess this client first.**
2. Refusing to eat hospital food should be discussed with the client, but the nurse could ask the unit secretary to have the dietitian see the client.
3. Clients diagnosed with pancreatitis have nasogastric tubes to rest the bowel. However, these tubes are typically uncomfortable. Regardless, the nurse should see this client after the client diagnosed with DVT has been assessed and appropriate interventions initiated. The nurse should discuss the importance of maintaining the tube with the client.
4. This is an expected symptom of osteoarthritis. This client does not need to be assessed first.

Surgical Nursing

3

ABBREVIATION LIST

AAA	Abdominal Aortic Aneurysm	**LPN**	Licensed Practical Nurse
ABG	Arterial Blood Gas	**MAR**	Medication Administration Record
ACS	American Cancer Society	**NCSBN**	National Council of State Boards of Nursing
AP	Apical Pulse		
BP	Blood Pressure	**NPO**	Nothing per (by) Os (Mouth)
COPD	Chronic Obstructive Pulmonary Disease	**OR**	Operating Room
D&C	Dilation and Curretage	**PACU**	Post-Anesthesia Care Unit
DNR	Do Not Resuscitate	**PDR**	Physician's Desk Reference
DVT	Deep Vein Thrombosis	**PICC**	Peripherally Inserted Central Catheter
ED	Emergency Department		
H&H	Hemoglobin and Hematocrit	**PRN**	As Needed
		R	Respiration
HCP	Health-Care Provider	**RN**	Registered Nurse
HIPPA	Health Information Privacy and Portability Act	**THR**	Total Hip Replacement
		TKR	Total Knee Replacement
ICU	Intensive Care Unit	**TURP**	Transurethral Resection of the Prostate
IV	Intravenous		
IVP	Intravenous Push	**UAP**	Unlicensed Assistive Personnel
IVPB	Intravenous Piggy Back		
K+	Potassium	**WBC**	White Blood Cell

PRACTICE QUESTIONS

Setting Priorities When Caring for Clients

1. The nurse has received the morning shift report on a surgical unit in a community hospital. Which client should the nurse assess first?
   1. The elderly client diagnosed with a left fractured hip who is crying and is frightened about the surgery.
   2. The school-aged client who has an open reduction and internal fixation of the right ulna with 1+ edema.
   3. The middle-aged client who is 1 day postoperative for abdominal surgery and who has a rigid, hard abdomen.
   4. The adolescent client who is 2 days postoperative for an emergency appendectomy and who is complaining of abdominal pain and rating it as an "8."

2. The client is diagnosed with laryngeal cancer and is scheduled for a laryngectomy next week. Which intervention would be priority for the clinic nurse?
   1. Assess the client's ability to swallow.
   2. Refer the client to a speech therapist.
   3. Order the client's preoperative lab work.
   4. Discuss the client's operative permit.

3. The client who is 2 days postoperative for a left pneumonectomy has an apical pulse (AP) of 128 and a blood pressure (BP) of 80/50. Which intervention should the nurse implement first?
   1. Notify the health-care provider (HCP) immediately.
   2. Assess the client's incisional wound.
   3. Prepare to administer dopamine, a vasopressor.
   4. Increase the client's intravenous (IV) rate.

4. The charge nurse is reviewing the morning laboratory results. Which data should the charge nurse report to the HCP via telephone?
   1. The client who is 4 hours postoperative for gastric lap banding with a white blood cell (WBC) count of 15,000 mm.
   2. The client who is 1 day postoperative for total knee replacement (TKR) with a hemoglobin and hematocrit (H&H) of 12/36.
   3. The client who is 4 days postoperative for coronary artery bypass surgery whose fasting glucose is 180 mg/dL.
   4. The client who is 8 hours postoperative for exploratory laparotomy whose potassium (K^+) is at 4.5 mEq/L.

5. The nurse is preparing clients for surgery. Which client has the greatest potential for experiencing complications?
   1. The 17-year-old client scheduled for left knee arthroscopy who reports chewing tobacco several times a day.
   2. The 48-year-old client scheduled for surgery for an abdominal aortic aneurysm (AAA) who has a history of high blood pressure.
   3. The 55-year-old client scheduled for an open cholecystectomy who smokes two packs of cigarettes per day.
   4. The 25-year-old client scheduled for a dilatation and curettage (D&C) who smokes marijuana on a daily basis.

6. The nurse is administering medications to clients on a surgical unit. Which medication should the nurse administer first?
    1. The narcotic analgesic morphine IV infusion to the client who is 8 hours postoperative and who is complaining of pain and rating it as a "7."
    2. The aminoglycoside antibiotic vancomycin intravenous piggy back (IVPB) to the client with an infected abdominal wound.
    3. The proton-pump inhibitor pantoprazole (Protonix) IVPB to the client who is at risk for developing a stress ulcer.
    4. The loop-diuretic furosemide (Lasix) intravenous push (IVP) to the client who has undergone surgical débridement of the right lower limb.

7. The night shift nurse is caring for clients on the surgical unit. Which client situation would warrant immediate notification of the surgeon?
    1. The client who is 2 days postoperative for bowel resection and who refuses to turn, cough, and deep breathe.
    2. The client who is 5 hours postoperative for abdominal hysterectomy who reported feeling a "pop" and then her pain went away.
    3. The client who is 2 hours postoperative for TKR and who has 400 mL in the cell-saver collection device.
    4. The client who is 1 day postoperative for bilateral thyroidectomy and who has a negative Chvostek sign.

8. The nurse is performing ostomy care for a client who had an abdominal-peritoneal resection with a permanent sigmoid colostomy. Rank the following interventions in order of priority.
    1. Cleanse the stomal site with mild soap and water.
    2. Assess the stoma for a pink, moist appearance.
    3. Monitor the drainage in the ostomy drainage bag.
    4. Apply stoma adhesive paste to the skin around the stoma.
    5. Attach the ostomy drainage bag to the abdomen.

9. The rehabilitation nurse is caring for a client who is 1 week postoperative for left carotid endarterectomy. The client's 11:30 A.M. bedside glucometer reading is 408 mg/dL. Based on the medication administration record (MAR), which intervention should the nurse implement first?

Client's Name:	Account Number: 123456		Allergies: NKDA
Height: 69 inches	**Weight:** 165 pounds		
Date	**Medication**	**2301–0700**	**0701–1500**	**1501–2300**
	Regular Insulin by bedside glucose subcu ac & hs			
	<60 notify HCP 150 0 units 151–200 2 units		0730 DN BG 142 0 units	
	201–250 4 units 251–300 6 units			
	301–350 8 units 351–400 10 units >400 notify HCP			
Signature/Initials		Day Nurse RN DN	

   1. Notify the health-care provider.
   2. Administer 10 units regular insulin.
   3. Notify the laboratory to draw a serum glucose level.
   4. Recheck the bedside glucometer reading.

10. The nurse is transcribing the HCP's orders for a client who is scheduled for an emergency appendectomy and who is being transferred from the emergency department (ED) to the surgical unit. Which order should the nurse implement first?
   1. Obtain the client's informed consent.
   2. Administer IV morphine 2 mg, every 4 hours, prn.
   3. Shave the lower right abdominal quadrant.
   4. Administer the on-call IVPB antibiotic.

Delegating and Assigning Tasks

11. The nurse and unlicensed assistive personnel (UAP) are caring for clients on a surgical unit. Which action by the UAP warrants immediate intervention?
   1. The UAP empties the indwelling catheter bag for the client with transurethral resection of the prostate (TURP).
   2. The UAP assists a client who received an IV narcotic analgesic 30 minutes ago to ambulate in the hall.
   3. The UAP provides apple juice to a client who has just been advanced to a clear liquid diet.
   4. The UAP applies moisture barrier cream to the elderly client who has an excoriated perianal area.

12. The charge nurse is making shift assignments to the surgical staff, which consists of two registered nurses (RNs), two licensed practical nurses (LPNs), and two UAPs. Which assignment would be most appropriate by the charge nurse?
    1. Instruct the RN to administer all prn medications.
    2. Instruct the UAP to clean the recently vacated room.
    3. Assign the LPN to administer routine medications.
    4. Request the LPN to complete the admission for a new client.

13. The nurse on the surgical unit is working with a UAP. Which task would be most appropriate for the nurse to delegate to the UAP?
    1. Change an abdominal dressing on a client who is 2 days postoperative.
    2. Check the client's IV insertion site on the right arm.
    3. Monitor vital signs on a client who has just returned from surgery.
    4. Escort a client who has been discharged to the client's vehicle.

14. The charge nurse is making assignments for the surgical unit. Which client should be assigned to the new graduate nurse?
    1. The 84-year-old client who has a chest tube that is draining bright red blood.
    2. The 38-year-old client who is 1 day postoperative with a temperature of 101.2°F.
    3. The 42-year-old client who has just returned to the unit after a breast biopsy.
    4. The 55-year-old client who is complaining of unrelenting abdominal pain.

15. The client is being prepared for a colonoscopy in the day surgery center. The charge nurse observes the primary nurse instructing the UAP to assist the client to the bathroom. Which action should the charge nurse implement?
    1. Take no action because this is appropriate delegation.
    2. Tell the UAP to obtain a bedside commode for the client.
    3. Discuss the inappropriate delegation of the nursing task.
    4. Document the situation in an adverse occurrence report.

16. The HCP writes an order for the client with a fractured right hip to ambulate with a walker four times per day. Which action should the nurse implement?
    1. Tell the UAP to ambulate the client with the walker.
    2. Request a referral to the physical therapy department.
    3. Obtain a walker that is appropriate for the client's height.
    4. Notify the social worker of the HCP's order for a walker.

17. Which task would be most appropriate for the nurse to delegate to the UAP working on a surgical unit?
    1. Escort the client to the smoking area outside.
    2. Obtain vital signs on a newly admitted client.
    3. Administer a feeding to the client with a gastrostomy tube.
    4. Check the toes of a client who just had a cast application.

18. The charge nurse is making assignments in the day surgery center. Which client should be assigned to the most experienced nurse?
    1. The client who had surgery for an inguinal hernia and who is being prepared for discharge.
    2. The client who is in the preoperative area and who is scheduled for laparoscopic cholecystectomy.
    3. The client who has completed scheduled chemotherapy treatment and who is receiving 2 units of blood.
    4. The client who has end-stage renal disease and who has had an arteriovenous fistula created.

19. The LPN is working in a surgical rehabilitation unit. Which nursing task would be most appropriate for the LPN to implement?
    1. Bathe the client who is incontinent of urine.
    2. Document the amount of food the client eats.
    3. Conduct the afternoon bingo game in the lobby.
    4. Perform routine dressing changes on assigned clients.

20. The nurse is completing the admission assessment on the client scheduled for cystectomy with creation of an ileal conduit. The client tells the nurse, "I am taking saw palmetto for my enlarged prostate." Which action should the nurse implement first?
    1. Notify the client's HCP to write an order for the herbal supplement.
    2. Ask the client why he is taking an herb for his enlarged prostate.
    3. Consult with the pharmacist to determine any potential drug interactions.
    4. Look up saw palmetto in the Physician's Desk Reference (PDR).

Managing Clients and Nursing Staff

21. The ED nurse is requesting a bed in the intensive care unit (ICU). The ICU charge nurse must request a transfer of one client from the ICU to the surgical unit to make room for the client coming into the ICU from the ED. Which client should the ICU charge nurse request to transfer to the surgical unit?
    1. The client diagnosed with flail chest who has just come from the operating room with a right-sided chest tube.
    2. The client diagnosed with acute diverticulitis who is 1 day postoperative for creation of a sigmoid colostomy.
    3. The client who is 1 day postoperative for total hip replacement (THR) whose incisional dressing is dry and intact.
    4. The client who is 2 days postoperative for repair of a fractured femur and who has had a fat embolism.

22. A terrible storm causes the electricity to go out in the hospital and the emergency generator lights come on. Which action should the charge nurse implement?
    1. Request all family members to leave the hospital as soon as possible.
    2. Instruct the staff to plug critical electrical equipment into the red outlets.
    3. Have the UAP place a portable flashlight on each bedside table.
    4. Contact the maintenance department to determine how long the electricity will be out.

23. The HCP is angry and yelling in the nurse's station because the client's laboratory data are not available. Which action should the charge nurse implement first?
    1. Contact the laboratory for the client's results.
    2. Ask the HCP to step into the nurse's office.
    3. Tell the HCP to discuss the issue with the laboratory.
    4. Report the HCP's behavior to the chief nursing officer.

24. The staff nurse is concerned about possible increasing infection rates among clients with peripherally inserted central catheters (PICCs). The nurse has noticed several clients with problems in the last few months. Which action would be appropriate for the staff nurse to implement first?
    1. Discuss the infections with the chief nursing officer.
    2. Contact the infection control nurse to discuss the problem.
    3. Assume the employee health nurse is monitoring the situation.
    4. Volunteer to be on an ad hoc committee to research the infection rate.

25. The charge nurse on the 30-bed surgical unit has been told to send one staff member to the medical unit. The surgical unit is full, with multiple clients who require custodial care. Which staff member would be most appropriate to send to the medical unit?
    1. Send the UAP who has worked on the surgical unit for 5 years.
    2. Send the RN who has worked in the hospital for 8 years in a variety of areas.
    3. Send the LPN who has 3 years experience, which includes 6 months on the medical unit.
    4. Send the new graduate nurse who is orienting to the surgical unit.

26. The nurse educator is discussing fire safety with new employees. List in order of performance the following actions the nurse should teach to ensure the safety of clients and employees in the case of fire on the unit.
    1. Extinguish.
    2. Rescue.
    3. Confine.
    4. Alert.

27. The client tells the nurse, "I am having surgery on my right knee." However, the operative permit is for surgery on the left knee. Which action should the nurse implement first?
    1. Notify the operating room team.
    2. Initiate the time-out procedure.
    3. Clarify the correct extremity with the client.
    4. Call the surgeon to discuss the discrepancy.

28. The elderly female client fell and fractured her left femur. The nurse finds the client crying, and she tells the nurse, "I don't want to go to the nursing home but my son says I have to." Which response would be most appropriate by the nurse?
    1. "Let me call a meeting of the health-care team and your son."
    2. "Has the social worker talked to you about this already?"
    3. "Why are you so upset about going to the nursing home?"
    4. "I can see you are upset. Would you like to talk about it?"

29. The primary nurse informs the shift manager that one of the UAPs is falsifying vital signs. Which action should the shift manager implement first?
    1. Notify the unit manager of the potential situation of falsifying vital signs.
    2. Take the assigned client's vital signs and compare with the UAP's results.
    3. Talk to the UAP about the primary nurse's allegation.
    4. Complete a counseling record and place in the UAP's file.

30. The client scheduled for a D&C is upset because the HCP told her she has syphilis. The client asks the nurse, "This is so embarrassing, do you have to tell anyone about this?" Which statement is the nurse's best response?
    1. "This must be reported to the Public Health Department and your sexual partners."
    2. "According to the Health Information Privacy and Portability Act (HIPPA), I cannot report this to anyone without your permission."
    3. "You really should tell your sexual partners so they can be treated for syphilis."
    4. "I realize you are embarrassed. Would you like to talk about the situation?"

Setting Priorities When Caring for Clients

1. 1. This client is experiencing a psychosocial need, which, although important, is not priority over a physiologic problem.
   2. One-plus edema would be expected in a client with a fractured ulna.
   3. A hard, rigid abdomen indicates peritonitis, which is a life-threatening emergency. This client should be assessed first.
   4. The client who is 2 days postoperative and who is complaining of and rating pain as an "8" should be assessed, but the pain is not life threatening and, therefore, does not take priority over the patient with probable peritonitis.

   MAKING NURSING DECISIONS: When deciding which client to assess first, the test taker should determine whether the signs/symptoms the client is exhibiting are normal or expected for the client's situation. After eliminating the expected options, the test taker should determine which situation is more life threatening.

2. 1. The client's ability to swallow is not impaired prior to the surgical procedure.
   2. The client will not be able to speak after the removal of the larynx; therefore, referral to a speech therapist who will be able to discuss an alternate means of communication is priority.
   3. The HCP, not the nurse, is responsible for ordering the preoperative laboratory work.
   4. The HCP, not the nurse, is responsible for discussing the operative permit.

   MAKING NURSING DECISIONS: The test taker must be aware of the setting that ultimately dictates the appropriate intervention. The adjectives will clue the test taker to the setting. In this question the words "clinic nurse" clue the test taker to the setting. The test taker must also remember the nurse's scope of practice and realize that options 3 and 4 are outside the nurse's scope of practice.

3. 1. The HCP should be notified, but this is not the first intervention. The HCP will require other information, such as what the incision looks like and whether there is any bleeding that can be seen, before making any decisions. The nurse, therefore, should first provide emergency care to the client—in this case, support the client's circulatory system by increasing the IV rate—and then assess the patient before reporting to the HCP.
   2. The incisional wound should be assessed, but the priority is maintaining circulatory status because the client's vital signs indicate shock.
   3. The client may require medication, such as dopamine, to increase the blood pressure, but the client's circulatory system needs immediate support, which increasing the IV rate will provide. That, then, is the priority.
   4. Increasing the IV rate will provide the client with circulatory volume immediately. Therefore, this is the first intervention.

   MAKING NURSING DECISIONS: Remember: "If the client is in distress, do not assess." Situations such as those in this question require the nurse to intervene to prevent the client's status from deteriorating. Before selecting "notify the HCP" as the correct answer, the test taker must examine the other three options. If information in any of the other options is data that will relieve the client's distress, prevent a life-threatening situation, or provide information the HCP will need to make an informed decision, then the test taker should eliminate the "notify the HCP" option.

4. 1. Because a client undergoing an elective procedure such as a gastric lap banding is usually healthy prior to the surgery, an elevated postoperative WBC count—which this client has—may indicate infection and, therefore, requires notifying the HCP.
   2. The H&H of 12/36 is within normal limits.
   3. The glucose level is elevated, but many clients with coronary artery disease have concurrent diabetes, so a glucose reading of 180 mg/dL would not require calling the HCP.
   4. A K^+ level of 4.5 mEq/L is within normal limits.

   MAKING NURSING DECISIONS: The test taker must know normal laboratory data. See Appendix A for normal laboratory data.

5. 1. Although chewing tobacco can produce long-term health effects, this client is only 17 years old; therefore, this habit should not complicate the knee surgery.
   2. The client's high blood pressure caused the AAA; therefore, a history of hypertension should not cause concern for the nurse.
   3. The location of the incision for a cholecystectomy, the general anesthesia needed, and a heavy smoking history makes this client high risk for pulmonary complications.
   4. Use of marijuana daily does not increase the risk of pulmonary complications.

6. 1. **The client who is in pain is priority. None of the other clients has a life-threatening condition. Pain is considered the fifth vital sign.**
   2. Routine antibiotics are not priority over a client who has postoperative pain.
   3. Risk for a stress ulcer is a potential, not an actual, problem, and proton-pump inhibitors are administered routinely to help prevent stress ulcers.
   4. The loop diuretic is a routine medication prescribed for a medical comorbid condition, not for surgical débridement.

   MAKING NURSING DECISIONS: When the test taker is making a decision about prioritizing medication administration, client comfort takes priority over regularly scheduled medications.

7. 1. The nurse would not need to notify the surgeon of the client's refusal because this is a situation the nurse should manage.
   2. **Feeling a "pop" after an abdominal hysterectomy may indicate possible wound dehiscence, which is a surgical emergency and requires the nurse to notify the surgeon via telephone.**
   3. This situation indicates that it is time for the nurse to reinfuse the lost blood.
   4. A negative Chvostek sign is normal and indicates the calcium level is within normal limits.

   MAKING NURSING DECISIONS: When the test taker is deciding when to notify an HCP immediately, the test taker should think, "Does this situation warrant calling the HCP in the middle of the night?" If the answer is yes, then this option is the correct answer.

8. In order of performance: 3, 2, 1, 4, 5.
   3. The nurse must first assess the drainage in the bag for color, consistency, and amount.
   2. After removing the bag, the nurse should assess the site to ensure circulation to the stoma. A pink, moist appearance indicates adequate circulation.
   1. The nurse should cleanse the area with a mild soap and water to ensure that the skin is prepared for the adhesive paste.
   4. The nurse should then apply adhesive paste to the clean, dry skin.
   5. The ostomy drainage bag is attached last.

9. 1. The HCP should be notified when the glucose level is verified by the laboratory.
   2. The sliding scale indicates that a blood glucose level of 351 to 400 mg/dL requires 10 units of regular insulin. There is no insulin dosage administered for 408 mg/dL.
   3. This should be done, but not until the nurse rechecks the blood glucose level at the bedside.
   4. **The nurse should first recheck the blood glucose level at the bedside prior to taking any further action.**

10. 1. **The nurse must first obtain the operative permit or determine whether it has been signed by the client prior to implementing any other orders.**
    2. The client cannot give informed consent after receiving pain medication; therefore, administration of morphine cannot be implemented first.
    3. The operating room staff usually performs shave preps, but the nurse would not implement this prior to medicating the client.
    4. The on-call IVPB is not administered until the operating room (OR) is prepared for the client. New standards recommend that the prophylactic IVPB antibiotic be administered within 1 hour of opening the skin during a surgical procedure.

Delegating and Assigning Tasks

11. 1. The UAP can empty an indwelling catheter drainage bag because this does not require judgment.
    2. **The client who received a narcotic analgesic 30 minutes ago is at risk for falling because of the effects of the medication; therefore, the UAP should not ambulate this client. The nurse should intervene.**

3. The UAP can provide juice to the client, and apple juice is part of the client's liquid diet.
4. Moisture barrier cream is not a medication; therefore, the UAP can apply such creams to an intact perianal area.

MAKING NURSING DECISIONS: The nurse cannot delegate to a UAP the assessment, evaluation, teaching, or administration of medications to any client or the care of an unstable client.

12. 1. The LPN can administer routine as well as some prn medications; assigning the RN to administer all prn medications is not appropriate.
2. The housekeeping department, not the UAP, is assigned to clean recently vacated rooms.
3. **The LPN can administer most routine medications; therefore, this would be the most appropriate assignment for the LPN.**
4. The RN would be the most appropriate staff member to complete the admission assessment.

MAKING NURSING DECISIONS: The nurse cannot assign assessment, evaluation, teaching, or any action that requires nursing judgment to an LPN. The nurse can, however, delegate the administration of routine medications to an LPN.

13. 1. The UAP cannot change abdominal dressings because the incision must be assessed for healing.
2. The UAP cannot check the client's IV site. Remember, check is "assess."
3. The nurse must monitor the vital signs on a client recently returned from surgery to determine whether the client is stable; the UAP can take vital signs and report results to the nurse.
4. **The UAP can escort the client to the vehicle after discharge.**

14. 1. This client is not stable and requires a more experienced nurse.
2. An elevated temperature indicates a potential complication of surgery; therefore, this client requires a more experienced nurse.
3. **Of the four clients, the one who is most stable is the client who has just undergone a breast biopsy; therefore, this client would be the most appropriate to assign to a new graduate nurse.**
4. Unrelenting pain requires further assessment; therefore, the client should be assigned to a more experienced nurse.

MAKE NURSING DECISIONS: When the test taker is deciding which client should be assigned to a new graduate, the most stable client should be assigned to the least experienced nurse.

15. 1. **The primary nurse's instruction to the UAP to assist the client to the bathroom is an appropriate delegation that ensures the safety of the client. It requires no action by the charge nurse.**
2. There is no information in the stem that indicates the client needs a bedside commode; therefore, this is not an appropriate action.
3. The UAP can assist a client who is stable to ambulate; therefore, this is not inappropriate delegation.
4. An adverse occurrence report is completed whenever potential or actual harm has come to the client. Ambulating the client with assistance is not harmful.

16. 1. The first time a client ambulates after hip surgery should be with a physical therapist or a nurse qualified to evaluate the client's ability to ambulate safely with a walker. The UAP does not have these qualifications.
2. **According to the National Council of State Boards of Nursing (NCSBN), collaboration with interdisciplinary team members is part of the management of care. Physical therapy is responsible for management of the client's ability to move and transfer.**
3. The physical therapist will measure and obtain the correct walker for the client.
4. The social worker is not responsible for assisting the client to ambulate, but may assist the client on discharge in obtaining needed medical equipment in the home.

17. 1. The UAP is being paid to assist the nurse to care for clients on the surgical unit, not take clients downstairs to smoke.
2. **The UAP can take vital signs on a newly admitted client.**
3. The client has a tube into the stomach via the abdominal wall that requires assessing the residual to determine whether the stomach is digesting the tube feeding. This task is not appropriate to delegate to the UAP.
4. If the toes are cold, have a capillary refill time of more than 3 seconds, or are pale, the nurse must make a judgment as to the circulatory status of the foot; therefore, the nurse would not delegate this task.

18. 1. The most experienced nurse should be assigned to the client who requires teaching and evaluation of knowledge for home health care, because the client is in the surgery center for less than 1 day.
    2. A routine preoperative client does not require the most experienced nurse.
    3. Any nurse can administer and monitor blood transfusion to the client.
    4. Although the creation of an arteriovenous fistula requires assessment and teaching on the part of the most experienced nurse, this client is not being discharged home at this time.

19. 1. The LPN can bathe a client, but this should be assigned to the UAP, thereby allowing the LPN to perform a higher-level task.
    2. The LPN can document the amount of food the client eats, but this should be assigned to the UAP, thereby allowing the LPN to perform a higher-level task.
    3. According to the NSCBN NCLEX-RN test plan, collaboration with interdisciplinary team members is part of the management of care. The activity director of the long-term care facility would be responsible for this activity.
    4. The LPN scope of practice allows routine sterile procedures on the client who is stable, such as clients in a surgical rehabilitation facility.

20. 1. If the HCP deems that the client can continue to take the herbal supplement, then an order must be written; however, this is not the first intervention.
    2. The nurse could ask for clarification of why he is taking the herbal supplement, but this is not the first intervention. Many clients use herbal supplements for a variety of health-care needs.
    3. According to the NSCBN NCLEX-RN test plan, collaboration with interdisciplinary team members is part of the management of care. The nurse should first consult with the pharmacist to determine whether the client is taking any medications that could interact with the saw palmetto.
    4. The PDR is available to research medications, not herbal supplements.

Managing Clients and Nursing Staff

21. 1. The client who has just returned from surgery should not be transferred from the ICU because he or she may not be stable.
    2. A sigmoid colonostomy is a surgical procedure that causes major fluid shifts and has the potential for multiple complications; therefore, this client should not be transferred to the surgical unit.
    3. Although the client is only 1 day postoperative for a total hip replacement, it is an elective procedure, which indicates that the client was stable prior to the surgery. The incision is also dry and intact. Of the four clients, this client is the most stable and should be transferred to the surgical unit.
    4. A fat embolism is a potentially life-threatening complication of a fracture; therefore, this client should not be transferred from the ICU.

22. 1. Family members should be asked to stay in the client's room until the lights come back on. This helps ensure safety of the family members.

2. During an electrical failure, the red outlets in the hospital run on the backup generator, and all IV pumps and necessary equipment should be plugged into these outlets.
3. The hospital may provide tap bells for contacting the hospital staff, but would not provide flashlights to all clients. The hospital staff would need the flashlights.
4. The charge nurse should not tie up the phone lines during an emergency situation; the phones may not even be working.

23. 1. The charge nurse should contact the laboratory, but the first action should be to address the HCP's behavior in a private area.
2. **This is the charge nurse's first action because it will diffuse the HCP's anger. Inappropriate behavior at the nurse's station should not be in an area where visitors, clients, or staff will observe the behavior.**
3. The HCP can call the laboratory and share his or her concerns, but it is not the first intervention.
4. The charge nurse has the option to report any HCP's inappropriate behavior, but the immediate situation must be dealt with first.

24. 1. The staff nurse should go through the chain of command when wanting to investigate a problem.
2. **Possibly increasing infection rates among clients with PICCs falls within the infection control nurse's scope of practice, and the infection control nursing staff will have data from all units in the hospital.**
3. The nurse should follow through with investigating a potential problem, but this problem does not fall within the scope of practice of the employee health nurse.
4. The staff nurse should be a part of the solution to a problem. Volunteering is a good action to effect change, but it is not the first action. More information—which the infection control nurse can provide—is necessary first.

25. 1. Because there are multiple surgical clients requiring custodial care, the charge nurse should not send an experienced UAP to the medical unit.
2. The charge nurse should not send the experienced RN to the medical unit because this nurse represents the strength of the staff.

3. **The LPN would be the most appropriate staff to send to the medical unit because the LPN has experience on the unit. His or her expertise is also not required to perform custodial care.**
4. A new orientee should not be sent to an unfamiliar area.

MAKING NURSING DECISIONS: The charge nurse must evaluate each of the staff member's qualifications and value to the unit. The charge nurse cannot deplete the staffing resources on his or her own unit to help staff another unit; however, the charge nurse must be fair when sending staff to another unit.

26. In order of performance: 2, 4, 3, 1. The nurse must remember the acronym RACE, which is a recognized national standard for fire safety in health-care facilities.
2. R is for rescue.
4. A is for alert.
3. C is for confine.
1. E is for extinguish.

MAKING NURSING DECISIONS: The nurse is responsible for knowing and complying with local, state, and federal standards of care. The nurse must be knowledgeable about hospital emergency preparedness. Students as well as new employees receive this information in hospital orientations and are responsible for implementing procedures correctly. The NCSBN NCLEX-RN blueprint includes questions on safe and effective care environment.

27. 1. The nurse should notify the operating room team, but according to the Joint Commission, the first intervention is to call a time-out, which stops the surgery until clarification is obtained.
2. **According to the Joint Commission, the first intervention is to call a time-out, which stops the surgery until clarification is obtained.**
3. The nurse should discuss this with the client but should first initiate the time-out procedure.
4. Calling the surgeon is a part of the time-out procedure, so the first intervention is to call the time-out.

28. 1. The nurse should initiate a client care conference to discuss the client's feelings, but at this time the most appropriate response is to allow the client to begin the grieving process.

2. The nurse could notify the social worker about the client's situation, but the most appropriate response is to allow the client to begin the grieving process, which the client often goes through when experiencing any type of loss. In this situation, the client is losing her independence and her home.

3. The client does not owe the nurse an explanation for "feelings."

4. According to the NSCBN NCLEX-RN test plan, advocacy is part of the management of care under the safe and effective care environment. Therapeutic communication involves being an advocate in this situation because sometimes the nurse cannot prevent a perceived "bad" situation from occurring.

29. 1. This should not be implemented until verification of the allegation is complete, and the shift manager has discussed the situation with the UAP.

2. The shift manager should have objective data prior to confronting the UAP about the allegation of falsifying vital signs; therefore, the shift manager should take the client's vital signs and compare them with the UAP's results before taking any other action.

3. The shift manager should not confront the UAP until objective data is obtained to support the allegation.

4. Written documentation should be the last action when resolving staff issues.

30. 1. HIPAA does not apply in some situations, including the reporting of sexually transmitted diseases to the Public Health Department. The Public Health Department will attempt to notify any sexual partners the client reports.

2. This is a false statement. HIPPA does not apply in certain situations, and the nurse must be knowledgeable of HIPPA guidelines.

3. The client should notify her sexual partners so they can be treated; however, in response to the client asking "does anyone have to know," the nurse's best response is to provide facts.

4. This is a therapeutic response aimed at encouraging the client to verbalize feelings, but the nurse should provide factual information in this situation.

COMPREHENSIVE EXAMINATION

1. The 24-year-old male client diagnosed with testicular cancer is scheduled for a unilateral orchiectomy. Which priority intervention should the clinic nurse implement?
   1. Teach the client to turn, cough, and deep breathe.
   2. Discuss the importance of sperm banking.
   3. Explain about the testicular prosthesis.
   4. Refer the client to the American Cancer Society (ACS).

2. The nurse is caring for clients on a surgical unit. Which client should the nurse assess first?
   1. The client who is 1 day postoperative for mastectomy and who is refusing to perform arm exercises.
   2. The client who is 8 hours postoperative for splenectomy and who is complaining of abdominal pain and rating it as a "5."
   3. The client who is 12 hours postoperative for adrenalectomy and who has vomited 100 mL of dark green bile.
   4. The client who is 2 days postoperative for hiatal hernia repair and who is complaining of feeling constipated.

3. The client is confused and pulling at the IV and indwelling catheter. Which order from the HCP should the nurse clarify concerning restraining the client?
   1. Restrain the client's wrists, as needed.
   2. Offer the client fluids every 2 hours.
   3. Apply a hand mitt to the arm opposite the IV site for 12 hours.
   4. Check circulation of the restrained limb every 2 hours.

4. The charge nurse on a 20-bed surgical unit has one RN, two LPNs, and two UAPs for a 12-hour shift. Which task would be an inappropriate delegation of assignments?
   1. The RN will perform the shift assessments.
   2. The LPN should administer all IVP medications.
   3. The UAP will complete all A.M. care.
   4. The RN will monitor laboratory values.

5. The client in the post-anesthesia care unit (PACU) has noisy and irregular respirations (Rs) with a pulse oximeter reading of 89%. Which intervention should the PACU nurse implement first?
   1. Increase the client's oxygen rate via nasal cannula.
   2. Notify the respiratory therapist to draw arterial blood gases.
   3. Tilt the head back and push forward on the angle of the lower jaw.
   4. Obtain an intubation tray and prepare for emergency intubation.

6. The day surgery admission nurse is obtaining operative permits for clients having surgery. Which client should the nurse question signing the consent form?
   1. The 84-year-old client diagnosed with chronic obstructive pulmonary disease (COPD).
   2. The 16-year-old married client who is diagnosed with an ectopic pregnancy.
   3. The 50-year-old client who admits to being a recovering alcoholic.
   4. The 39-year-old client diagnosed with paranoid schizophrenia.

7. The female client in the preoperative holding area tells the nurse that she had a reaction to a latex diaphragm. Which intervention should the nurse perform first?
   1. Notify the operating room personnel.
   2. Label the client's chart with the allergy.
   3. Place a red allergy band on the client.
   4. Inform the client to tell all HCPs of the allergy.

8. Which task would be most appropriate for the nurse to delegate/assign when caring for clients on a surgical unit?
   1. Instruct the LPN to feed the client who is 1 day postoperative for vaginal hysterectomy.
   2. Ask another RN to administer an IVP pain medication to a client in severe pain.
   3. Request the UAP to check the client whose AP was 112, R was 26, and BP was 92/58.
   4. Instruct the LPN to obtain the pre-transfusion assessment on a postoperative client.

9. The client is being prepared for emergency surgery and is asking to complete an Advance Directive. Which type of Advance Directive should the nurse recommend the client complete at this time?
   1. Power of Attorney.
   2. Living Will.
   3. Do Not Resuscitate (DNR) Order.
   4. Durable Power of Attorney for Health Care.

10. The nurse is caring for clients in the PACU. Which client would require immediate intervention by the PACU nurse?
    1. The client who is exhibiting masseter rigidity.
    2. The client who has not urinated for 2 hours after surgery.
    3. The client who is sleepy but arouses easily to verbal stimuli.
    4. The client who has hypoactive bowel sounds.

11. The charge nurse on a busy 20-bed surgical unit must send one staff member to the nursery. Which staff member would be most appropriate to send to the nursery?
    1. The nurse who has worked on the surgical unit for 4 years.
    2. The graduate nurse who has been on the surgical unit for 6 months.
    3. The LPN who has maternal child area experience.
    4. The UAP who has six small children of her own.

12. The surgical unit has a low census and is overstaffed. Which staff member should the house supervisor notify first and request to stay home?
    1. The nurse who has the most vacation time.
    2. The nurse who asked to be requested off.
    3. The nurse who has the least experience on the unit.
    4. The nurse who has called in sick the previous 2 days.

13. The night nurse walks into the client's room and finds the client crying. The client asks the nurse "Am I dying? I think something bad is wrong but they aren't telling me." The nurse knows the client has cancer and has less than 6 months to live. Which response is an example of the ethical principle of veracity?
    1. "You are concerned they are not telling you something is wrong."
    2. "I am sorry to tell you but you have cancer and less than 6 months to live."
    3. "If you think something is wrong you should speak with your doctor in the morning."
    4. "What makes you think there is something wrong and you are dying?"

14. The female client tells the clinic nurse her stomach hurts after she takes her morning medications. The MAR indicates the client is taking an antibiotic, a daily aspirin, and a stool softener. Which intervention should the nurse implement first?
    1. Assess the client for abnormal bleeding.
    2. Instruct the client to quit taking the aspirin.
    3. Recommend the client take an enteric-coated aspirin.
    4. Instruct the client to notify the HCP.

15. The nurse educator is discussing delegation guidelines to a group of new graduates. Which statement from the group indicates the need for more teaching?
    1. "The UAP will be practicing on my brand new nursing license."
    2. "I will still retain accountability for what I delegate to the UAP."
    3. "I must make sure the UAP to whom I delegate is competent to perform the task."
    4. "When I delegate, I must follow up with the UAP and evaluate the task."

16. The nurse is reviewing the literature to identify evidenced-based practice research that supports a new procedure using a new product when changing the central line catheter dressing. Which research article would best support the nurse's proposal for a change in the procedure?
    1. The article in which the study was conducted by the manufacturer of the product used.
    2. The research article that included 10 subjects participating in the study.
    3. The review-of-literature article that cited ambiguous statistics about the product.
    4. The review-of-literature article that cited numerous studies supporting the product.

17. The head nurse is completing the yearly performance evaluation on a nurse. Which data regarding the nurse's performance should be included in the evaluation?
    1. The number of times the nurse has been tardy.
    2. The attitude of the nurse at the client's bedside.
    3. The thank you notes the nurse received from clients.
    4. The chart audits of the clients for whom the nurse cared.

18. The nurse is discharging the 72-year-old client who is 5 days postoperative for repair of a fractured hip with comorbid medical conditions. At this time, which referral would be the most appropriate for the nurse to make for this client?
    1. To a home health-care agency.
    2. To a senior citizen center.
    3. To a rehabilitation facility.
    4. To an outpatient physical therapist.

19. The nurse is caring for clients on a 12-bed intermediate care surgical unit. Which task should the nurse implement first?
    1. Reinsert the nasogastric tube for the client who has pulled it out.
    2. Complete the preoperative checklist for the client scheduled for surgery.
    3. Instruct the client who is being discharged home about colostomy care.
    4. Change the client's surgical dressing that has a 20-cm area of drainage.

20. The nurse is preparing to administer medications to clients on a surgical unit. Which medication should the nurse question administering?
    1. The antiplatelet, clopidogrel (Plavix), to a client scheduled for surgery.
    2. The anticoagulant, enoxaparin (Lovenox), to a client who had a TKR.
    3. The sliding scale insulin, Humalog, to a client who had a Whipple procedure.
    4. The aminoglycoside, vancomycin, to a client allergic to the antibiotic penicillin.

1. 1. The client must be taught postoperative care, but this is not the priority intervention of the clinic nurse.
   2. Sperm banking will allow the client's sperm to be kept until the time the client wants to conceive a child. This is priority because it must be done between the clinic visit and admission to the hospital for the procedure. The unilateral orchiectomy will not result in sterility, but the subsequent treatments may cause sterility.
   3. The nurse can discuss the testicular prosthesis, but this is not priority over sperm banking because the prosthesis may or may not be inserted at the time of surgery.
   4. A referral to the ACS is appropriate, but is not the most important information a 24-year-old male client needs at this time.

2. 1. The client should perform arm exercises to prevent potential complications, but this client is not priority over a client with a physiologic complication.
   2. The client's pain should be assessed by the nurse, but a pain rating of "5" is considered moderate pain and would be expected in a client 8 hours postoperative for abdominal surgery.
   3. The client who has had nothing by mouth (NPO) at least 20 hours (8 hours before surgery and 12 hours postoperative) and has started vomiting dark green bile is priority. If the nurse were to rate nausea on a 1 to 10 scale, the active vomiting would be a "10" and this client would be seen first.
   4. The client who is complaining of being constipated would not be priority over a client with active vomiting.

3. 1. The client cannot be restrained as needed. The nurse must have documentation for the need and an HCP's specific order that includes reason for restraint and time limited to no more than 24 hours. This HCP order should be clarified.
   2. The client in restraints should be offered fluids at least every 2 hours.
   3. Hand mitts are the least restrictive limb restraints and can be used to help prevent the client from pulling out lines.
   4. The nurse must check to ensure that restrained limbs have adequate circulation at least every 2 hours.

4. 1. The RN is responsible for assessing clients; therefore, this is an appropriate assignment.
   2. The LPN may be allowed administer some IVP medications in some facilities, but the word "all" makes this an inappropriate assignment. Many IVP medications are considered high risk, and only RNs should administer such IVP medications.
   3. This option has the word "all," but it is within the scope of the UAP to complete the A.M. care. The RN and LPN can perform A.M. care, but it should be assigned to the UAP.
   4. The RN should monitor laboratory values because this requires interpretation, evaluation, and notification of the HCP in some instances.

5. 1. Increasing the oxygen rate will not help open the client's airway, which is the first intervention. Oxygen can be increased after the airway is patent.
   2. The respiratory therapist could be notified and arterial blood gases (ABGs) drawn if positioning does not increase the pulse oximeter reading, but this is not the first intervention.
   3. The client is exhibiting signs/symptoms of hypopharyngeal obstruction, and this maneuver pulls the tongue forward and opens the air passage. The ABC of cardiopulmonary resuscitation is Airway, Breathing, and Circulation.
   4. The client may need to be intubated if positioning does not open the airway, but this is not the first intervention.

6. 1. The elderly client is considered competent until deemed incompetent in a court of law or meets the criteria to be considered incompetent.
   2. An emancipated minor who is under the age of 18, but is married or independently earning his or her own living, would not warrant the nurse's questioning this client signing the permit. "Married" indicates an independently functioning individual.
   3. A recovering alcoholic is not considered incapacitated. If the client is currently under the influence of alcohol, then the permit could not legally be signed by the client.
   4. An incompetent client cannot sign the consent form. An incompetent client is an individual who is not autonomous and cannot give or withhold consent, for example, individuals who are cognitively

impaired, mentally ill, neurologically incapacitated, or under the influence of mind-altering drugs. The client may be able to sign the permit, but the nurse should question the client's ability to sign the permit because paranoid schizophrenia is a mental illness.

7. 1. Because the client is in the preoperative holding area, the immediate safety need for the client is to inform the operating room personnel so that no latex gloves or equipment will come into contact with the client. Person-to-person communication for a safety issue ensures that the information is not overlooked.
   2. The nurse should label the chart with the allergy, but because the client is in the preoperative holding area, this is not the first intervention.
   3. The nurse should place a red allergy band on the client, but because the client is in the preoperative holding area, this is not the first intervention.
   4. The nurse should always teach the client, but at this time the first intervention is the client's safety, which is why the OR team should be notified.

8. 1. This would be an inappropriate assignment because the UAP, not the LPN, could feed this stable client.
   2. **The nurse could request that another RN administer pain medication so that the client obtains immediate pain relief.**
   3. This client's vital signs indicate that the client is unstable; therefore, the nurse should check on this client and not delegate the assessment to a UAP.
   4. The client who requires a blood transfusion is unstable. The nurse should complete the pre-transfusion assessment. The RN, not the LPN, assesses.

9. 1. A Power of Attorney is a legal document authorizing an individual to conduct business for the client. The nurse should not recommend this type of document for a health-care situation.
   2. The Living Will usually requests the client's refusal of life-sustaining treatment. General anesthesia requires the client to be intubated and placed on a ventilator; therefore, the client's request to deny this type of life-sustaining efforts will not be honored in the OR. The nurse should not recommend this type of Advance Directive.

3. A DNR order must be written in the client's chart by the HCP and may reflect the client's wishes, but it is not an Advance Directive.
4. **This document would be most appropriate for the nurse to recommend because it names an individual to be responsible in the event the client cannot make health-care decisions for himself or herself.**

10. 1. Masseter rigidity is a sign of malignant hyperthermia, which is a life-threatening complication of surgery. The client will also exhibit tachycardia (a heart rate greater than 150 bpm), hypotension, decreased cardiac output, and oliguria. It is a rare muscle disorder chemically induced by anesthesia.
    2. The client was NPO after midnight and during surgery; therefore, not urinating for 2 hours after surgery would not warrant immediate intervention.
    3. The client should be sleepy after surgery and easy to arouse; therefore, this client would not warrant immediate intervention.
    4. As long as the client has bowel sounds after surgery, hypoactive or hyperactive, then this client would not warrant immediate intervention.

11. 1. The nurse who has worked on the unit for 4 years should not be sent because the nurse's expertise is needed on the unit.
    2. The graduate nurse, while knowledgeable of the surgical unit with 6 months experience, would not be sent because he or she does not have experience in the maternal child area.
    3. **The LPN with maternal child area experience would be most helpful to the nursery.**
    4. The charge nurse should not make assignments based on a staff member's personal life.

12. 1. Vacation time is a benefit that the nurse has earned so that the nurse's salary is protected when the nurse chooses to take time off at his or her request. It would be inappropriate to force staff to use vacation time because of low census when another nurse has requested to stay home.
    2. **This nurse who has requested to be allowed time off—because of low census—should be the first person the house supervisor notifies to stay home.**

3. This should not be a consideration when making decisions about which nurse should stay at home as a result of low census because this affects the nurse's financial security.
4. The house supervisor should not assume because the nurse was sick the previous 2 days that he or she requires a third day off. The house supervisor may choose to wait to see whether this nurse will be calling in for a third day prior to notifying the nurse in option 2.

13. 1. This statement is a therapeutic response, but it is not telling the client the truth.
2. **The ethical principle of veracity is the duty to tell the truth.**
3. This statement is "passing the buck," which the nurse should not do if at all possible.
4. This is attempting to obtain more information about the situation, but it is not telling the truth.

14. 1. Because the client is on a daily aspirin, the nurse could assess for bleeding, but the complaint of stomach discomfort would not cause the nurse to implement this intervention first.
2. Because aspirin can cause gastric distress, the nurse could instruct the client to quit taking it; however, because this is a daily medication being used as an antiplatelet agent, the nurse should provide information that would allow the client to continue the medication.
3. **After assessing the MAR, the nurse should realize the stomach discomfort is probably secondary to daily aspirin, and enteric-coated aspirin would be most helpful to decrease the stomach discomfort and allow the client to stay on the medication.**
4. Because aspirin is not a prescription medication, the nurse can recommend a different form of aspirin, such as one that is enteric coated. However, if the enteric-coated aspirin does not relieve the pain, the HCP should then be notified.

15. 1. **This statement indicates the new graduate needs more teaching because the nurse is responsible for delegating the right task to the right individual. Absolutely no one works on the nurse's license but the nurse holding the license.**
2. The nurse does retain accountability for the task delegated; therefore, the new graduate does not need more teaching.

3. The nurse must make sure the UAP is able to perform the task safely and competently; therefore, the new graduate does not need more teaching.
4. The nurse must make sure the delegated task was completed correctly; therefore, the new graduate does not need more teaching.

16. 1. The manufacturer of a product would provide biased information and would not provide the best data to support a change proposal.
2. Research studies with a limited number of participants indicate the need for further research and would not be the best research to support a change proposal.
3. Research should provide clear statistical data that support the research problem or hypothesis.
4. **The more research articles that support a change proposal, the more valid the information, which increases the possibility for change to be considered by the health-care facility.**

17. 1. Tardiness information is objective data obtained for all employees in the facility, but it does not specifically provide information about the nurse's performance.
2. The attitude of the nurse is very subjective to evaluate and does not specifically provide information about the nurse's performance.
3. Thank you notes from the clients are nice for the nurse to receive, but they are not taken into consideration during the evaluation process of the nurse.
4. **The nurse's ability to document client care directly correlates with the nurse's performance; therefore, these data should be included in the yearly evaluation.**

18. 1. The home health-care agency would not be the best referral because comorbid conditions increase the client's recovery time. The client at home does not have access to health care 24 hours a day.
2. A senior citizen center may help the client's psychosocial needs but not the client's rehabilitation needs.
3. **The rehabilitation facility will provide intensive therapy and address the comorbid conditions 24 hours a day. This will assist in the client's recovery.**
4. An outpatient physical therapist does not have the education to address and care for the comorbid issues. The physical therapist is focused on the hip fracture only,

and the client may have transportation problems going to an outpatient clinic.

19. 1. The nasogastric tube should be replaced, but this task will require more time and obtaining new equipment; therefore, it should not be done first.
    2. **The client scheduled for surgery is priority and must be ready when the OR calls; therefore, completing the preoperative checklist is the first task the nurse should implement. The preoperative checklist ensures the client's safety.**
    3. The client being discharged can wait until the safety needs of the client going to surgery have been addressed.
    4. This is a minimal to moderate amount of drainage, which requires a dressing change, but not prior to making sure the client going to surgery is ready.

20. 1. Antiplatelet medication will increase the client's bleeding time and should be held 5 days prior to surgery; therefore, this medication should be questioned.
    2. A client with a TKR is at risk for developing deep vein thrombosis (DVT); therefore, an anticoagulant medication would not be questioned.
    3. The client with a Whipple procedure has had part of the pancreas removed and is placed on insulin; therefore, the nurse would not question administering Humalog.
    4. An aminoglycoside antibiotic is not in the penicillin family; therefore, the nurse would not question administering this medication.

Critical Care Nursing 4

"If a man does his best, what else is there?"

—General George S. Patton

ABBREVIATION LIST

ABG	Arterial Blood Gas
ADLs	Activities of Daily Living
AP	Apical Pulse
ARD	Acute Respiratory Distress Syndrome
BP	Blood Pressure
CCB	Calcium Channel Blocker
CKD	Chronic Kidney Disease
COPD	Chronic Obstructive Pulmonary Disease
CPK-MB	Creatinine Phosphokinase-Cardiac Muscle
CPR	Cardiopulmonary Resuscitation
CVA	Cerebrovascular Accident (stroke)
DIC	Disseminated Intravascular Coagulation
DNR	Do Not Resuscitate
ED	Emergency Department
ESRD	End-Stage Renal Disease
H&H	Hemoglobin and Hematocrit
HCP	Health-Care Provider
ICP	Intracranial Pressure
ICU	Intensive Care Unit
INR	International Normalized Ratio
IV	Intravenous
IVP	Intravenous Push
IVPB	Intravenous Piggy Back
K+	Potassium
LPN	Licensed Practical Nurse
MAR	Medication Administration Record
MG	Myasthenia gravis
NSAID	Nonsteroidal Anti-Inflammatory Drug
P	Pulse
PVC	Premature Ventricular Contraction
R	Respiration
ROM	Range of Motion
RN	Registered Nurse
SCD	Sequential Compression Device
SCI	Spinal Cord Injury
THR	Total Hip Replacement
TKR	Total Knee Replacement
UAP	Unlicensed Assistive Personnel

PRACTICE QUESTIONS

Setting Priorities When Caring for Clients

1. The charge nurse, along with the registered nurse (RN) staff, in the critical care unit is caring for clients with a spinal cord injury (SCI). Which client should the charge nurse assess first after receiving the change-of-shift report?
   1. The client with a C-6 SCI who is complaining of dyspnea and has a respiratory rate of 12 breaths/minute.
   2. The client with an L-4 SCI who is frightened about being transferred to the rehabilitation unit.
   3. The client with an L-2 SCI who is complaining of a headache and feeling very hot all of a sudden.
   4. The client with a C-4 SCI who is on a ventilator and has a pulse oximeter reading of 98%.

2. The intensive care unit (ICU) nurse is caring for a client on a ventilator who is exhibiting respiratory distress. The ventilator alarms are going off. Which intervention should the nurse implement first?
   1. Notify the respiratory therapist immediately.
   2. Ventilate with a manual resuscitation bag.
   3. Check the ventilator to resolve the problem.
   4. Auscultate the client's lung sounds.

3. The charge nurse in the critical care unit is making rounds. Which client should the nurse see first?
   1. The client who is complaining that the nurses are being rude and won't answer the call lights.
   2. The client diagnosed with an acute myocardial infarction who has an elevated creatinine phosphokinase-cardiac muscle (CPK-MB) level.
   3. The client diagnosed with diabetic ketoacidosis who has a blood glucose reading of 189 mg/dL.
   4. The client who is being transferred to the medical unit to make room for a client from the emergency department (ED).

4. The nurse is caring for clients in a surgical intensive care unit. Which client should the nurse assess first?
   1. The client who is 4 hours postoperative for abdominal surgery who is complaining of abdominal pain and has hypoactive bowel sounds.
   2. The client who is 1 day postoperative for total hip replacement (THR) who has voided 550 mL of clear amber urine in the last 8 hours.
   3. The client who is 8 hours postoperative for open cholecystectomy who has a T-tube draining green bile.
   4. The client who is 12 hours postoperative for total knee replacement (TKR) who is complaining of numbness and tingling in the foot.

5. The critical care nurse has just received the A.M. shift report on a client diagnosed with heart failure and who has preexisting type 2 diabetes. The client has the following medication administration record (MAR). Which medication should the nurse administer first?

Client's Name:	Account Number: 123456		Allergies: Penicillin
Height: 67 inches	Weight: 148 pounds		
Date	Medication	2301–0700	0701–1500	1501–2300
	Lasix 60 mg IVP qd		0800	
	70/30 insulin 24 units subcu		0730	
	Digoxin 1.25 mg IVP qd		0800	
	Rocephin 100 mg IVPB	0700		
Signature/Initials		Day Nurse RN DN	Night Nurse RN NN	

    1. Lasix (furosemide) 60 mg IVP.
    2. Digoxin 1.25 mg IVP.
    3. Rocephin (ceftriaxone) 100 mg IVPB.
    4. 70/30 insulin subcutaneously.

6. The nurse is preparing to administer digoxin 0.25 mg IVP to a client in severe congestive heart failure who is receiving $D_5W/0.9$ NaCL at 25 mL/hr. Rank the following interventions in order of importance.
    1. Administer the medication over 5 minutes.
    2. Dilute the medication with normal saline.
    3. Draw up the medication in a tuberculin syringe.
    4. Check the client's identification band.
    5. Clamp the primary tubing distal to the port.

7. The charge nurse has received laboratory data on clients in the critical care unit. Which situation requires the charge nurse's intervention first?
    1. The client with COPD who has the following arterial blood gas (ABG) values: pH, 7.35; PaO_2, 75; $PaCO_2$, 50; HCO_3, 26.
    2. The client with inflammatory bowel disease who has a potassium (K^+) level of 3.4 mEq/L.
    3. The client who is 1 day postoperative for thyroidectomy who has a calcium level of 9.4 mg/dL.
    4. The client who has a chest tube for a hemothorax whose hemoglobin and hematocrit (H&H) is 8/24.

8. The primary nurse in the critical care unit is very busy. Which nursing task should be implemented first?
    1. Assist the HCP with a sterile dressing change for a client with an amputation.
    2. Obtain a tracheostomy tray for a client who is exhibiting air hunger.
    3. Transcribe orders for a client who was transferred from the ED.
    4. Administer sliding scale insulin to a client who has type 1 diabetes mellitus.

9. Which situation should the charge nurse in the critical care unit address first after receiving the shift report?
   1. Talk to the family member who is irate over their loved one's nursing care.
   2. Complete the 90-day probationary evaluation for a new ICU graduate intern.
   3. Call the laboratory concerning the type and crossmatch for a client who needs blood.
   4. Arrange for a client to be transferred to the telemetry step-down unit.

10. The nurse is caring for a client diagnosed with flail chest who has had a chest tube for 3 days. The nurse notes there is no fluctuation or tidaling in the water-seal compartment. Which intervention should the nurse implement first?
    1. Check the tubing for any dependent loops.
    2. Auscultate the client's posterior breath sounds.
    3. Prepare to remove the client's chest tubes.
    4. Notify the HCP that the lungs have re-expanded.

Delegating and Assigning Nursing Tasks

11. The ICU nurse and unlicensed assistive personnel (UAP) are caring for a client with right-sided paralysis secondary to a cerebrovascular accident (CVA). Which action by the UAP requires the nurse to intervene?
    1. The UAP performs passive range-of-motion (ROM) exercises for the client.
    2. The UAP places the client on the abdomen with the head to the side.
    3. The UAP uses a lift sheet when moving the client up in bed.
    4. The UAP praises the client for attempting to feed self.

12. The UAP is bathing the client diagnosed with adult acute respiratory distress syndrome (ARDS) who is on a ventilator. The bed is in the high position with the opposite side rail elevated. Which action should the ICU nurse take?
    1. Demonstrate the correct technique when giving a bed bath.
    2. Encourage the UAP to put the bed in the lowest position.
    3. Explain that the client on a ventilator should not be bathed.
    4. Give the UAP praise for performing the bath safely.

13. The charge nurse is making client assignments in the critical care unit. Which client should be assigned to the most experienced nurse?
    1. The client with type 2 diabetes who has a blood glucose level of 308 mg/dL.
    2. The client who has the following ABG values: pH, 7.35; PaO_2, 88; $PaCO_2$, 44; HCO_3, 22.
    3. The client who is showing multifocal premature ventricular contractions (PVCs).
    4. The client diagnosed with angina who is scheduled for a cardiac catheterization.

14. The nurse, a licensed practical nurse (LPN), and the UAP are caring for clients in a critical care unit. Which task would be most appropriate for the nurse to assign/delegate?
    1. Instruct the UAP to obtain the client's serum glucose level.
    2. Request the LPN to change the central line dressing.
    3. Ask the LPN to bathe the client and change the bed linens.
    4. Tell the UAP to obtain urine output for the 12-hour shift.

15. The nurse and the UAP are caring for clients in a critical care unit. Which task would be most appropriate for the nurse to delegate?
    1. Provide indwelling catheter care to a client on bed rest.
    2. Evaluate the client's 8-hour intake and output.
    3. Give a bath to the client who is third-spacing.
    4. Administer a cation-exchange resin enema.

16. The critical care nurse asks the female UAP to apply the sequential compression devices (SCDs) to the client who is on strict bed rest. The UAP tells the nurse that she has never done this procedure. Which action would be priority for the nurse to take?
    1. Tell another UAP to put the SCDs on the client.
    2. Demonstrate the procedure for applying the SCDs.
    3. Perform the task and apply the SCDs to the client.
    4. Request the UAP to watch the video demonstrating this task.

17. The nurse in the critical care unit is working with an LPN who was pulled to the unit as a result of high census. Which task would be most appropriate for the nurse to assign to the LPN?
    1. Assess the client who will be transferred to the medical unit in the morning.
    2. Administer a unit of blood to the client who is 1 day postoperative.
    3. Hang the bag of heparin to a client diagnosed with a pulmonary embolus.
    4. Assist the HCP with the insertion of a client's Swan-Ganz line.

18. Which delegation to the UAP by the primary nurse in the critical care unit would warrant intervention by the charge nurse?
    1. The UAP is instructed to bathe the client who is on telemetry.
    2. The UAP is requested to obtain a bedside glucometer reading.
    3. The UAP is asked to assist with a portable chest x-ray.
    4. The UAP is told to feed a client who is dysphagic.

19. The nurse is caring for clients in the ICU. Which task would be most appropriate for the nurse to delegate to a UAP?
    1. Instruct the UAP to empty the client's chest tube drainage.
    2. Request the UAP to double check a unit of blood that is being hung.
    3. Change the surgical dressing on the client with a Syme amputation.
    4. Ask the UAP to transfer the client from the ICU to the medical unit.

20. The charge nurse of a critical care unit is making assignments for the night shift. Which client should be assigned to the graduate nurse who has just completed an internship?
    1. The client diagnosed with a head injury resulting from a motor vehicle accident whose Glasgow Coma Scale score is 13.
    2. The client diagnosed with inflammatory bowel disease who has severe diarrhea and has a serum K^+ level of 3.2 mEq/L.
    3. The client diagnosed with Addison's disease who is lethargic and has a BP of 80/45, P of 124, and R rate of 28.
    4. The client diagnosed with hyperthyroidism who has undergone a thyroidectomy and has a positive Trousseau's sign.

Managing Clients and Nursing Staff

21. The critical care nurse is caring for a client with a head injury secondary to a motorcycle accident who, on morning rounds, is responsive to painful stimuli and assumes decorticate posturing. Two hours later, which data would warrant immediate intervention by the nurse?
    1. The client has purposeful movement when the nurse rubs the sternum.
    2. The client extends the upper and lower extremities in response to painful stimuli.
    3. The client is aimlessly thrashing in the bed when a noxious stimulus is applied.
    4. The client is able to squeeze the nurse's hand on a verbal request.

22. The nurse is administering medications to clients in the critical care area. Which client should the nurse question administering the medication?
    1. The client receiving a calcium channel blocker (CCB) who is drinking grapefruit juice.
    2. The client receiving a beta-adrenergic blocker who has an apical heart rate of 62 beats/minute.
    3. The client receiving nonsteroidal anti-inflammatory drugs (NSAIDs) who has just finished eating breakfast.
    4. The client receiving an oral anticoagulant who has an international normalized ratio (INR) of 2.8.

23. The nurse in the critical care area is administering 1 unit of packed red blood cells to a client. Fifteen minutes after initiation of the blood transfusion, the client becomes restless and complains of itching on the trunk and arms. Which intervention should the nurse implement first?
    1. Assess the client's vital signs.
    2. Notify the HCP.
    3. Maintain a patent IV line.
    4. Stop the transfusion at the hub.

24. The charge nurse is counseling a female staff nurse because the nurse has clocked in late multiple times for the 7:00 A.M to 7:00 P.M. shift. Which conflict resolution utilizes the win-win strategy?
    1. The charge nurse terminates the staff nurse as per the hospital policy so that a new nurse can be transferred to the unit.
    2. The charge nurse discovers that the staff nurse is having problems with child care; therefore, the charge nurse allows the staff nurse to work a 9:00 A.M. to 9:00 P.M. shift.
    3. The charge nurse puts the staff nurse on probation with the understanding that the next time the staff nurse is late to work she will be terminated.
    4. The staff nurse asks another staff member to talk to the charge nurse to explain that she is a valuable part of the team.

25. The staff nurse asks the charge nurse, "What should I be looking for when I read a research article?" Which response indicates the charge nurse does not understand how to read a nursing research article?
    1. "You should be able to determine why the research was done."
    2. "You should look to find out how much money was used for the study."
    3. "You should evaluate which research method was used for the study."
    4. "You should read the method section to find out what setting was used."

26. The female charge nurse tells the male nurse, "You are really cute and have a great body. Do you work out?" Which action should the male nurse implement first if he thinks he is being sexually harassed?
    1. Document the comment in writing and tell another staff nurse.
    2. Ask the charge nurse to stop making comments like this.
    3. Notify the clinical manager of the sexual harassment.
    4. Report this to the corporate headquarter's office.

27. The UAP in the critical care unit tells the primary nurse angrily, "You are the worst nurse I have ever worked with and I really hate working with you." Which action should the primary nurse implement first?
    1. Don't respond to the comment, and appraise the situation.
    2. Tell the UAP to leave the critical care unit immediately.
    3. Report this comment and behavior to the charge nurse.
    4. Explain that the UAP cannot talk to the primary nurse like this.

28. The charge nurse is making rounds and notices that the sharps container in the client's room is above the fill line. Which action should the charge nurse implement?
    1. Complete an adverse occurrence report.
    2. Discuss the situation with the primary nurse.
    3. Instruct the UAP to change the sharps container.
    4. Notify the infection control nurse immediately.

29. Which client should the charge nurse in the critical care unit not assign to a nurse who is 3 months pregnant?
    1. The client who is receiving outpatient chemotherapy who is immunosuppressed.
    2. The client who has been on antituberculosis medication for 3 months.
    3. The client who has gastroenteritis and is experiencing vomiting and diarrhea.
    4. The client diagnosed with AIDS who has cytomegalovirus.

30. The charge nurse in the ICU is making client assignments. Which client should the charge nurse assign to the graduate nurse who has just finished the 3-month orientation?
    1. The client with a cystectomy who had a creation of an ileal conduit.
    2. The client on continuous hemodialysis who is awaiting a kidney transplant.
    3. The client with a head injury who is developing DIC.
    4. The client who has had abdominal surgery whose wound has eviscerated.

Setting Priorities When Caring for Clients

1. 1. This client with dyspnea and a respiration rate of 12 has signs/symptoms of a respiratory complication and should be assessed first because ascending paralysis at the C-6 level could cause the client to stop breathing.
   2. This is a psychosocial need and should be addressed, but it is not priority over a physiologic problem.
   3. A client with a lower SCI would not be at risk for autonomic dysreflexia; therefore, a complaint of headache and feeling hot would not be priority over an airway problem.
   4. The client with a pulse oximeter reading greater than 93% is receiving adequate oxygenation.

   MAKING NURSING DECISIONS: When deciding which client to assess first, the test taker should determine whether the signs/symptoms the client is exhibiting are normal or expected for the situation. After eliminating the expected options, the test taker should determine which situation is more life threatening.

2. 1. The nurse must first address the client's acute respiratory distress and then notify other members of the multidisciplinary team.
   2. If the ventilator system malfunctions, the nurse must ventilate the client with a manual resuscitation bag (Ambu) until the problem is resolved. The nurse should determine whether the nurse can remedy the situation by assessing the ventilator before beginning manual ventilations.
   3. The client is having respiratory distress and the ventilator is sounding an alarm; therefore, the nurse should first assess the ventilator to determine the cause of the problem and correct it because the client is totally dependent on the ventilator for breathing. This is one of the few situations where the nurse would assess the equipment before assessing the client.
   4. In most situations, assessing the client is the first intervention, but because the client is totally dependent on the ventilator for breathing, the nurse should first assess the ventilator to determine the cause of the alarms.

3. 1. The charge nurse is responsible for all clients. At times it is necessary to see clients with a psychosocial need before other clients who have situations that are expected and are not life threatening.
   2. An elevated CPK-MB, cardiac isoenzyme, level is expected in a client with an acute myocardial infarction; therefore, the charge nurse would not see this client first.
   3. Although a blood glucose reading of 189 mg/dL is not within normal range, it is also not in a range that indicates the client is catabolizing fats and proteins in the body; therefore, the nurse would not need to see this client first.
   4. This client is being transferred to the medical unit; therefore, the client is stable and would not require the charge nurse to see this client first.

4. 1. A client who is 4 hours postoperative for abdominal surgery would be expected to have abdominal pain and hypoactive bowel sounds secondary to general anesthesia. This client would not be assessed first.
   2. This output indicates the client is voiding at least 30 mL an hour; therefore, the nurse would not assess this client first.
   3. The client with an open cholecystectomy frequently has a T-tube that would normally drain green bile. This client would not be assessed first.
   4. The client is exhibiting signs of compromised circulation; therefore, the nurse should assess this client first. The nurse should assess for the 6 Ps: pain, pulse, paresthesia, paralysis, pallor, and polar (cold).

   MAKING NURSING DECISIONS: When deciding which client to assess first, the test taker should determine whether the signs/symptoms the client is exhibiting are normal or expected for the situation. After eliminating the expected options, the test taker should determine which situation is more life threatening.

5. 1. After the A.M. shift report, the priority medication should be the insulin prior to the breakfast meal, not Lasix.
   2. After the A.M. shift report, the priority medication should be the insulin prior to the breakfast meal, not digoxin.

3. An antibiotic IVPB is a routine, scheduled medication and should have been administered by the night nurse; there's also a 1-hour leeway when administering this medication. The nurse would have to see whether the IVPB apparatus was hanging at the client's bedside or contact the night nurse before administering this medication.

4. Insulin is a medication that must be administered prior to the meal; therefore, this medication is priority.

6. In order: 3, 2, 4, 5, 1.
   3. Because this is less than 1 mL, the nurse should draw this medication up in a 1-mL tuberculin syringe to ensure accuracy of dosage.
   2. The nurse should dilute the medication with normal saline to a 5- to 10-mL bolus to help decrease pain during administration and maintain the IV site longer. Administering 0.25 mg of digoxin in 0.5 mL is very difficult, if not impossible, to push over 5 full minutes, which is the manufacturer's recommended administration rate. If the medication is diluted to a 5- to 10-mL bolus, it is easier for the nurse to administer the medication over 5 minutes.
   4. The nurse must check two identifiers according to the Joint Commission safety guidelines.
   5. The nurse should clamp the tubing between the port and the primary IV line so that the medication will enter the vein, not ascend up the IV tubing.
   1. Cardiovascular and narcotic medications are administered over 5 minutes.

7. 1. Although these are abnormal ABG values, they would be expected in a client with COPD; therefore, the nurse would not need to see this client first.
   2. This is a slightly decreased K^+ level, but it would not be unexpected in a client with severe diarrhea, which occurs with inflammatory bowel disease. This client would not need to be seen first.
   3. This calcium level is within normal range; therefore, this client would not need to be seen first.
   4. A client with a hemothorax will be bleeding into the chest tube drainage system. Because the client's H&H are becoming critically low, the nurse would see this client first.

   MAKING NURSING DECISIONS: The test taker must know normal laboratory data. See Appendix A for normal laboratory data.

8. 1. Changing the dressing is not priority over a client who is in respiratory distress.
   2. **The client who is exhibiting air hunger indicates respiratory distress; therefore, a tracheostomy tray should be obtained first.**
   3. The transcribing of orders is important, but not more important than a client in respiratory distress.
   4. The sliding scale insulin must be administered, but the client in respiratory distress is priority.

9. 1. This situation should be addressed first because the charge nurse is responsible for family/client complaints. If the family contacts the administration, the charge nurse must be aware of the situation.
   2. The evaluation needs to be completed, but it does not take priority over handling an irate family member.
   3. The charge nurse could assign this task to another nurse or ward clerk. Dealing appropriately with an irate family member takes priority over calling the laboratory.
   4. The charge nurse could assign this task to another nurse or ward clerk. Dealing appropriately with an irate family member takes priority over transferring a client.

10. 1. After 3 days, the nurse should suspect that the lung has re-expanded. The nurse should not expect dependent loops to have caused this situation.
    2. After 3 days, the nurse should assess the lung sounds to determine whether the lungs have re-expanded. This would be the nurse's first intervention.
    3. This will be done if it is determined the lungs have re-expanded, but it is not the first intervention.
    4. The nurse should notify the HCP if it is determined the lungs have re-expanded; a chest x-ray can be taken prior to removing the chest tubes.

Delegating and Assigning Nursing Tasks

11. 1. It would be appropriate for the UAP to perform ROM exercises to help prevent contractures; therefore, this action would not require the nurse to intervene.
    2. This would be an appropriate intervention for the client not at risk for increased intracranial pressure (ICP). However, in the ICU, the client should

never be placed on the abdomen; therefore, this action requires the nurse to intervene. The prone position helps promote hyperextension of the hip joints, which is essential for normal gait and helps prevent knee and hip flexion contractures.

3. The client should be pulled up in bed by placing the arm underneath the back or using a lift sheet; therefore, the nurse would not need to intervene.

4. The client should be encouraged and praised for attempting to perform any activities independently, such as combing hair, brushing teeth, or feeding self. The nurse would not need to intervene.

12. 1. This is the correct technique when bathing a client; therefore, the nurse does not need to demonstrate the correct technique to give a bath.

2. The bed should be at a comfortable height for the UAP to bathe the client, not in the lowest position.

3. All clients should receive a bath; therefore, this would not be an appropriate action for the nurse to take.

4. Part of the delegation process is to evaluate the UAP's performance, and the nurse should praise any action on the part of the UAP that ensures the client's safety.

13. 1. Although this blood glucose level is indeed elevated, it's not life threatening in the client with type 2 diabetes; therefore, a less experienced nurse could care for this client.

2. These ABG values are within normal limits; therefore, a less experienced nurse could care for this client.

3. Multifocal PVCs are an emergency and are possibly life threatening. An experienced nurse should care for this client.

4. A cardiac catheterization is a routine procedure and would not require the most experienced nurse.

MAKING NURSING DECISIONS: The test taker must determine which client is the most unstable, thus making this type of question an "except" question. Three clients are either stable or have non–life-threatening conditions.

14. 1. The serum blood glucose level requires a venipuncture, which is not within the scope of the UAP's expertise. The laboratory technician would be responsible for obtaining a venipuncture.

2. This is a sterile dressing change and requires assessing the insertion site for infection; therefore, this would not be the most appropriate task to assign to the LPN.

3. The nurse should ask the UAP to bathe the client and change bed linens because this is a task the UAP can perform. The LPN could be assigned higher-level tasks.

4. The UAP can add up the urine output for the 12-hour shift; however, the nurse is responsible for evaluating whether the urine output is what is expected for the client.

MAKING NURSING DECISIONS: When the test taker is deciding which option is the most appropriate task to delegate/assign, the test taker should choose the task that allows each member of the staff to function at his or her full scope of practice. Do not assign a task to a staff member that requires a higher level of expertise than the staff member has, and do not assign a task to a staff member when another staff member with a lower level of expertise can do it.

15. 1. The UAP can clean the perineal area of a client who is on bed rest and who has an indwelling catheter. Because the client is stable, this nursing task could be delegated to the UAP.

2. The assistant can obtain the client's intake and output, but the nurse must evaluate the data to determine whether interventions are needed or whether interventions are effective.

3. A client who is third-spacing is unstable and in a life-threatening situation; therefore, the nurse cannot delegate the UAP to give this client a bath.

4. This is a medication enema, and the UAP cannot administer medications. In addition, if a cation-exchange resin enema is ordered, the client is unstable and has an excessively high serum potassium (K^+) level.

16. 1. Although the nurse could request another UAP to perform the task, this is not the best action because the nurse should demonstrate applying SCDs so that the UAP can learn how to complete the task.

2. This is the priority action because the nurse will ensure that the UAP knows how to apply SCDs correctly, thereby enabling the nurse to delegate (to the UAP) the task successfully in the future.

3. The nurse could do the task, but if the UAP is not shown how to do it, then the UAP will not be able to perform the task the next time it is delegated.
4. The UAP could watch a video demonstrating this task, but the priority action is that the nurse should demonstrate SCD application to the UAP.

17. 1. The nurse should not assign assessment to an LPN even if the client is stable.
2. The LPN cannot initiate administration; therefore, this task must be completed by the nurse.
3. **The LPN can administer medications; therefore, the LPN could hang a bag of heparin on an IV pump to this client.**
4. The nurse must assess for dysrhythmias during the insertion, and the nurse assisting the HCP should be experienced in inserting the line. An LPN pulled from another unit should not be assigned this task.

18. 1. All clients in the ICU are on telemetry, and the UAP could bathe the client. This would not warrant intervention by the charge nurse.
2. The UAP can perform glucometer checks at the bedside, and there is nothing that indicates the client is unstable. This would not warrant intervention by the charge nurse.
3. The UAP can assist with helping the client sit up for a portable chest x-ray as long as the UAP is not pregnant and wears a shield.
4. **This client is at risk for choking and is not stable; therefore, the charge nurse should intervene and not allow the UAP to feed this client.**

19. 1. The drainage in the client's chest tube system is not emptied. The drainage chamber should be marked for output, but not emptied.
2. An RN must double check a unit of blood prior to infusing the blood; therefore, this task cannot be delegated.
3. The surgical dressing for a Syme amputation must be changed by the surgeon or the nurse; this task cannot be delegated to personnel with a lower level of expertise.
4. **The UAP could transfer the client from the ICU because the client is stable and is being transferred to the medical unit.**

20. 1. **The Glasgow Coma Scale ranges from 0 to 15, with 15 indicating the client's neurologic status is intact. A Glasgow Coma Scale score of 13 indicates the client is stable and would be the most appropriate client to assign to the graduate nurse.**
2. This client's K^+ level is low, and the client is at risk for developing cardiac dysrhythmias; therefore, the client should be assigned to a more experienced nurse.
3. This client has a low blood pressure and evidence of tachycardia and could possibly go into an addisonian crisis, which is a potentially life-threatening condition. A more experienced nurse should be assigned to this client.
4. A positive Trousseau sign indicates the client is hypocalcemic and is experiencing a complication of the surgery; therefore, this client should be assigned to a more experienced nurse.

MAKE NURSING DECISIONS: When the test taker is deciding which client should be assigned to a new graduate, the most stable client should be assigned to the least experienced nurse.

Managing Clients and Nursing Staff

21. 1. Purposeful movement following painful stimuli would indicate an improvement in the client's condition and would not warrant intervention by the nurse.
2. **Extension of the upper and lower extremities is assuming a decerebrate posture, which indicates the client's ICP is increasing. This would warrant immediate intervention by the nurse.**
3. Aimless thrashing would indicate an improvement in the client's condition and would not warrant intervention by the nurse.
4. If the client is able to follow simple commands, then the client's condition is improving and would not warrant intervention by the nurse.

22. 1. The client receiving a CCB should avoid grapefruit juice because it can cause the CCB to rise to toxic levels. Grapefruit juice inhibits cytochrome P450-3A4 found in the liver and the intestinal wall. This inhibition affects the metabolism of some drugs and can,

as is the case with CCBs, lead to toxic levels of the drug. For this reason, the nurse should investigate any medications the client is taking if the client drinks grapefruit juice.

2. The apical heart rate should be greater than 60 beats/minute before administering the medication; therefore, the nurse would not question administering this medication.

3. Nonsteroidal anti-inflammatory drugs (NSAIDs) should be taken with foods to prevent gastric upset; therefore, the nurse would not question administering this medication.

4. The INR therapeutic level for warfarin (Coumadin), an anticoagulant, is 2 to 3; therefore, the nurse would not question administering this medication.

23. 1. The client is having signs/symptoms of a blood transfusion reaction. The nurse must stop the transfusion immediately and then assess the client's vital signs.

2. The HCP needs to be notified, but not before the nurse stops the blood transfusion.

3. The nurse should maintain a patent IV so that medications can be administered, but this is not the first intervention.

4. **Any time the nurse suspects the client is having a reaction to blood or blood products, the nurse should stop the infusion at the spot closest to the client and not allow any more of the blood to enter the client's body. This is the nurse's first intervention.**

24. 1. This is a win-lose strategy where, during the conflict, one party (charge nurse) exerts dominance and the other (staff nurse) submits.

2. **This is a win-win strategy that focuses on goals and attempts to meet the needs of both parties. The charge nurse keeps an experienced nurse and the staff nurse keeps her position. Both parties win.**

3. This is negotiation in which the conflicting parties give and take on the issue. The staff nurse gets one more chance and the charge nurse's authority is still intact.

4. This is not an example of a win-win strategy and is not an appropriate action for the staff nurse to take. The opinion of the staff should not influence the charge nurse's action.

25. 1. A research article should answer the question "why": Why was the research done?

This statement indicates the charge nurse understands how to read a research article.

2. The cost of the research is not pertinent when reading a research article and determining whether the research supports evidence-based practice. This statement indicates the charge nurse does not understand how to read a research article.

3. A research article should answer the question "how": What research method was used? This statement indicates the charge nurse understands how to read a research article.

4. A research article should answer the question "where": In what setting was the research conducted? This statement indicates the charge nurse understands how to read a research article.

26. 1. The male nurse should document the comment and tell other people, such as family, friends, and staff, but this is not the nurse's first intervention.

2. **The first action is to ask the person directly to stop. The harasser needs to be told in clear terms that the behavior makes the nurse uncomfortable and that he wants it to stop immediately.**

3. The male nurse could take this action, but it is not the first action.

4. This male nurse could take this action, but only if direct contact and the chain of command at the hospital do not stop the charge nurse's behavior.

27. 1. **The nurse should first appraise the situation and not do anything. This is the pivotal point where the nurse can get angry back or reappraise the situation. The important thing is to empathize with the UAP and to try to find out the provocation for the behavior.**

2. The primary nurse could tell the UAP to leave the unit, but this is responding to the anger and not the reason for the anger.

3. The comment may need to be reported to the charge nurse, but not until the primary nurse can determine what caused the comment. The UAP may be upset about something else entirely.

4. This is not the first action when dealing with someone who is angry. This comment may cause further angry behavior by the UAP and will not diffuse the situation. The nurse is the professional person and should control the situation.

28. 1. An adverse occurrence report is completed for incidents occurring to clients.
    2. The nurse should talk to the primary nurse, but the sharps container should be changed immediately.
    3. The UAP can change a sharps container. This must be done because a sharps container above the fill line is a violation of Occupational Safety Health Administration Rules (OSHA) and can result in a financial fine.
    4. The infection control nurse does not need to be notified of this situation.

    MAKING NURSING DECISIONS: The nurse is responsible for knowing and complying with local, state, and federal standards of care.

29. 1. The pregnant nurse can administer antineoplastic medications to clients. The nurse should not be exposed to antineoplastic agents outside of the administration bags and tubing. The nurse can care for a client who is immunosuppressed.
    2. The client who has been taking antituberculosis medication for 3 months is no longer communicable; therefore, the pregnant nurse could care for this client safely.
    3. As long as the nurse uses Standard Precautions, the nurse who is pregnant could care for a client with gastroenteritis. Nothing indicates the client has a communicable or contagious disease.
    4. The client has the cytomegalovirus, which crosses the placental barrier. Therefore, a pregnant nurse should not be assigned this client. Any client with a communicable disease that crosses the placental barrier should not be assigned to a nurse who is pregnant.

30. 1. Although cystectomy is a major surgical procedure, it has a predictable course, and no complications were identified. After removing the bladder, the client must have an ileal conduit. This is expected with this type of surgery, and the new graduate nurse could be assigned this client.
    2. A client on continuous hemodialysis would require a nurse trained in this area of nursing; therefore, this client should be assigned to a more experienced nurse.
    3. DIC is life threatening; the client is unstable and should be assigned to a more experienced nurse.
    4. An eviscerated wound indicates the client's incision has opened and the bowels are out of the abdomen. This client is critically ill and should not be assigned to an inexperienced nurse.

    MAKE NURSING DECISIONS: When the test taker is deciding which client should be assigned to a new graduate, the most stable client should be assigned to the least experienced nurse.

COMPREHENSIVE EXAMINATION

1. The nurse in the critical care unit of a medical center answers the phone and the person says, "There is a bomb in the hospital kitchen." Which action should the nurse take?
   1. Notify the kitchen that there is a bomb.
   2. Call the operator to trace the phone call.
   3. Notify the hospital security department.
   4. Call the local police department.

2. The critical care unit is having problems with staff members clocking in late and clocking out early from the shift. Which statement by the male charge nurse indicates he has a democratic leadership style?
   1. "You cannot clock out 1 minute before your shift is complete."
   2. "As long as your work is done you can clock out any time you want."
   3. "We are going to have a meeting to discuss the clocking in procedure."
   4. "The clinical manager will take care of anyone who clocks out early."

3. The husband of a client diagnosed with a brain tumor asks the nurse, "How am I going to take care of my wife when we go home?" Which intervention would be most appropriate for the ICU nurse to implement?
   1. Notify the social worker about the husband's concerns.
   2. Contact the hospital chaplain to talk to the husband.
   3. Leave a note on the chart for the HCP to talk to the husband.
   4. Reassure the husband that everything will be all right.

4. The nurse is caring for a client on a ventilator when the high alarm indicates that there is an increase in the peak airway pressure. Which intervention should the nurse implement first?
   1. Determine whether the airway tubing is plugged.
   2. Prepare to perform in-line suctioning.
   3. Check the client's pulse oximeter reading.
   4. Sedate the client with a muscle relaxant.

5. The client with hypothyroidism and a diagnosis of myxedema coma is admitted to the critical care unit. Which assessment data would warrant immediate intervention by the nurse?
   1. The client's blood glucose level is 74 mg/dL.
   2. The client's temperature is 96.2°F; AP, 54; R, 12; and BP, 90/58.
   3. The client's ABG values are pH, 7.33; PaO$_2$, 78; PaCO$_2$, 48; HCO$_3$, 25.
   4. The client is lethargic and sleeps all the time.

6. The client is admitted to the critical care unit after a motor vehicle accident. The client asks the nurse, "Do you know if the person in the other car is all right?" The nurse knows the person died. Which statement does not support the ethical principle of beneficence?
   1. "I am not sure how the other person is doing."
   2. "I will try to find out how the other person is doing."
   3. "You should rest now and try not worry about it."
   4. "I am sorry to have to tell you, but the person died."

7. The client admitted to the critical care unit tells the nurse, "I have a Living Will and I do not want to have cardiopulmonary resuscitation (CPR)." Which action should the nurse implement first?
   1. Ask the client for a copy of the Living Will so that it can be placed in the chart.
   2. Inform the HCP of the client's request as soon as possible.
   3. Determine whether the client has a Durable Power of Attorney for Health Care.
   4. Request the hospital chaplain to come and talk to the client about this request.

8. The client diagnosed with end-stage renal disease (ESRD), also known as chronic kidney disease (CKD), who is on peritoneal dialysis is admitted to the critical care unit. Which assessment data warrants immediate intervention by the nurse?
   1. The client's serum creatinine level is 2.4 mg/dL.
   2. The client's abdomen is soft to touch and nontender.
   3. The dialysate being removed from the abdomen is cloudy.
   4. The dialysate instilled was 1500 mL and removed was 2100 mL.

9. The charge nurse in the ICU is notified of a bus accident with multiple injuries, and clients are being brought to the ED. The hospital is implementing the disaster policy. Which intervention should the nurse implement first?
   1. Determine which clients could be transferred out of the ICU.
   2. Call any off-duty nurses to notify them to come in to work.
   3. Assess the staffing to determine which staff could be sent to ED.
   4. Request all visitors to leave the hospital as soon as possible.

10. The 18-year-old client is admitted to the critical care unit after a serious motor vehicle accident resulting from driving under the influence. The mother comes to the unit and starts yelling at her son about "driving drunk." Which action should the nurse implement?
    1. Allow the mother to continue talking to her son.
    2. Notify the hospital security to remove the mother.
    3. Escort the mother to a private area and talk to her.
    4. Tell the mother if she wants to stay, she must be quiet.

11. The nurse calls the HCP for an order for pain medication for a client. The HCP gives the nurse an order for "Demerol 50 mg IVP now and then every 4 hours as needed." Which action should the nurse implement first?
    1. Write the order in the chart with the words per telephone order.
    2. Request another nurse to verify the HCP's order on the phone.
    3. Read back the order to the HCP before hanging up the phone.
    4. Transcribe the order to the medication administration record.

12. The charge nurse is reviewing laboratory blood work. Which results warrant intervention by the charge nurse?
    1. The client whose INR is 2.3.
    2. The client whose H&H is 11 g/dL and 36%.
    3. The client whose platelet count is 65,000 per milliliter of blood.
    4. The client whose red blood cell count is $4.8 \times 10 \text{ mm}^6$.

13. The client in the critical care unit tells the day shift primary nurse that the night nurse did not answer the call light for almost 1 hour. Which statement would be most appropriate by the day shift primary nurse?
    1. "The night shift often has trouble answering the lights promptly."
    2. "I am sorry that happened and I will answer your lights promptly today."
    3. "I will notify my charge nurse to come and talk to you about the situation."
    4. "There might have been an emergency situation so your light was not answered."

14. Which priority client problem should be included in the care plan for the client diagnosed with Guillian-Barré syndrome who is admitted to the critical care unit?
    1. Decreased cardiac output.
    2. Fear and anxiety.
    3. Complications of immobility.
    4. Ineffective breathing pattern.

15. To which collaborative health-care team member should the critical care nurse refer the client in the late stages of myasthenia gravis?
    1. Occupational therapist.
    2. Physical therapist.
    3. Social worker.
    4. Speech therapist.

16. The nurse is caring for a client and is accidentally stuck with the stylet used to start an IV infusion. The nurse flushes the skin with water and tries to get the area to bleed. Which action should the nurse implement next?
    1. Have the laboratory draw the client's blood.
    2. Notify the charge nurse and complete the incident report.
    3. Contact the employee health nurse to start prophylactic medication.
    4. Follow up with the employee health nurse to have lab work drawn.

17. A client diagnosed with AIDS dementia is angry and yells at everyone entering the room. None of the critical care staff wants to be assigned to this client. Which intervention would be most appropriate for the nurse manager to use in resolving this situation?
    1. Explain that this attitude is a violation of the client's rights.
    2. Request the HCP to transfer the client to the medical unit.
    3. Discuss some possible options with the nursing staff.
    4. Try to find a nurse who does not mind being assigned to the client.

18. Which situation would prompt the health-care team to utilize the client's Advance Directive when needing to make decisions for the client?
    1. The client with a head injury who is exhibiting decerebrate posturing.
    2. The client with a C-6 SCI who is on a ventilator.
    3. The client in ESRD who is being placed on dialysis.
    4. The client diagnosed with terminal cancer who is mentally retarded.

19. Which staff nurse should the charge nurse in the critical care unit send to the medical unit?
    1. The nurse who has worked in the unit for 18 months.
    2. The nurse who is orienting to the critical care unit.
    3. The nurse who has been working at the hospital for 2 months.
    4. The nurse who has 12 years' experience in this ICU unit.

20. The confused client in the critical care unit is attempting to pull out the IV line and the indwelling urinary catheter. Which action should the nurse implement first?
    1. Ask a family member to stay with the client.
    2. Request the UAP to stay with the client.
    3. Place the client in a chest restraint.
    4. Notify the HCP to obtain a restraint order.

1. 1. Notifying the kitchen will only scare the kitchen personnel and will not alert the bomb squad as to the situation.
   2. The operator would not be able to trace a phone call that has been disconnected.
   3. **The chain of command in a hospital is to notify the security department, and they will institute the hospital procedure for the bomb threat.**
   4. The nurse should not directly call the local police department because the hospital security department is responsible for implementing the procedure for a bomb scare.

2. 1. Autocratic managers use an authoritarian approach to direct the activities of others.
   2. Laissez-faire managers maintain a permissive climate with little direction or control.
   3. **A democratic manager is people oriented and emphasizes efficient group functioning. The environment is open and communication flows both ways, and this includes having meetings to discuss concerns.**
   4. This statement reflects shirking of responsibility, thus letting someone else address the problem, and is not characteristic of a democratic manager.

3. 1. **A social worker is qualified to assist the client with referrals to any agency or personnel that may be needed after the client is discharged home.**
   2. The chaplain should be referred to if spiritual guidance is required, but the stem did not specify this need.
   3. The HCP can talk to the husband but will not be able to address his concerns of taking care of his wife when she is discharged home.
   4. This is false reassurance and does not address the husband's concern after his wife is discharged home. The nurse does not know whether everything is going to be all right.

4. 1. **When peak airway pressure is increased, the nurse should implement the intervention that is less invasive for the client. The high alarm indicates there is a problem with the client that may include a plugged airway, "bucking" of the ventilator, decreasing lung compliance, kinked tubing, or pneumothorax.**
   2. The ventilator high alarm may indicate the client needs suctioning, but the nurse should always implement the least invasive procedure when troubleshooting a ventilator alarm; therefore, this is not the first intervention.
   3. The nurse should check to determine whether the client is being oxygenated, but the first intervention should be to determine what is causing the high alarm to go off, which is to check for kinks in the tubing.
   4. This may be needed, but the nurse should not sedate the client unless absolutely necessary; therefore, this is not the first intervention.

5. 1. This is within the normal range of 70 to 120 mg/dL. Hypoglycemia is expected in a client with myxedema; therefore, a 74 mg/dL blood glucose level would be expected.
   2. The client's metabolism is slowed in myxedema coma, which would result in these vital signs.
   3. **These ABGs indicate respiratory acidosis (ph <7.35, $PaCO_2$ >45) and hypoxemia (O_2 <80); therefore, this client would warrant immediate intervention by the nurse. Untreated respiratory acidosis can result in death if not treated immediately.**
   4. Lethargy is an expected symptom in a client diagnosed with myxedema; therefore, this would not warrant immediate intervention.

6. 1. Beneficence is the ethical principle to do good actively for the client. Because the client is in the ICU, the client is critically ill and does not need any type of news that will further upset the client. This statement supports the ethical principle of beneficence.
   2. The statement supports beneficence, but the stem asks which option does not support beneficence.
   3. This statement avoids directly telling the client the other individual is dead.
   4. **This statement supports the ethical principle of veracity, which is the duty to tell the truth. This statement will probably further upset the client and cause psychological distress that may hinder the recovery period.**

7. 1. A copy of the Living Will should be placed in the client's chart, but it is not the nurse's first intervention.
   2. **The nurse should first inform the HCP so the order can be written in the client's chart. The HCP must write the do not resuscitate (DNR) order before the client's wishes can be honored.**

3. The person with the Durable Power of Attorney for Health Care can make healthcare choices for the client if the client is unable to verbalize his or her wishes, but the first intervention is to have the HCP write a DNR order.
4. The client has a right to make this request, and the chaplain does not need to talk to the client about the Living Will.

8. 1. The client in ESRD, chronic kidney disease (CKD), would have an elevated creatinine level. The normal creatinine level is 0.7 to 1.8 mg/dL. This data would not warrant immediate intervention.
   2. Peritonitis, inflammation of the peritoneum, is a serious complication that would result in a hard, rigid abdomen; therefore, a soft abdomen would not warrant immediate intervention.
   3. **The dialysate return should be colorless or straw colored but should never be cloudy, which indicates an infection; therefore, this data warrants immediate intervention.**
   4. Because the client is in ESRD, fluid must be removed from the body, so the output should be more than the amount instilled; therefore, this indicates the peritoneal dialysis is effective and does not warrant intervention.

9. 1. The charge nurse should have as many beds as possible available for any clients who must be transferred to the ICU. The charge nurse should send a nurse to ED and then assess the bed situation.
   2. This may need to be done, but it is not the first intervention, and the charge nurse could assign this to a staff member who is not providing direct client care.
   3. **Most disaster policies require one nurse to be sent immediately from each area; therefore, this intervention should be implemented first. The charge must determine which staff nurse would be most helpful in the ED without compromising the staffing in the ICU.**
   4. The charge nurse should not request any one to leave the hospital. This is not typical protocol for a disaster.

10. 1. The nurse must diffuse the situation and remove the mother from the client's room because a seriously ill client does not need to be yelled at.
   2. Hospital security does not need to be called unless the mother refuses to leave the client's room in the critical care unit.
   3. **The nurse should remove the mother from the room and allow her to ventilate her feelings about the accident her son sustained while he was under the influence.**

4. The nurse should remove the mother because she is upset and let her ventilate. Telling the mother she must be quiet is condescending, and when someone is upset, telling the person to be quiet is not helpful.

11. 1. The nurse should write the order on the HCP's order and write "per telephone order" (TO), but this is not the nurse's first intervention.
   2. The nurse does not need to have another nurse verify the HCP's telephone order.
   3. **The Joint Commission has implemented this requirement for all telephone orders. The nurse should document on the HCP's order "repeat order verified."**
   4. The nurse should transcribe the order to the MAR, but it is not the first intervention.

12. 1. The therapeutic level for a client on warfarin (Coumadin) is an INR of 2 to 3; therefore, this client does not warrant intervention.
   2. These hemoglobin/hematocrit levels are a little low but not so critical that this would warrant intervention by the charge nurse.
   3. **A platelet count of less than 100,000 per milliliter of blood indicates thrombocytopenia; therefore, this client warrants intervention by the charge nurse.**
   4. This is a normal red blood cell count; therefore, the charge nurse would not need to intervene.

13. 1. This statement is not supporting the night shift and makes the unit look bad. The nurse should not "bad-mouth" the night shift.
   2. The nurse has no idea what happened that delayed answering the call light, it could have been a code or other type of life-threatening situation. The day shift primary nurse may not be able to answer the light in some certain situations and should not falsely reassure the client.
   3. **The nurse should have someone come talk to the client who is in a position to then investigate what happened on the night shift and determine why this happened. The day shift primary nurse does not have this authority.**
   4. This is negating the client's feeling, and the client does not need to know what was going on in the critical care unit.

14. 1. The client with Guillain-Barré syndrome is at risk for airway compromise resulting from the ascending paralysis. Cardiac output is not a priority.
   2. The client's psychological needs are important, but psychosocial problems are not priority.

3. Complications of immobility are pertinent but do not take priority over the airway.
4. **Guillain-Barré syndrome produces ascending paralysis that will cause respiratory failure; therefore, breathing pattern is priority.**

15. 1. The occupational therapist addresses assisting the client with ADLs, but with MG the client has no problems with ADLs if the client takes the medication correctly, 30 minutes prior to performing ADLs.
2. A physical therapist addresses transfer and movement issues with the client, but this would not be priority in the critical care unit.
3. The social worker assists the client with discharge issues or financial issues, but this would not be appropriate for the client in the critical care unit.
4. **Speech therapists address swallowing problems, and clients with MG are dysphagic and are at risk for aspiration; the speech therapist can help match food consistency to the client's ability to swallow and thus help enhance client safety. This referral would be appropriate in the critical care unit.**

16. 1. This should be done but not prior to notifying the charge nurse and reporting the incident.
2. **The nurse should notify the charge nurse first so that the hospital protocol can be followed, including notifying the infection control nurse, completing an incident report, obtaining blood from the client, and starting prophylactic medication if warranted.**
3. This should be done within 4 hours of the stick, but the charge nurse should be notified first so that proper hospital protocol can be initiated.
4. This is done at 3 months and 6 months.

17. 1. The feelings of the staff are not a violation of the client's rights. Refusing to care for the client is a violation of the client's rights.
2. Transferring the client to the medical unit solves the problem for the critical care unit, but the client's behavior should be addressed by the health-care team. This is not the most appropriate intervention for the nurse manager.
3. **This would be the most appropriate intervention because it allows the staff to have input into resolving the problem. When staff have input into resolving the situation, then there is ownership of the problem.**
4. One nurse cannot be on duty 24 hours a day. The nurse manager should try to allow the staff to identify options to address the client's behavior.

18. 1. **The client must have lost decision-making capacity because of a condition that is not reversible or must be in a condition that is specified under state law, such as a terminal, persistent vegetative state, irreversible coma, or as specified in the Advance Directive. A client who is exhibiting decerebrate posturing is unconscious and unable to make decisions.**
2. The client on a ventilator has not lost the ability to make health-care decisions. The nurse can communicate by asking the client to blink his or her eyes to yes/no questions.
3. The client receiving dialysis is alert and does not lose the ability to make decisions; therefore, the Advance Directive should not be consulted to make decisions for the client.
4. Mental retardation does not mean the client cannot make decisions for himself or herself unless the client has a legal guardian who has a Durable Power of Attorney for Health Care. If the client has a legal guardian, then the client cannot complete an Advance Directive.

19. 1. **This nurse should be sent to the medical unit because, with 18 months' experience, the nurse is familiar with the hospital routine and would be helpful to the medical unit but is not the most experienced ICU nurse on duty.**
2. The nurse who is still orienting to the unit should not be sent to the medical unit. The nurse in orientation should be kept with the nurse preceptor.
3. The nurse who is new to the hospital should not be sent to a new unit with which he or she is unfamiliar.
4. The nurse with 12 years' experience should be kept on in the ICU because his or her expertise would be more helpful for client care than a nurse with 18 months' experience.

20. 1. The family may or may not be able to control the client's behavior but the nurse should not ask a family member first. The CCU usually has mandated visiting hours.
   2. **The nurse should first ensure the client's safety by having someone stay at the bedside with the client, and then call the HCP, and finally apply mitt restraints.**
   3. This is a form of restraint and is against the law unless the nurse has a health-care provider's order. This is the least restrictive form of restraint but would not be helpful if the client is pulling at tubes.
   4. The nurse must notify the health-care provider before putting the client in restraints; restraints must be used only in an emergency situation, for a limited time, and for the protection of the client.

Pediatric Nursing

5

"Let whoever is in charge keep this simple question in her head (NOT how can I always do the right thing myself but) how can I provide for this right thing always to be done."

—Florence Nightingale

ABBREVIATION LIST

ADHD	Attention-Deficit Hyperactivity Disorder	**MRSA**	Methicillin-Resistant *Staphylococcus aureus*
CNO	Chief Nursing Officer	**NCSBN**	National Council of State Boards of Nursing
CT	Computed Tomography	**NICU**	Neonatal Intensive Care Unit
CVA	Cerebrovascular Accident	**NPO**	Nothing per (by) Os (Mouth)
ED	Emergency Department		
HCP	Health-Care Provider	**PO**	Orally
HIPAA	Health Insurance Portability and Accountability Act	**PRN**	As Needed
		RN	Registered Nurse
HOB	Head of Bed	**ROM**	Range of Motion
IM	Intramuscular	**UAP**	Unlicensed Assistive Personnel
IV	Intravenous		
IVP	Intravenous Push		
LPN	Licensed Practical Nurse		

PRACTICE QUESTIONS

Setting Priorities When Caring for Clients

1. The nurse is working in the emergency department (ED) of a children's medical center. Which client should the nurse assess first?
   1. The 1-month-old infant who has developed colic and is crying.
   2. The 2-year-old toddler who was bitten by another child at the day care center.
   3. The 6-year-old school-age child who was hit by a car while riding a bicycle.
   4. The 14-year-old adolescent whose mother suspects her child is sexually active.

2. The 8-year-old client diagnosed with a vaso-occlusive sickle cell crisis is complaining of a severe headache. Which intervention should the nurse implement first?
   1. Administer 6 L of oxygen via nasal cannula.
   2. Assess the client's neurologic status.
   3. Administer a narcotic analgesic by intravenous push (IVP).
   4. Increase the client's intravenous (IV) rate.

3. The 6-year-old client who has undergone abdominal surgery is attempting to make a pinwheel spin by blowing on it with the nurse's assistance. The child starts crying because the pinwheel won't spin. Which action should the nurse implement first?
   1. Praise the child for the attempt to make the pinwheel spin.
   2. Notify the respiratory therapist to implement incentive spirometry.
   3. Encourage the child to turn from side to side and cough.
   4. Demonstrate how to make the pinwheel spin by blowing on it.

4. The nurse is caring for clients on the pediatric medical unit. Which client should the nurse assess first?
   1. The child diagnosed with type 1 diabetes who has a blood glucose level of 180 mg/dL.
   2. The child diagnosed with pneumonia who is coughing and has a temperature of 100°F.
   3. The child diagnosed with gastroenteritis who has a potassium (K^+) level of 3.9 mEq/L.
   4. The child diagnosed with cystic fibrosis who has a pulse oximeter reading of 90%.

5. The nurse has received the A.M. shift report for clients on a pediatric unit. Which medication should the nurse administer first?
   1. The third dose of the aminoglycoside antibiotic to the child diagnosed with methicillin-resistant *Staphylococcus aureus* (MRSA).
   2. The IVP steroid methylprednisolone (Solumedrol) to the child diagnosed with asthma.
   3. The sliding scale insulin to the child diagnosed with type 1 diabetes mellitus.
   4. The stimulant methylphenidate (Ritalin) to a child diagnosed with attention-deficit hyperactivity disorder (ADHD).

6. The nurse enters the client's room and realizes the 9-month-old infant is not breathing. Rank in order of priority. Which interventions should the nurse implement?
   1. Perform cardiac compression 30:2.
   2. Check the infant's brachial pulse.
   3. Administer two puffs to the infant.
   4. Determine unresponsiveness.
   5. Open the infant's airway.

7. The 3-year-old client has been admitted to the pediatric unit. Which task should the nurse instruct the unlicensed assistive personnel (UAP) to perform first?
   1. Orient the parents and child to the room.
   2. Obtain an admission kit for the child.
   3. Post the child's height and weight at the HOB.
   4. Provide the child with a meal tray.

8. The clinic nurse is preparing to administer an intramuscular (IM) injection to the 2-year-old toddler. Which intervention should the nurse implement first?
   1. Immobilize the child's leg.
   2. Explain the procedure to the child.
   3. Cleanse the area with an alcohol swab.
   4. Administer the medication in the thigh.

9. The nurse is writing a care plan for the 5-year-old child diagnosed with gastroenteritis. Which client problem is priority?
   1. Imbalanced nutrition.
   2. Fluid volume deficit.
   3. Knowledge deficit.
   4. Risk for infection.

10. Which data would warrant immediate intervention from the pediatric nurse?
   1. Proteinuria for the child diagnosed with nephrotic syndrome.
   2. Petechiae for the child diagnosed with leukemia.
   3. Drooling for a child diagnosed with acute epiglottitis.
   4. Elevated temperature in a child diagnosed with otitis media.

Delegating and Assigning Nursing Tasks

11. The charge nurse has assigned a staff nurse to care for an 8-year-old client diagnosed with cerebral palsy. Which nursing action by the staff nurse would warrant immediate intervention by the charge nurse?
    1. The staff nurse performs gentle range-of-motion (ROM) exercises to extremities.
    2. The staff nurse puts the client's bed in the lowest position possible.
    3. The staff nurse takes the client in a wheelchair to the activity room.
    4. The staff nurse places the child in semi-Fowler's position to eat lunch.

12. The nurse and the UAP are caring for clients on the pediatric unit. Which action by the nurse indicates appropriate delegation?
    1. The nurse requests the UAP to check the circulation on the child with a cast.
    2. The nurse asks the UAP to feed an infant who has just had a cleft palate repair.
    3. The nurse has the UAP demonstrate a catheterization for a child with a neurogenic bladder.
    4. The nurse checks to make sure the UAP's delegated tasks have been completed.

13. The nurse on a pediatric unit has received the A.M. shift report and tells the UAP to keep the 2-year-old child NPO for a procedure. At 0830, the nurse observes the mother feeding the child. Which action should the nurse implement first?
    1. Determine what the UAP did not understand about the instruction.
    2. Tell the HCP that the UAP did not follow the nurse's direction.
    3. Ask the mother why she was feeding her child if the child was NPO.
    4. Notify the dietary department to hold the child's meal trays.

14. The charge nurse on the six-bed pediatric burn unit is making shift assignments and has one registered nurse (RN), one scrub technician, one UAP, and a unit secretary. Which client care assignment indicates the best use of the hospital personnel?
    1. The RN performs daily whirlpool dressing changes.
    2. The unit secretary transcribes the HCP's orders.
    3. The scrub technician medicates the client prior to dressing changes.
    4. The UAP places the current laboratory results on the chart.

15. The RN and the UAP are caring for clients on a pediatric surgical unit. Which tasks would be most appropriate to delegate to the UAP? Select all that apply.
    1. Pass dietary trays to the clients.
    2. Obtain routine vital signs on the clients.
    3. Complete the preoperative checklist.
    4. Change linens on the client's beds.
    5. Document the client's intake and output.

16. Which client should the charge nurse on the pediatric unit assign to the most experienced nurse?
    1. The 4-year-old child diagnosed with hemophilia receiving factor VIII.
    2. The 8-year-old child with headaches who is scheduled for a CT scan.
    3. The 6-year-old child recovering from a sickle cell crisis.
    4. The 11-year-old child newly diagnosed with rheumatoid arthritis.

17. The charge nurse is making shift assignments on a pediatric oncology unit. Which delegation/assignment would be most appropriate?
    1. Delegate the UAP to obtain routine blood work from the central line.
    2. Instruct the licensed practical nurse (LPN) to contact the leukemia support group.
    3. Assign the chemotherapy certified RN to administer chemotherapeutic medication.
    4. Have the dietitian check the meal trays for the amount eaten.

18. The nurse observes the UAP bringing a cartoon video to a 6-year-old female child on bed rest so that she can watch it on the VCR. Which action should the nurse take?
    1. Tell the UAP that the child should not be watching videos.
    2. Explain that this is the responsibility of the child life therapist.
    3. Praise the UAP for providing the child with an appropriate activity.
    4. Notify the charge nurse that the UAP gave the child videos to watch.

19. Which newborn should the nurse in the neonatal intensive care unit (NICU) assign to a new graduate who has just completed an NICU internship?
    1. The 1-day-old infant diagnosed with a myelomeningocele.
    2. The 2-week-old infant who was born 6 weeks premature.
    3. The 3-hour-old infant who is being evaluated for esophageal atresia.
    4. The 1-week-old infant diagnosed with tetralogy of Fallot.

20. The newly hired nurse is working on a pediatric unit and needs the UAP to obtain a urine specimen on an 11-month-old infant. Which statement made to the UAP indicates the nurse understands the delegation process?
    1. "Be sure to weigh the diaper when obtaining the urine specimen."
    2. "Do you know how to apply the urine collection bag?"
    3. "Use a small indwelling catheter when obtaining the urine specimen."
    4. "I need for you to get a urine specimen on the infant."

Managing Clients and Nursing Staff

21. The 8-year-old male child in the pediatric unit is refusing to ambulate postoperatively. Which intervention would be most appropriate?
    1. Give the child the option to ambulate now or after lunch.
    2. Ask the parents to insist the child ambulate in the hall.
    3. Refer the child to the child developmental therapist.
    4. Tell the child he can watch a video game if he cooperates.

22. The clinic nurse overhears a mother in the waiting room tell her 6-year-old son, "If you don't sit down and be quiet, I am going to get the nurse to give you a shot." Which action should the nurse implement?
    1. Do not take any action because the mother is attempting to discipline her son.
    2. Tell the child the nurse would not give him a shot because the mother said to.
    3. Report this verbally abusive behavior to Child Protective Services.
    4. Tell the mother this behavior will cause her son to be afraid of the nurses.

23. The parents of an infant born with Down syndrome are holding their infant and crying. The father asks, "I have heard children like this are hard to take care of at home." Which referral would be most appropriate for the parents?
    1. The Web site for the National Association for Down syndrome.
    2. The hospital chaplain.
    3. A Down syndrome support group.
    4. A geneticist.

24. The charge nurse on the pediatric unit hears the overhead announcement Code Pink (infant abduction), newborn nursery. Which action should the charge nurse implement?
    1. Send a staff member to the newborn nursery.
    2. Explain the situation to the clients and visitors.
    3. Continue with the charge nurse's responsibilities.
    4. Station a staff member at all the unit exits.

25. The mother of a 4-year-old child diagnosed with Duchenne's muscular dystrophy is overwhelmed and asks the nurse, "I have been told a case manager will come and talk to me. What will they do for me?" Which statement indicates the nurse understands the role of the case manager?
    1. "You will have a case manager so that the hospital can save money."
    2. "She will make sure your child gets the right medication for muscular dystrophy."
    3. "She will help you find the resources you need to care for your child."
    4. "The case manager helps your child to have a normal life expectancy."

26. The nurse is assigned to the pediatric unit performance improvement committee. The unit is concerned with IV infection rates. Which action should the nurse implement first when investigating the problem?
    1. Contact central supply for samples of IV start kits.
    2. Obtain research to determine the best length for IV dwell time.
    3. Identify how many IV infections have occurred in the last year.
    4. Audit the charts to determine if hospital policy is being followed.

27. The clinic nurse is discussing a tubal ligation with a 17-year-old adolescent with Down syndrome. The adolescent does not want the surgery, but her parents (who are also in the room) are telling her she must have it. Which statement by the nurse would be an example of the ethical principle of justice?
    1. "I think this requires further discussion before scheduling this procedure."
    2. "You will not be able to have children after you have this procedure."
    3. "You should have this procedure because you could not care for a child."
    4. "You can refuse this procedure and your parents can't make you have it."

28. The school nurse has referred an 8-year-old student for further evaluation of vision. The single mother has told the school nurse she does not have the money for the evaluation or glasses. Which action by the nurse would be an example of client advocacy?
    1. Tell the mother the child cannot read the board.
    2. Refer the mother to a local service organization.
    3. Ask the mother if the family is on Medicaid.
    4. Loan the mother money for the examination.

29. The ED nurse is scheduling the 16-year-old client for an emergency appendectomy. Which intervention should the nurse implement when obtaining permission for the surgery?
    1. Withhold the narcotic pain medication until the client signs the permit.
    2. Have the client's parent or legal guardian sign the operative permit.
    3. Explain the procedure to the client and the parents in simple terms.
    4. Get a visitor from the ED waiting area to witness the parent's signature.

30. The unit manager has been notified by central supply that many client items are missing from stock and have not been charged to the client. Which action should the nurse manager implement in regards to the lost charges?
    1. Send out a memo telling the staff to follow the charge procedures.
    2. Form a performance improvement committee to study the problem.
    3. Determine whether the items in question are being restocked daily.
    4. Schedule a staff meeting to discuss how to prevent further lost charges.

Setting Priorities When Caring for Clients

1. 1. The main sign of colic is intense crying; therefore, this is expected and would not warrant the nurse's assessing the child first.
   2. A human bite is dangerous, but it is not life threatening.
   3. The child hit by a car should be assessed first because he or she may have life-threatening injuries that must be assessed and treated promptly.
   4. This client is not priority over a client with a physiologic problem.

2. 1. Administering oxygen may help decrease the sickling of the cells, but this should not be the first intervention to address the client's headache.
   2. Because the client is complaining of a headache, the nurse should first rule out cerebrovascular accident (CVA) by assessing the client's neurologic status and then determine whether it is a headache that can be treated with medication.
   3. Prior to administering any pain medication to a client, the nurse must first assess the client to determine whether the pain is what is expected with the disease process or whether it is a complication that requires further nursing intervention.
   4. Only after CVA has been ruled out should the nurse medicate the client. Adequate hydration will help decrease sickling of the cells, but this is not the first intervention to address the client's pain.

3. 1. The nurse should always praise the child for attempts at cooperation even if the child did not accomplish what the nurse asked.
   2. This action can be taken by the nurse after praising the child for the attempt.
   3. This action is appropriate and should be implemented, but not before the nurse praises the child for the attempt.
   4. The nurse can demonstrate the correct technique for the child but not before praising the child for the attempt.

4. 1. A 180 mg/dL glucose level for a child with type 1 diabetes is not life threatening, and the nurse would not assess this child first.
   2. The nurse would expect the child with pneumonia to have these signs and

symptoms; therefore, the nurse would not assess this child first.
   3. This is a normal potassium level; therefore, the nurse would not assess this child first.
   4. A pulse oximeter reading of less than 93% is significant and indicates hypoxia, which is life threatening; therefore, this child should be assessed first.

MAKING NURSING DECISIONS: When deciding which client to assess first, the test taker should determine whether the signs/symptoms the client is exhibiting are normal or expected for the client situation. After eliminating the expected options, the test taker should determine which situation is more life threatening.

5. 1. The third dose of an antibiotic would not be priority over sliding scale insulin because insulin must be administered prior to the breakfast meal.
   2. Routine medications have a 1-hour leeway before and after the scheduled time; therefore, this medication does not have to be administered first.
   3. Sliding scale insulin is ordered ac, which is before meals; therefore, this medication must be administered first after receiving the A.M. shift report.
   4. Routine medications have a 1-hour leeway before and after the scheduled time; therefore, this medication does not have to be administered first.

6. In order of priority: 4, 5, 3, 2, 1.
   4. The nurse must first determine the infant's responsiveness by thumping the baby's feet.
   5. The nurse should then open the child's airway using the head-tilt chin-lift technique, with care taken not to hyperextend the neck. Then the nurse should look, listen, and feel for respirations.
   3. The nurse then administers quick puffs of air while covering the child's mouth and nose, preferably with a rescue mask.
   2. The nurse should determine whether the infant has a pulse by checking the brachial artery.
   1. If the infant has no pulse, the nurse should begin chest compressions using two fingers at a rate of 30:2.

7. 1. The first intervention after the child is admitted to the unit is to orient the parents and child to the room, the call system, and the hospital rules, such as not leaving the child alone in the room.
   2. This task is within the scope of the UAP, but it is not priority over orienting the child/parents to the room.
   3. The height/weight should be posted in case the client codes, but this can be done after the child/parents are oriented to the room.
   4. The child should receive a meal tray, but not before orientation to the room.

8. 1. The nurse should immobilize the child's leg, but it is not the first intervention.
   2. **The nurse must explain any procedure in words the child can understand. It does not matter how old the child is.**
   3. This is an appropriate intervention, but it is not the first intervention.
   4. This is an appropriate intervention, but it is not the first intervention.

9. 1. This is not the priority problem because lack of fluids is more life threatening to a child than lack of food.
   2. **The child diagnosed with gastroenteritis is at high risk for hypovolemic shock resulting from vomiting and diarrhea; therefore, maintaining fluid and electrolyte homeostasis is priority.**
   3. Knowledge deficit is a psychosocial diagnosis, and although it is important to teach the parents and child, it is not priority over a physiologic problem.
   4. The child already has an infection; thus there is no risk.

   MAKING NURSING DECISIONS: The test taker should use Maslow's Hierarchy of Needs to determine the client's priority problem. Physiologic problems are priority.

10. 1. The child diagnosed with nephrotic syndrome would be expected to have proteinuria.
    2. The child diagnosed with leukemia would be expected to have petechaie.
    3. **Drooling indicates the child is having trouble swallowing, and the epiglottis is at risk of completely occluding the airway. This warrants immediate intervention. The nurse should notify the HCP and obtain an emergency tracheostomy tray for the bedside.**
    4. A child with an ear infection would be expected to have an elevated temperature.

    MAKING NURSING DECISIONS: When deciding which client to assess first, the test taker should determine whether the signs/symptoms the client is exhibiting are normal or expected for the client situation. After eliminating the expected options, the test taker should determine which situation is more life threatening.

Delegating and Assigning Nursing Tasks

11. 1. It is appropriate for the nurse to perform ROM exercises to help prevent contractures, specifically, scissoring of the legs. This action would not require intervention.
    2. Safety issues should always be addressed, and keeping the bed in the lowest position may prevent injury to the child.
    3. Taking the child to the activity room is being a client advocate and would not warrant intervention.
    4. **The child should be positioned upright to prevent aspiration during meals; therefore, this action would require the charge nurse to intervene.**

12. 1. The UAP cannot assess a client; therefore, this is an inappropriate delegation.
    2. The child with a cleft palate repair is at risk for choking or damaging the incision site; therefore, this task should not be delegated to a UAP.
    3. Demonstrating is teaching, and the UAP cannot teach a client.
    4. **The last step of delegating to a UAP is for the nurse to evaluate and determine whether the delegated tasks have been completed and performed correctly. This indicates the nurse has delegated appropriately.**

    MAKING NURSING DECISIONS: When delegating to a UAP, the nurse must follow the four rights of clinical delegation: the right task, to the right person, using the right communication, and providing the right feedback. The right feedback includes determining whether the delegated tasks were performed correctly.

13. 1. **Communication to the UAP must be clear, concise, correct, and complete. The nurse must determine why there was a lack of communication, which resulted in the child's receiving food; therefore, this action should be implemented first.**

2. The nurse retains ultimate accountability for any delegated tasks and cannot blame the UAP for the child's being fed by the mother. The HCP needs to be notified to cancel the procedure.
3. The nurse should talk to the mother about why the child was being fed, but the nurse must first determine whether the UAP told the mother not to feed the child and that the child was to be given nothing by mouth.
4. This action is too late to take care of the situation.

14. 1. The scrub technician is assigned to perform daily whirlpool dressing changes, which is a lengthy procedure. Therefore, assigning the one RN to this task would be inappropriate because he or she cannot be unavailable for an extended period of time.
2. **One of the responsibilities of the unit secretary is to transcribe the HCP's orders, but the licensed nurse retains total responsibility for the correctness and accuracy of the transcribed orders.**
3. The scrub technician cannot administer medications.
4. The unit secretary and laboratory personnel are responsible for posting laboratory data into the client's charts. The UAP should be on the unit taking care of the clients.

15. 1, 2, 4, and 5 are correct.
1. **The UAP can pass the dietary trays to the clients because it does not require judgment.**
2. **One of the responsibilities of the UAP is taking routine vital signs on clients.**
3. The nurse must complete the preoperative check list because it requires nursing judgment to determine whether the client is ready for surgery.
4. **One of the responsibilities of the UAP is changing bed linens.**
5. **The UAP can document the client's intake and output, but the UAP cannot evaluate the numbers.**

16. 1. The administration of blood products does not require the most experienced nurse.
2. Preparing a child for a routine procedure does not require the most experienced nurse.
3. The child recovering from a sickle cell crisis would not require the most experienced nurse.
4. **The child newly diagnosed with a chronic disease, which will have acute**

exacerbations, requires extensive teaching; therefore, the most experienced nurse should be assigned to this child and family.

17. 1. Only a nurse can withdraw blood from a central line.
2. The social worker or case manager is responsible for referring clients to support groups. This is not an expected responsibility of a floor nurse/LPN.
3. **Only chemotherapy certified RNs can administer antineoplastic, chemotherapeutic medications. This is a national minimal standard of care according to the Oncology Nursing Society.**
4. The dietitian is responsible for ensuring that the proper food is provided along with evaluating the child's nutritional intake, not checking the amount of food eaten—this is the responsibility of the nursing staff.

18. 1. A 6-year-old child on bed rest needs an appropriate activity to help with distraction; a cartoon video would be an age-appropriate activity.
2. The child life therapist is responsible for recreational and developmental activity for the hospitalized child, but any staff member should address the child's psychosocial needs.
3. **Part of the delegation process is to evaluate the UAP's performance of duties, and the nurse should praise any initiative on the part of the UAP in being a client advocate.**
4. Videos are one of the few age-appropriate activities to occupy a 6-year-old on bed rest; therefore, there is no reason to notify the charge nurse.

19. 1. The newborn with the myelomeningocele has a portion of the spinal cord and membranes protruding through the back and is at risk for hydrocephalus and meningitis and should be assigned to a more experienced nurse.
2. **The new graduate who has completed the NICU internship should be able to care for a premature infant because care is primarily supportive.**
3. Esophageal atresia, a congenital anomaly in which the esophagus does not completely develop, is a clinical and surgical emergency. It puts the newborn at risk for aspiration because the upper esophagus ends in a blind pouch with the lower part of the esophagus connected to the trachea.

This newborn should be assigned to a more experienced nurse.

4. Tetralogy of Fallot is a cyanotic, congenital anomaly. It includes a combination of four defects of the heart, all of which result in unoxygenated blood's being pumped into the systemic circulation. This newborn must be assigned to an experienced nurse.

MAKING NURSING DECISIONS: The test taker must determine which client is the most stable, which makes this an "except" question. Three clients are either unstable or have potentially life-threatening conditions.

20. 1. Weighing the diaper is the procedure for determining the infant's urinary output and is not part of the procedure for obtaining a urine specimen.
   2. **The NCSBN position paper in 1995 defined delegation as transferring to a competent individual the authority to perform a selected nursing task in a selected situation. The nurse retains the accountability for the delegation. The nurse must determine whether the UAP has the ability and knowledge to perform a task. This question clarifies whether the UAP has the ability to obtain a urine specimen.**
   3. Obtaining a urine specimen with an indwelling catheter on an 11-month-old infant would require more expertise than a UAP would have on the pediatric unit. Furthermore, it does not determine whether the UAP understands how to do the procedure.
   4. This statement does not determine whether the UAP understands how to perform the procedure of obtaining a urine specimen from an 11-month-old infant.

Managing Clients and Nursing Staff

21. 1. The nurse should offer the child choices that ensure cooperation with the therapeutic regimen. The choices are when the child will ambulate, not whether the child will ambulate.
   2. The nurse could ask the parents for help in making sure the client ambulates, but this may cause a rift in the nurse/parent/child relationship. This is not the most appropriate intervention.
   3. The child development therapist could assist with activities that would encourage

the client to ambulate, but the nurse should take control of the situation and ensure the client ambulates. This is not the most appropriate intervention.
   4. This is bribery, and the nurse should not use this technique to ensure cooperation with the therapeutic regimen.

22. 1. The nurse must take action or the child will be afraid of the nurse.
   2. The nurse should discuss the inappropriate comment with the mother, not with the child.
   3. If every nurse who overheard this type of comment reported it to Child Protective Services, it would only unnecessarily increase the workload in an already overloaded system. Furthermore, reporting perceived potential abuse to Child Protective Services is a very serious accusation.
   4. **The nurse should explain to the mother that threatening the child with a shot will cause the child to be frightened of health-care professionals. This type of comment is inappropriate and should not be used to discipline a child.**

23. 1. There is a Web site to obtain information about Down syndrome, but this type of referral would not be the most appropriate for parents who need to deal with emotional aspects of having a child with special needs.
   2. The hospital chaplain is an important part of the multidisciplinary health-care team but would not have specialized knowledge regarding caring for a special needs child.
   3. **According to the NCSBN NCLEX-RN test plan, referrals are included in management of care. The most appropriate referral would be to a support group where other parents who have special needs children can share their feelings and provide advice on how to care for their child in the home.**
   4. Although Down syndrome results from a trisomy chromosome 21, it is primarily associated with maternal age over 35 years. Furthermore, a geneticist would not have specialized knowledge regarding caring for a special needs child.

24. 1. The newborn nursery does not need any more people in the area. Personnel are needed to monitor any and all exits.
   2. The purpose of using code names to alert hospital personnel of emergency situations is to avoid panic among the clients and visitors; therefore, the nurse should not

explain the situation to the clients and visitors.

3. Any time there is an overhead emergency announcement, the charge nurse is responsible for following the hospital emergency plan.

4. **Code Pink means an infant has been abducted from the newborn nursery. The priority intervention is to prevent the abductor from taking the child from the hospital, which can be prevented by placing a staff member at all the unit exits.**

MAKING NURSING DECISIONS: The nurse must be knowledgeable of hospital emergency preparedness. Students as well as new employees receive this information in hospital orientations and are responsible for implementing procedures correctly. The NCSBN NCLEX-RN blueprint includes questions on safe and effective care environment.

25. 1. Even though case management is a strategy to ensure coordination of care while reducing costs, the nurse should not share this with the mother.

2. The case manager is not responsible for ensuring that the client receives the correct medication; it is the responsibility of the HCP.

3. **According to the NSCBN NCLEX-RN test blueprint, questions on case management are included. The case manager will coordinate the care for a client with a chronic illness with other members of the multidisciplinary health-care team. This attempts to prevent duplication of services and allows the mother to have a specific individual to coordinate services to meet the child's needs.**

4. The life expectancy of a child with Duchenne's muscular dystrophy is approximately 25 years. The case manager is not responsible for helping the child have a normal life expectancy.

26. 1. Although this would not be the first step in investigating a problem, this action may be initiated if it is determined to be the cause for the increase in infection rates.

2. The nurse should utilize evidenced-based practice research when proposing changes because it is part of the performance improvement process, but it is not the first intervention when investigating the problem.

3. **The first intervention is to determine the extent of the problem and who owns the problem. The NCSBN NCLEX-RN test blueprint includes performance improvement (quality improvement) in the management of care content.**

4. This action may need to be implemented once it is determined whether there is a problem with IV infection rates. However, this would be the second step in the process.

27. 1. The ethical principle of justice is to treat all clients fairly, without regard to age, socioeconomic status, or any other variable, including clients with special needs. This statement supports the adolescent's right to her opinion even though she has Down syndrome.

2. If the adolescent needs clarification of the procedure, this would be an appropriate response, which is an example of the ethical principle of veracity or truth telling.

3. This statement is an example of the ethical principle of paternalism, in which the nurse knows what is best for the client.

4. **This is an example of autonomy, in which the client has the right to self-determination. The Nuremburg code of ethics specifically supports the right of individuals with special needs against being forced to participate in procedures against their will.**

28. 1. Although this may be the case, this is not client advocacy, and doing so may make the mother feel guilty about not being able to afford glasses for her child.

2. **This is an example of client advocacy because many local service organizations, such as the Lions Club or the Rotary Club, will subsidize the cost of the vision test and glasses.**

3. Medicaid does not pay for glasses, and it is not the school nurse's business if the family is on Medicaid.

4. The nurse should not loan the mother money because this crosses professional boundaries.

29. 1. The 16-year-old client is not old enough to sign the permit; therefore, pain medication would not be withheld.

2. Legally, a child under the age of 18 must have a parent or legal guardian sign for informed consent. The nurse should determine whether the child is

aware of the situation and assents to the procedure.

3. The surgeon is responsible for explaining the procedure; the nurse is responsible for witnessing the signature on the operative permit.

4. The nurse is responsible for witnessing the signature. Having a visitor sign the operative permit is a violation of HIPAA.

30. 1. A written memo does not allow the staff to have input into how to correct the problem. This memo might lead to blaming and arguments among the staff.

2. The performance improvement committee is designed to improve client care, not to address management issues.

3. This is implying that the unit manager does not believe the central supply lost charges. If the unit manager has this concern, it should be addressed directly with the central supply supervisor.

4. **Because the staff is responsible for following the hospital procedure for charging for items used in client care, the unit manager should discuss this with staff to determine what should be done to correct the problem.**

COMPREHENSIVE EXAMINATION

1. The nurse is caring for clients on the pediatric unit. Which child would warrant a referral to the early childhood development specialist?
   1. The 9-month-old child who says only "mama" or "dada."
   2. The 11-month-old child who walks hanging onto furniture.
   3. The 8-month-old child who sits by leaning forward on both hands.
   4. The 4-month-old infant who turns from the abdomen to the back.

2. The 10-year-old child diagnosed with leukemia is scheduled for a bone marrow aspiration. Which intervention is most important when obtaining informed consent for the procedure?
   1. Obtain assent from the child.
   2. Have the parent sign the permit.
   3. Refer any questions to the HCP.
   4. Witness the signature on the permit.

3. The 13-year-old client has just delivered a 4-pound baby boy. The stepfather of the client becomes verbally abusive to the nurse when he is asked to leave the room. The client is withdrawn and silent. Which legal action should the nurse implement?
   1. Call hospital security to come to the room.
   2. Contact Child Protective Services.
   3. Refer the child to the social worker.
   4. Ask the client whether she feels safe at home.

4. The fire alarm on the pediatric unit has just started sounding. Which action should the charge nurse implement first?
   1. Call the hospital operator to find out the location of the fire.
   2. Ensure that all visitors and clients are in the room with the door closed.
   3. Prepare to evacuate the clients and visitors down the stairs.
   4. Make a list of which clients are not currently on the unit.

5. A nurse overhears two other nurses talking about a client in the hospital dining room. Which action should the nurse implement first?
   1. Notify the HIPAA officer about the breach of confidentiality.
   2. Immediately report the two nurses to their clinical manager.
   3. Document the situation in writing and submit to the Chief Nursing Officer (CNO).
   4. Tell the two nurses they are violating the client's confidentiality.

6. The nurse is caring for newborns in the nursery. Which newborn warrants immediate intervention by the nurse?
   1. The 8-hour-old newborn who has not passed meconium.
   2. The 15-hour-old newborn who is slightly jaundiced.
   3. The 4-hour-old newborn who is jittery and irritable.
   4. The 10-hour-old newborn who will not stop crying.

7. At 1300, the nurse is assessing a 12-year-old child who is complaining of abdominal pain and rating it as a "5" on a scale of 1 to 10. Which intervention should the nurse implement?

Client's Name:	Account Number: 123456		Allergies: NKDA	
Height: 60 inches	Weight: 98 pounds			
Date	Medication	2301–0700	0701–1500	1501–2300
	Maalox 30 mL q 1 hour prn			
	Acetominophen (Tylenol) 650 mg PO q 6 hrs prn			
	Hydrocodone (Vicodin) 5 mg PO prn pain q 4–6 hours	0600 NN		
	Morphine 2 mg IVP prn pain q 4 hours			
Signature/Initials		Day Nurse RN DN	Night Nurse RN NN	

1. Administer 30 mL of Maalox PO.
2. Administer 650 mg of Tylenol PO.
3. Administer 5 mg of hydrocodone PO.
4. Administer 2 mg of morphine IVP.

8. The nurse who has never worked on the maternity ward has been pulled from the surgical unit to work in the newborn nursery. Which assignment would be most appropriate for the nurse to accept?
   1. Perform an assessment on the newborn.
   2. Assist the pediatrician with a circumcision.
   3. Gavage feed a newborn who is 8 hours old.
   4. Transport newborns to the mothers' room.

9. The nurse is instructing the UAP on gross motor skill activity that is appropriate for a developmentally delayed 9-month-old infant. Which activity should the nurse delegate to the UAP?
   1. Help the child to sit without support.
   2. Teach the child to catch the beach ball.
   3. Reward the child with food for sitting up.
   4. Teach the child to blow a kiss.

10. Which incident should the primary nurse report to the clinical manager concerning a violation of information technology guidelines?
    1. The nurse keeps the computer screen turned away from public view.
    2. The nurse researches medications using the online formulary.
    3. The nurse shares the computer access code with another nurse.
    4. The nurse logs off the computer when leaving the terminal.

11. The nurse is caring for clients in a pediatric ED. Which client should the nurse assess first?
    1. The child with a dog bite on the left hand who is bleeding.
    2. The child who has a laceration on the right side of the forehead.
    3. The child with a fractured tibia who will not move the foot.
    4. The child who has ingested a bottle of prenatal vitamins.

12. The nurse is caring for a client in a children's medical center. Which behavior indicates the nurse understands the pediatric client's rights?
    1. The nurse administers an injection without talking to the child.
    2. The nurse covers the 5-year-old child's genitalia during a code.
    3. The nurse discusses the child's condition with the grandparents.
    4. The nurse leaves an uncapped needle at the client's bedside.

13. The home health nurse is planning the care of a 14-year-old client diagnosed with leukemia who is receiving chemotherapy. Which psychosocial problem is priority for this client?
    1. Diversional activity deficit.
    2. High risk for infection.
    3. Social isolation.
    4. Hopelessness.

14. The nurse is administering IV fluids to a 3-year-old client. Which action by the nurse would warrant intervention by the charge nurse?
    1. The nurse places the IV on an infusion pump.
    2. The nurse does not use a volume-controlled chamber.
    3. The nurse checks the child's IV site every hour.
    4. The nurse labels the IV tubing with date and time.

15. The nurse is caring for clients on a psychiatric pediatric unit. Which action by the nurse is reportable to the state board of nursing?
    1. The nurse leaves for lunch and does not return to complete the shift.
    2. The nurse fails to check the ID band when administering medications.
    3. The nurse has had three documented medication errors in the last 3 months.
    4. The nurse has admitted to having an affair with another staff member.

16. The nurse is working in a free health-care clinic. Which client situation warrants further investigation?
    1. The child diagnosed with rheumatoid arthritis who is wearing a copper bracelet.
    2. The mother of a child with a sunburn who is using juice from an aloe vera plant on the burn.
    3. The grandmother who reports rubbing Vick's Vapo-Rub on the child's chest for a cold.
    4. The father who tells the nurse that the child receives a variety of herbs every day.

17. The UAP tells the primary nurse that the 4-year-old child is alone in the room because the mother went to the cafeteria to get something to eat. Which action should the nurse implement first?
    1. Arrange for the mother to have a tray sent to the room.
    2. Go to the cafeteria and ask the mother to return to the room.
    3. Tell the UAP to stay with the child until the mother returns.
    4. Notify social services that the mother left the child alone.

18. The nurse is evaluating an 18-month-old child in the pediatric clinic. Which data would indicate to the nurse that the child is not meeting task according to Erikson's Stages of Psychosocial development?
    1. The child stamps his or her foot and says "no" frequently.
    2. The child does not interact with the mother.
    3. The child cries when the mother leaves the room.
    4. The child responds when called by name.

19. Which statement by the female charge nurse indicates she has an autocratic leadership style?
    1. "You must complete all the A.M. care before you take your morning break."
    2. "I don't care how the work is done as long as it is completed on time."
    3. "I would like to talk to you about your ideas on a new staffing mix."
    4. "I think we should have a pot luck lunch tomorrow because it is Saturday."

20. The nurse is evaluating the care of a 5-year-old client with a cyanotic congenital heart defect. Which client outcome would support that discharge teaching has been effective?
    1. The mother makes the child get up when squatting.
    2. The child is playing in the dayroom without oxygen.
    3. The father buys the child a baseball and a bat.
    4. The nurse finds unopened packs of salt on the meal tray.

1. 1. The 9-month-old infant's language and cognitive skills include imitating sounds, saying single syllables, and beginning to put syllables together. Using "mama" and "dada" indicates this child is developmentally on target.
   2. The 10- to-12-month-old infant can walk with one hand held or cruise the furniture, but will usually crawl to get places more rapidly. This behavior indicates the child is developmentally on target.
   3. **The 8-month-old infant should be able to sit steadily unsupported; therefore, this child is developmentally delayed and warrants a referral to the early childhood development specialist. Leaning forward on both hands to sit is normal for a 6-month-old.**
   4. The 4-month-old infant should be able to turn from the abdomen to back; therefore, this child is developmentally on target.

2. 1. **The most important intervention for this child is to make sure the child has some control and input into the decision-making. It is customary to obtain assent from children 7 years and older. Assent means the child has been fully informed about the procedure and concurs with those giving the informed consent.**
   2. The parents must sign the permit because the child is under age 18, but the most important intervention is to make sure the child is included and aware of decisions being made about his or her body.
   3. The nurse may be able to clarify some of the child's or parent's questions and does not need to refer all questions to the HCP.
   4. Witnessing the signature on the permit is required prior to the child's having surgery, but it is not the most important intervention.

3. 1. The nurse should call hospital security when a client or visitor is being abusive, but this is not a legal action.
   2. **Legally, the nurse is required to report any suspected child abuse. A 13-year-old child who is having a baby and is withdrawn and silent along with a potential abuser who is trying to control access to the child should make the nurse suspect child abuse.**
   3. Referring the client to a social worker is not a legal action.
   4. Asking the client whether she feels safe at home is an appropriate assessment question, but it is not a legal action.

4. 1. The charge nurse must first make sure that clients and visitors are safe. Someone will notify the charge nurse about the location of the fire.
   2. **Safety of the clients and visitors is priority; therefore, ensuring that they are in a room with the door closed is the first intervention.**
   3. The charge nurse may need to prepare for evacuation, but it is not the first intervention.
   4. Although making a list of clients not currently on the unit is an appropriate intervention, the charge nurse must first ensure the safety of the clients and visitors that are on the pediatric unit.

5. 1. The HIPPA officer can be notified of the breach of confidentiality, but the nurse must first confront the two nurses and correct the behavior.
   2. The nurses can be reported to their clinical manager, but the nurse must first confront the two nurses and correct the behavior.
   3. The situation can be documented in writing and turned into the HIPPA officer (not the CNO), but the nurse must first confront the two nurses and correct the behavior.
   4. **This is a violation of HIPPA; therefore, the nurse must first confront the two nurses and correct the behavior.**

6. 1. The nurse would not be concerned about not passing meconium until at least 24 hours after delivery.
   2. The nurse would not be concerned about a newborn who is slightly jaundiced until after 24 hours after delivery, at which point the HCP would investigate to determine whether the jaundice is pathologic.
   3. **A newborn who is jittery and irritable needs to be assessed first for possible hypoglycemia. The nurse could feed the newborn glucose water or provide more frequent regular feedings.**
   4. Although the nurse should determine why the newborn will not stop crying, the newborn who is showing signs of hypoglycemia warrants immediate intervention.

7. 1. An antacid is administered to neutralize gastric acidity and help with heartburn, not abdominal pain.
   2. A non-narcotic analgesic is used to treat mild pain, a "2 to 4" on a pain scale.
   3. **A narcotic analgesic is used for moderate to severe pain; a "5" is considered moderate pain. The child received a dose at**

0600, which relieved the pain for 7 hours; therefore, this would be the most appropriate medication.

4. An IVP narcotic analgesic should be administered for severe pain, that is, pain greater than "7" on the 1-to-10 pain scale.

8. 1. The nurse should not accept any assignment for which he or she is unqualified. A newborn assessment requires specialized knowledge and skills to detect potential complications.

2. The nurse who is not familiar with the procedure or the unit should not be assigned to assist a pediatrician to perform a procedure.

3. This is a dangerous procedure because the nurse must insert a tube into the newborn's stomach. A nurse who is not familiar with this procedure should refuse the assignment.

4. **Any nurse can take an infant to the mother's room and check the bands to ensure the right infant is with the right mother. This is an appropriate task for a nurse who has never worked in the nursery.**

9. 1. **The 9-month-old infant should be able to sit without support. Therefore, the nurse should instruct the UAP to perform the developmental task of helping the child sit without support.**

2. Teaching a child to catch a beach ball would be appropriate for a 15- to 18-month-old child, so the nurse should not instruct the UAP to perform this task.

3. The UAP should not use food as a reward or comfort measure because it may lead to childhood obesity.

4. Teaching a child how to blow a kiss is a language/cognitive activity and will not help the child's gross motor development.

10. 1. Making sure no one can view the screen is an appropriate information technology guideline.

2. Researching medication online is ensuring safe and effective nursing care and shows that the nurse is keeping abreast of new medications.

3. **According to the NSCBN NCLEX-RN test blueprint, the nurse must be knowledgeable of information technology. Giving another nurse his or her access code is a very serious violation of information technology guidelines and should be reported.**

4. Logging off the computer is an appropriate information technology guideline.

11. 1. A dog bite is an emergency, but it is not life threatening; therefore, this child would not be assessed first.

2. The child with a head laceration must be assessed, but not before a child who might die of medication poisoning.

3. The child with a fractured tibia would not be expected to move the foot.

4. **A child who ingested a bottle of prenatal vitamins presents a medication poisoning that is a potentially life-threatening situation. This child must be assessed first to determine how many vitamins were taken, how long ago they were taken, and whether or not the vitamins contained iron. The child's neurologic status must also be assessed.**

12. 1. The pediatric client has the right to an explanation of procedures being done to his or her body.

2. **The pediatric client has a right to be treated with dignity and respect. Just because the child is being coded does not mean the nurse should allow the child's body to be exposed to everyone in the room.**

3. The pediatric client has a right to confidentiality, and the parents/legal guardians are the only individuals who have a right to the child's health information. Talking to the grandparents is a violation of HIPPA unless the parents have approved.

4. The nurse is responsible and accountable to protect the health, safety, and rights of the pediatric client. Leaving an uncapped needle at the bedside could cause serious harm to the child.

13. 1. Diversional activity deficit would be appropriate if the client did not have sufficient activities to keep him or her occupied. Most children of this age will watch television, play video games, or read books.

2. The client has leukemia and is receiving chemotherapy, which leads to an increased risk of infection; however, this is a physiologic problem, not a psychosocial problem.

3. The client will be isolated from peers and schools because of the high risk of infection resulting from the immunosuppression secondary to chemotherapy and the disease process. At this stage, the child needs to be developing peer relationships and independence from

parents. Therefore, social isolation is the priority psychosocial problem for this client.

4. The nurse should not identify hopelessness because childhood leukemia has a good prognosis.

14. 1. Placing the IV line on an infusion pump helps to make sure the client does not receive an overload of IV fluid. Most facilities require an IV pump and volume-controlled chamber when administering fluids in a pediatric clinic.

2. **A volume-controlled chamber (Buretrol) is a device that is used with children when administering IV fluids. The chamber is filled with 1 hour's amount of fluid so that the child will not inadvertently receive an overload of fluid. Fluid volume overload is a potentially life-threatening situation in children.**

3. The site should be checked frequently to ensure that the IV does not infiltrate; therefore, this does not warrant intervention.

4. The IV tubing should not be used longer than 72 hours; therefore, labeling the tubing with the date and time would not warrant intervention.

15. 1. **Abandonment is a reportable offense to the state board of nursing in every state. Reportable offenses could result in stipulations made to the nurse's license.**

2. This is failure to follow the five rights of medication administration, but it is not a reportable offense.

3. Multiple medication errors are a management issue, not a reportable offense.

4. Having an affair with a fellow employee is not a reportable offense.

16. 1. A copper bracelet may or may not help the child with rheumatoid arthritis, but because it will not hurt the child, it does not warrant further investigation.

2. Aloe vera is used in many topical burn preparations; therefore, this practice would not warrant further investigation.

3. Vick's VapoRub may or may not help the child's cold, but, because it will not hurt the child, it does not warrant further investigation.

4. **Herbal products are not regulated by the Food and Drug Administration, and there is very little (if any) research on herbal use with children. The nurse should at least investigate which herbs the child is receiving before taking further action.**

17. 1. This is an appropriate nursing intervention so that the mother will not have to leave her child, but it is not the first intervention. The child's safety is priority.

2. The nurse could go to the cafeteria and tell the mother to return to the room, but during this time the UAP should stay with the child.

3. **The child's safety is priority; therefore, the nurse should have the UAP stay with the child until the mother returns.**

4. Social services would not need to be notified at this time. If the mother continually leaves the child alone, then this would be an appropriate action.

18. 1. An 18-month-old child should be throwing temper tantrums. This indicates the child is developing a sense of autonomy.

2. **An 18-month-old child should cling to the mother and interact continuously with the primary caregiver. A child not interacting with the mother is not meeting the task of developing a sense of autonomy.**

3. The child has met the task of trust when he or she cries if the mother leaves the room.

4. When a child responds to his or her name, it indicates a sense of identity; therefore, the task is met.

19. 1. **An autocratic manager uses an authoritarian approach to direct the activities of others. This individual makes most of the decisions alone without input from other staff members.**

2. A laissez-faire manager maintains a permissive climate with little direction or control.

3. A democratic manager is people oriented and emphasizes efficient group functioning. The environment is open, and communication flows both ways.

4. A democratic manager is people oriented and emphasizes efficient group functioning.

20. 1. Squatting relieves the hypoxic episodes, and the child should be able to remain in the squatting position.

2. The child with a cyanotic, congenital heart defect should have oxygen when being active.

3. This indicates the father does not understand that the child will not be able to participate in active sports because of the stress that is placed on the heart.

4. **This behavior indicates the child understands the importance of salt restriction because of potential congestive heart failure.**

Geriatric Nursing

6

"You are the people who are shaping a better world. One of the secrets of inner peace is the practice of compassion."

—Dalai Lama

ABBREVIATION LIST

CNO	Chief Nursing Officer	MRI	Magnetic Resonance Imaging
CPR	Cardiopulmonary Resuscitation	NCSBN	National Council of State Boards of Nursing
CVA	Cerebrovascular Accident (Stroke)	NPO	Nothing per (by) Os (Mouth)
DVT	Deep Vein Thrombosis	PEG	Percutaneous Endoscopic Gastrostomy
ECG	Electrocardiogram	PTT	Partial Thromboplastin Time
ED	Emergency Department	RN	Registered Nurse
H&H	Hemoglobin and Hematocrit	TURP	Transurethral Resection of the Prostate
HCP	Health-Care provider	UAP	Unlicensed Assistive Personnel
HIPAA	Health Insurance Portability and Accountability Act	WBC	White Blood Cell
IV	Intravenous		
LPN	Licensed Practical Nurse		
MAR	Medication Administration Record		

PRACTICE QUESTIONS

Setting Priorities When Caring for Clients

1. The nurse is caring for clients in a long-term care facility. Which client should the nurse assess first after receiving morning report?
   1. The client diagnosed with Parkinson's disease who began to hallucinate during the night.
   2. The client diagnosed with congestive heart failure who has 3+ pitting edema of both feet.
   3. The client diagnosed with Alzheimer's disease who was found wandering in the hall at 0200 in the morning.
   4. The client diagnosed with terminal cancer who has lost 8 pounds since the last weight 4 weeks ago.

2. The nurse in a long-term care facility is administering medications to a group of clients. Which medication should the nurse administer first?
   1. Acetylsalicylic acid (aspirin), an antiplatelet, to a client newly diagnosed with coronary disease.
   2. Neostigmine (Prostigmin), an anticholinesterase, to a client diagnosed with myasthenia gravis.
   3. Cephalexin (Keflex), an antibiotic, to a client diagnosed with an acute urinary tract infection.
   4. Erythropoeitin (Epogen), a biologic response modifier, to a client diagnosed with end-stage renal disease.

3. The nurse is caring for an 84-year-old male client diagnosed with benign prostatic hypertrophy who has undergone a transurethral resection of the prostate (TURP) and is complaining of bladder spasms. Which intervention should the nurse implement first?
   1. Administer an antispasmodic medication for bladder spasms.
   2. Calculate the client's urinary output.
   3. Palpate the client's abdomen for bladder distention.
   4. Assess the client's three-way urinary catheter for patency.

4. The nurse is preparing to administer a unit of packed red blood cells to an elderly client diagnosed with anemia. Which interventions should the nurse implement? List in order of performance.
   1. Obtain the unit of blood from the blood bank.
   2. Start an IV access with normal saline at a keep-open rate.
   3. Have the client sign the permit to receive blood products.
   4. Check the unit of blood with another nurse at the bedside.
   5. Initiate the transfusion at a slow rate for 15 minutes.

5. The nurse in a long-term care facility is developing the plan of care for a client diagnosed with end-stage Alzheimer's disease. Which client problem is priority for this client?
   1. Inability to do activities of daily living.
   2. Increased risk for injury.
   3. Potential for constipation.
   4. Ineffective family coping.

6. The clinic nurse is providing discharge instructions to an elderly client diagnosed with cataracts. Which intervention is most important for the nurse to implement?
   1. Teach the client to increase the light in the home.
   2. Encourage the client to wear dark glasses outside.
   3. Discuss the need to have the cataracts removed.
   4. Tell the family not to rearrange furniture in the home.

7. The nurse is caring for clients on a surgical unit. Which client should the nurse assess first after shift report?
   1. The 68-year-old client diagnosed with diverticulitis who has a hard abdomen.
   2. The 75-year-old client who cannot void after inguinal hernia surgery.
   3. The 84-year-old client diagnosed with renal calculi who thinks he passed a stone.
   4. The 86-year-old client who refuses to ambulate with the UAP after a lung biopsy.

8. Which client should the charge nurse of a long-term care facility see first after receiving shift report?
   1. The client who is unhappy about being placed in a long-term care facility.
   2. The client who wants to have the HCP to order a nightly glass of wine.
   3. The client who is upset because the call light was not answered for 30 minutes.
   4. The client whose son is being discharged from the hospital after heart surgery.

9. The nurse is preparing to administer morning medications. Which medication should the nurse administer first?
   1. The levothyroxine (Synthroid), a thyroid hormone, to a client diagnosed with hypothyroidism.
   2. The Humulin N insulin, a pancreatic hormone, to a client diagnosed with type 2 diabetes.
   3. The prednisone, a glucocorticoid, to a client diagnosed with chronic obstructive pulmonary disease.
   4. The tiotropium (Spiriva) inhaler, a bronchodilator, to a client diagnosed with chronic asthma.

10. The elderly client diagnosed with deep vein thrombosis is complaining of chest pain during inhalation. Which intervention should the nurse implement first?
   1. Ask the HCP to order a stat lung scan.
   2. Place oxygen on the client via nasal cannula.
   3. Prepare to administer intravenous heparin.
   4. Tell the client not to ambulate and remain in bed.

Delegating and Assigning Nursing Tasks

11. The nurse and the UAP are caring for residents in a long-term care facility. Which task should the nurse delegate to the UAP?
   1. Apply a sterile dressing to a stage IV pressure wound.
   2. Check the blood glucose level of a resident who is weak and shaky.
   3. Document the amount of food the residents ate after a meal.
   4. Teach the residents how to play different types of bingo.

12. The UAP working in a long-term care facility notifies the nurse that the client on a low-sodium diet is complaining that the food is inedible. Which intervention should the nurse implement first?
   1. Have the family bring food from home for the client.
   2. Check to see what the client has eaten in the last 24 hours.
   3. Tell the client that a low-sodium diet is important for his or her health.
   4. Ask the dietitian to discuss food preferences with the client.

13. The RN is the charge nurse of a skilled nursing unit in a long-term care facility. Which task should the RN delegate to the UAP?
   1. Get the resident up in a wheelchair for meals.
   2. Check the incontinent client's perianal area.
   3. Discuss requirements for when the client goes on a pass.
   4. Explain diabetes care to the resident and family.

14. The director of nurses in a long-term care facility observes the LPN charge nurse explaining to a UAP how to calculate the amount of food a resident has eaten from the food tray. Which action should the director of nurses implement?
   1. Ask the charge nurse to teach all the other UAPs.
   2. Encourage the nurse to continue to work with the UAP.
   3. Tell the charge nurse to discuss this in a private area.
   4. Give the UAP a better explanation of the procedure.

15. The wound care nurse in a long-term care facility asks the UAP for assistance. Which task should not be delegated to the UAP?
   1. Apply the wound débriding paste to the wound.
   2. Keep the resident's heels off the surface of the bed.
   3. Turn the resident at least every 2 hours.
   4. Encourage the resident to drink a high-protein shake.

16. The charge nurse observes the nurse telling the UAP to feed an elderly client diagnosed with a CVA. Which question should the charge nurse ask the nurse?
    1. "How does the client swallow the medications?"
    2. "Did you complete your head to toe assessment?"
    3. "Does the client have some Thick It in the room?"
    4. "Why would you delegate feeding to a UAP?"

17. The charge nurse is making shift assignments. Which client should be assigned to the most experienced nurse?
    1. The 56-year-old client diagnosed with acute cellulitis of the right forearm.
    2. The 64-year-old client diagnosed with chronic alcoholic pancreatitis.
    3. The 70-year-old client diagnosed with fulminant pulmonary edema.
    4. The 72-year-old client diagnosed with inflammatory bowel disease.

18. The nurse and the UAP are caring for a client on a medical unit who has difficulty swallowing and is incontinent of urine and feces. Which task should the nurse delegate to the UAP?
    1. Check the client's PEG feeding tube for patency.
    2. Place DuoDERM wound care patches on the client's coccyx.
    3. Apply nonmedicated ointment to the client's perineum.
    4. Suction the client during feeding to prevent aspiration.

19. The UAP tells the nurse that the female client is crying and upset because the client has been told that her husband has just died. Which intervention should the nurse implement?
    1. Tell the UAP to go and sit with the client.
    2. Make a referral for the chaplain to see the client.
    3. Ask the HCP to prescribe a mild sedative.
    4. Leave the client alone in the room to grieve.

20. The UAP in a long-term care facility asks the nurse, "What do I do if the client refuses to have a bath?" Which statement is the nurse's best response?
    1. "The client does not need to take a bath if he or she does not want one."
    2. "Offer to take the resident to the shower room for the bath."
    3. "You should give the client a choice of when to have a bath."
    4. "Insist the resident take a bath because of the possible body odor."

Managing Clients and Nursing Staff

21. The male client in a long-term care facility complains that the staff does not listen to his complaints unless a family member also complains. Which action should the director of nurses implement?
    1. Call a staff meeting and tell the staff to listen to the resident when he talks to them.
    2. Determine who neglected to listen to the resident and place the staff member on leave.
    3. Ignore the situation because a resident in long-term care cannot determine his needs.
    4. Talk with the resident about his concerns and then initiate a plan of action.

22. The client diagnosed with a CVA is confined to a wheelchair for most of the waking hours. Which intervention is priority for the nurse to implement?
    1. Encourage the client to move the buttocks every 2 hours.
    2. Order a high-protein diet to prevent skin breakdown.
    3. Get a pressure-relieving cushion to place in the wheelchair.
    4. Refer the client to physical therapy for transfer teaching.

23. The newly admitted client in a long-term care facility stays in the room and refuses to participate in client activities. Which statement is priority for the nurse to discuss with the client?
    1. "You have to get out of this room or you will never make friends here at the home."
    2. "It is not so bad living here, you are lucky that we care about what happens to you."
    3. "You seem sad; would you like to talk about how you are feeling about being here?"
    4. "The activities director can arrange for someone to come and visit you in your room."

24. The charge nurse overhears two UAPs discussing a client in the hallway. Which action should the charge nurse implement first?
    1. Remind the UAPs that clients should not be discussed in a public area.
    2. Tell the unit manager that the UAPs might have been overheard.
    3. Have the UAPs review policies on client confidentiality and HIPPA.
    4. Find some nursing tasks the UAPs can be performing at this time.

25. The family member of a client in a long-term care facility is unhappy with the care being provided for the loved one. Which person would be most appropriate to investigate the complaint and report the findings during a client care conference?
    1. The ombudsman for the facility.
    2. The social worker for the facility.
    3. The family member who is unhappy.
    4. The director of nurses.

26. The 65-year-old client is being discharged from the hospital following major abdominal surgery and is unable to drive. Which referral should the nurse make to ensure continuity of care?
    1. A church that can provide transportation.
    2. A home health agency.
    3. An outpatient clinic.
    4. The health-care provider's office.

27. The nurse in an assisted living facility notes that the male client has several new bruises on both of his arms and hands. Which intervention should the nurse implement first?
    1. File an elder abuse report with the Department of Human Services.
    2. Ask the client whether he has fallen and hurt himself during the night.
    3. Check the MAR to determine which medications the client is receiving.
    4. Notify the client's family of the bruises so they are not surprised on their visit.

28. The resident in a long-term care facility tells the nurse, "I think my family just put me here to die because they think I am too much trouble." Which statement is the nurse's best response?
    1. "Can you tell me more about how you feel since your family placed you here?"
    2. "Your family did what they felt was best for your safety."
    3. "Why would you think that about your family? They care for you."
    4. "Tell me, how much trouble were you when you were at home?"

29. The elderly client receiving chemotherapy complains that food just does not taste like it used to. Which intervention should the medical unit nurse implement first?
    1. Ask the dietitian to consult with the client on food preferences.
    2. Medicate the client before meals with an antiemetic medication.
    3. Ask the HCP to suggest an over-the-counter nutritional supplement.
    4. Check the client's current weight with the client's usual weight.

30. The nurse is assigned to a quality improvement committee to decide on a quality improvement project for the unit. Which issue should the nurse discuss at the committee meetings?
    1. Systems that make it difficult for the nurses to do their job.
    2. How unhappy the nurses are with their current pay scale.
    3. Collective bargaining activity at a nearby hospital.
    4. The number of medication errors committed by a nurse.

Setting Priorities When Caring for Clients

1. 1. The client diagnosed with Parkinson's disease who has begun to hallucinate may be experiencing an adverse reaction to one of the medications used to treat the disease. The nurse should assess this client first.
   2. Peripheral edema is expected in a client diagnosed with heart failure. This client does not need to be assessed first.
   3. Wandering and lack of sleeping are expected in a client diagnosed with Alzheimer's disease. This client does not need to be assessed first.
   4. Weight loss in a client diagnosed with terminal cancer is expected. The nurse should review the client's intake, food preferences, and pain control before making an intervention. Weight loss does not occur in a matter of minutes to hours, and this client's needs do not merit assessment before the client with a new problem.

   MAKING NURSING DECISIONS: The test taker should first determine whether a new problem is occurring or whether the problem is expected for the disease process. If the symptom is expected for the disease process and is not life threatening, then that client does not have priority.

2. 1. A daily aspirin is not a priority medication. This medication can be administered within 30 minutes before or 30 minutes after the scheduled time.
   2. Prostigmin promotes muscle function in clients diagnosed with myasthenia gravis. This medication should always be administered on time to prevent loss of muscle tone, especially the muscles of the upper respiratory tract. This is the priority medication to administer at this time.
   3. An oral antibiotic can be administered within 30 minutes before or after the scheduled time frame.
   4. Epogen works by stimulating the bone marrow to produce red blood cells. It can take days to weeks to see a response in the client. This medication is not the priority medication to administer.

   MAKING NURSING DECISIONS: When the test taker is deciding on a priority medication, the test taker must first decide on the expected response of the client. If the expected response prevents or treats an emergency situation, then that medication becomes the priority medication to administer.

3. 1. The nurse may need to administer an antispasmodic medication but not before assessment of the client. Bladder spasms in a client who has had a TURP are usually caused by clots remaining in the bladder. A three-way indwelling catheter that is working properly will flush the clots from the bladder.
   2. The nurse should calculate the client's urine output, but that is not the first intervention and will not address the client's pain.
   3. The nurse could palpate the client's bladder for distention, but this will not help decrease the client's pain.
   4. The three-way indwelling catheter is placed during surgery to keep blood clots from remaining in the bladder and causing bladder spasms and increasing bleeding. The nurse should first assess the drainage system to make sure that it has not become obstructed with a clot.

   MAKING NURSING DECISIONS: The test taker should use a systematic guide whenever deciding on a priority intervention. The nursing process is an excellent tool for the test taker to use in this question. Assessment is the first step of the nursing process, and the option is assessing the correct area.

4. In order of performance: 3, 2, 1, 4, 5.
   3. The client must agree to the risks and benefits of a blood transfusion before the nurse can administer the blood product. This is the first intervention.
   2. The nurse has only 30 minutes from the time the blood is retrieved from the blood bank until the transfusion is initiated. The nurse should make sure the client has a patent IV access before obtaining the blood from the blood bank.
   1. The nurse can obtain the unit of packed cells when the client has signed the permit and has a patent IV access.
   4. The nurse should always check the blood product with another nurse at the client's bedside against the client's hospital identification band and blood bank crossmatch band.
   5. After the nurse has followed the procedure to ensure the correct blood

product is being administered, with a second nurse, then the transfusion of packed cells can be initiated. The blood is initiated at a slow rate—10 mL per hour for the first 15 minutes—so that the nurse can observe the client for potential complications.

MAKING NURSING DECISIONS: The nurse must be aware of standards of care when performing nursing tasks.

5. 1. Clients diagnosed with Alzheimer's disease may have problems with completing activities of daily living, but this is not the client's priority problem.
   2. Safety is the highest priority for clients diagnosed with end-stage Alzheimer's disease because the client is unaware of his or her own surroundings and can easily wander from an area of safety.
   3. The client in end-stage disease may have an increased risk for constipation, but this is not priority over safety of the client.
   4. The client's family is often distraught over seeing their loved one deteriorate because of Alzheimer's, but it is not priority over the safety of the client.

MAKING NURSING DECISIONS: The test taker can use Maslow's Hierarchy of Needs to determine the correct answer. On the pyramid of needs, beginning at the bottom, physiologic needs have priority, followed by safety.

6. 1. Cataracts cause less light to be filtered through an opaque lens to the retina. The client should have as much light as possible in the home to prevent falls.
   2. Dark glasses protect the eyes from the sun's rays when outside, as they do for anyone, but this client needs more light indoors.
   3. This is the responsibility of the HCP, not the nurse.
   4. The furniture in the client's house should not be moved. If the furniture is left in its usual position, the client will be less likely to fall or stumble. However, the priority intervention is safety when walking; therefore, increasing light in the home is priority.

MAKING NURSING DECISIONS: This question requires the test taker to use knowledge of the disease process and Maslow's Hierarchy of Needs. Cataracts cause opacity of the lens of the eye, and safety is a high priority according to Maslow.

7. 1. The nurse should assess this client first. A hard abdomen may indicate peritonitis, a medical emergency. The signs of peritonitis are a hard, rigid abdomen; tenderness; and fever.
   2. Clients frequently have difficulty voiding after inguinal surgery. This is expected.
   3. The nurse should check to determine whether the client has passed a stone, but this is a desired outcome and could wait until the client with an emergency has been assessed and appropriate interventions initiated.
   4. Refusing to ambulate is a problem that can wait until the client with an emergency has been assessed and appropriate interventions initiated.

MAKING NURSING DECISIONS: The test taker must read all the options to determine whether an option contains a life-threatening situation. If the option contains information that is expected or within normal limits, then that client does not have priority.

8. 1. This client will require time to adjust to living in an extended care facility. This would be an expected reaction.
   2. This client may or may not be allowed a glass of wine at night. Some long-term care facilities do allow the client to have a controlled amount of alcohol with an HCP order and the family supplying the alcohol, but this client is not priority.
   3. This client may or may not have a valid complaint. The nurse should investigate whether or not the complaint is true. Failure to answer a call light can result in the client's attempting to ambulate without assistance and could be a safety issue. The nurse should speak with this client first.
   4. The nurse is not in control of the client's son and his discharge, but if the son is being discharged, it can be assumed that the son is in a stable condition, and it is not a priority for the charge nurse to see this client.

MAKING NURSING DECISIONS: This question has options that do not have a physiologic reason to set a priority. The test taker must decide whether one or more of the options could result in a problem for the client. Safety is always considered a priority.

9. 1. Synthroid is a daily medication and can be administered within the 1-hour time frame (30 minutes before and 30 minutes after the dosing time).

2. Insulin should be administered before a meal for best effects. This medication should be administered first.
3. Prednisone is a routine medication and can be administered within the 1-hour time frame (30 minutes before and 30 minutes after the dosing time).
4. Spiriva is a routine daily medication and can be administered within the 1-hour time frame (30 minutes before and 30 minutes after the dosing time).

MAKING NURSING DECISIONS: The nurse must be aware of the actions and uses of medications when setting priorities.

10. 1. This should be an anticipated order if the nurse suspects a pulmonary embolus, but it is not the first intervention.
2. The nurse should suspect the client has a pulmonary embolus, a complication of the thrombophlebitis. Pulmonary emboli decrease the oxygen supply to the body, and the nurse should immediately administer oxygen to the client.
3. An anticoagulant infusion will be ordered for the client once it is determined that the client is experiencing a pulmonary embolus.
4. Getting oxygen to the body is priority; telling the client not to ambulate can be done after initiating the oxygen.

MAKING NURSING DECISIONS: Physiologic problems have the highest priority when deciding on a course of action. If the client is in distress, then the nurse must intervene with a nursing action that attempts to alleviate or control the problem. The test taker should not choose a diagnostic test if there is an option that directly treats the client.

Delegating and Assigning Nursing Tasks

11. 1. A nurse, not the UAP, should perform sterile dressing changes.
2. This client is unstable, and a nurse should perform this task.
3. The UAP can check to see the amount of food the residents consumed and document the information.
4. This is the job of the activity director and volunteers working with the activities department. Staffing is limited in any nursing area; the UAP should be assigned a nursing task.

MAKING NURSING DECISIONS: The nurse should be knowledgeable about the roles of different members of the multidisciplinary

health-care team in the long-term care facility. The nurse should not delegate tasks to the UAP that are the responsibility of another department.

12. 1. The family may be allowed to bring in food occasionally from home, but this may not adhere to a low-sodium diet, and the family should not be required to provide three meals per day for the client. This is the facility's responsibility.
2. Assessing the client's intake will help the nurse to determine the extent of the client's complaints. This is the first intervention.
3. This may be true but does not help the client adjust to a lack of sodium in the diet.
4. A referral to the dietitian should be made after the nurse fully assesses the situation.

MAKING NURSING DECISIONS: Assessment is the first step of the nursing process, and the test taker should use the nursing process or some other systematic process to assist in determining priorities.

13. 1. Getting a resident up in a wheelchair for meals is an appropriate delegation to a UAP. This task does not require nursing judgment.
2. Checking an incontinent client's perianal area requires nursing judgment and cannot be delegated to the UAP.
3. Discussing requirements for client going out on a pass should be done by the nurse responsible for completing the required documentation and providing the resident's medication that should go with the resident.
4. Explaining diabetes care is teaching, and the RN cannot ask the UAP to teach.

MAKING NURSING DECISIONS: The nurse cannot delegate assessment, evaluation, teaching, administering medications, or the care of an unstable client to a UAP.

14. 1. The charge nurse is not the nurse educator but is responsible for the UAPs working under him or her. This is adding additional duties to the charge nurse.
2. The director of nurses should encourage responsible behavior on the part of all staff. The charge nurse is performing a part of the responsibility of the charge nurse and should be encouraged to work with the UAP.
3. Because this is not a private conversation about a client, there is no reason for the charge nurse to be told to go to a private area. The charge nurse is not reprimanding the UAP.

4. The director of nurses should not interfere with a "better explanation." This could intimidate the charge nurse and make it difficult for the charge nurse to perform his or her duties.

15. 1. Wound débriding formulations are medications, and a UAP cannot administer medications.
2. The UAP can position the resident so that pressure is not placed on the resident's heels.
3. The UAP can turn the resident.
4. The UAP can give the resident a protein shake to drink.

MAKING NURSING DECISIONS: **The nurse cannot delegate assessment, evaluation, teaching, administering medications, or the care of an unstable client to a UAP.**

16. 1. This question will determine whether the nurse has assessed the client's ability to swallow. The nurse cannot delegate unstable clients, and a client newly diagnosed with a CVA may be unstable and have difficulty swallowing.
2. This question does not address the client's ability to swallow.
3. Thick It might be needed if the client has difficulty swallowing, but the charge nurse has not established that the client has swallowing difficulty.
4. A UAP can feed clients who are stable and do not require nursing judgment during the process.

MAKING NURSING DECISIONS: **The nurse cannot delegate assessment, evaluation, teaching, administering medications, or an unstable client to a UAP.**

17. 1. A client with cellulitis of the forearm requires IV medications and possibly hot packs to the arm; a less experienced nurse can care for this client.
2. A client with chronic alcoholic pancreatitis is kept NPO and often requires pain medication. A less experienced nurse can care for this client.
3. A client with fulminant pulmonary edema is experiencing an acute, life-threatening problem. The most experienced nurse should be assigned to this client.
4. A client with inflammatory bowel disease should be kept NPO and on IV fluids. A less experienced nurse can care for this client.

MAKING NURSING DECISIONS: **When the test taker is deciding which client should be assigned to the most experienced nurse, the test taker should decide which client is the most unstable or requires knowledge that a more experienced nurse would have.**

18. 1. Checking the patency of a PEG feeding tube requires nursing judgment, and feeding the client through the tube is based on this judgment. The UAP should not be asked to perform this task.
2. The nurse should assess the coccyx and where the DuoDERM should be placed. The UAP should not be asked to perform this task.
3. The UAP can apply nonmedicated ointment to protect the client's perineum when bathing and changing the client's incontinence pads. This will protect the client from skin breakdown.
4. The nurse should not delegate suctioning during feeding to a UAP.

MAKING NURSING DECISIONS: **When the test taker is deciding which option is the most appropriate task to delegate/assign, the test taker should choose the task that allows each member of the staff to function within his or her full scope of practice. Do not assign a task to a staff member that requires a higher level of expertise than that staff member has; similarly, do not assign a task to a staff member that could be assigned to a staff member with a lower level of expertise.**

19. 1. The UAP cannot sit for an extended period of time with a grieving client.
2. A chaplain is a spiritual advisor who can stay with the client until a family member or the client's personal spiritual advisor can come to the hospital to be with the client.
3. The client should not be sedated. Grieving is a natural process that must be worked through. Sedating the client will delay the grieving process. The nurse should allow the client to ventilate feelings to foster the grieving process and not numb the client.
4. The client may request to be left alone, but the nurse should refer the client for spiritual support first and not assume that the client wants to be left alone. Most clients feel the need for someone's presence.

20. 1. Refusing hygiene is a right within limits in a shared environment or in a situation where the resident has soiled himself or herself. There are times when the resident must be encouraged to participate in personal hygiene.

2. This is still personal hygiene and still requiring the resident to participate.
3. **Giving the resident a choice of times gives some control to the resident but still requires that personal hygiene is completed. This is the best response by the nurse.**
4. Insisting that a resident take a bath involves taking control over the resident's life and choices. It is much better to allow the resident to have the feeling of control.

MAKING NURSING DECISIONS: The test taker should look for an opportunity to turn the situation into a win-win situation. The correct option gives some control to the resident while accomplishing the desired outcome.

Managing Clients and Nursing Staff

21. 1. The director of nurses must first understand the extent of the complaint. Telling staff to ignore preconceived ideas about the elderly does not work. The director of nurses should have valid information to discuss with the staff.
2. The client has a general complaint, and so more than one staff member may have ignored the client's statements. Neglect was not mentioned in the stem of the question. Not treating the client with the dignity that the client deserves is implied.
3. This is a false statement. Some residents in a long-term care facility may not be able to determine their needs, but this is not true of all residents.
4. **The director of nurses should discuss the resident's complaints with the resident and then determine a plan of action to remedy the situation.**

22. 1. The client should be encouraged to move the buttocks to increase blood circulation to the area, but a wheelchair cushion used every time the client is in the wheelchair will help prevent pressure ulcers.
2. A high-protein diet will assist with maintaining a positive nitrogen balance that will support would healing, but it will not prevent pressure from causing a breakdown of the skin.
3. **All clients remaining in a wheelchair for extended periods of time should have a wheelchair cushion that relieves pressure to prevent skin breakdown.**

4. The more the client can move from the wheelchair to a chair to the bed, the more it will help decrease the possibility of a pressure ulcer, but a wheelchair cushion helps relieve pressure continuously.

23. 1. This may be a true statement, but this client is exhibiting symptoms of depression. The client may or may not wish to make friends at the facility.
2. This is not acknowledging the client's feelings.
3. **This client is exhibiting symptoms of depression. Therapeutic conversation is implemented to help the client ventilate feelings. This statement acknowledges the client's feeling and offers self.**
4. This action may get the client to interact with other people, but it does not acknowledge the client's feelings.

24. 1. **The charge nurse should remind the UAPs not to discuss confidential information in a public place. This is the first action.**
2. The charge nurse may need to inform the manager of the breach of confidentiality, but the first action is to stop the conversation.
3. The charge nurse and/or the manager may need to make sure the UAPs are familiar with confidentiality, but the conversation should be terminated first.
4. This might be a better activity for the UAPs, but the first action is to stop the conversation.

MAKING NURSING DECISIONS: In any business, confidential discussions should not occur among staff of any level where the customers can hear it or see it.

25. 1. **An ombudsman is a representative appointed to receive and investigate complaints made by individuals of abuses or capricious acts. All Medicare and Medicaid long-term care facilities must have an ombudsman to act as a neutral party in matters of dispute with the facility. This is the best person to investigate a complaint.**
2. The social worker is employed by the facility and is not the best person to investigate the complaint.
3. The upset family member should attend the conference but should have the ombudsman investigate the complaint.
4. The director will be biased; the best person to investigate the validity of the complaint is the ombudsman.

26. 1. The nurse should not refer the client to a church or volunteer organization to ensure

continuity of care. The organization's work may depend on unpaid individuals, and a volunteer may or may not be available to transport the client when needed.

2. The nurse should refer the client to a home health agency for follow-up care. The nurse will go to the client's home to assess the client and perform dressing changes. The home health agency will also assess the client and the client's home for further needs.

3. The client is unable to drive and would not be able to get to an outpatient clinic.

4. The client is unable to drive and would not be able to get to the HCP's office.

MAKING NURSING DECISIONS: The nurse must be knowledgeable about appropriate referrals for continuity of care. The NCSBN NCLEX-RN blueprint includes questions on management of care.

27. 1. The nurse must assess the cause of the bruises before filing a report of abuse. The nurse would file a report of elder abuse only if it is determined that the client has been abused.

2. The nurse should ask the client whether there is a reason for the bruises that the nurse should be aware of. This is the first intervention and can be done while the nurse is currently with the client.

3. The nurse should check the client's MAR to see whether he is currently on a medication, such as warfarin (Coumadin) or a systemic steroid, that would increase the risk for bruising; however, this would be done after talking with the client because the bruising is "new," and bruising from the medications can take several days to weeks to develop.

4. The family may need to be notified but not until the nurse assesses the situation.

28. 1. The client is expressing negative feelings about being placed in the nursing home. Asking about the client's feelings is a therapeutic response that encourages the client to discuss his or her feelings.

2. This is not acknowledging the client's feelings and is nontherapeutic because it is a judgmental statement.

3. The client does not owe the nurse an explanation. "Why" is never therapeutic.

4. This is assuming the client is correct in being "trouble at home" and agreeing that the family would punish the client for being a problem.

MAKING NURSING DECISIONS: The test taker must first decide whether the client is asking for information or is expressing feelings. If the client is asking for information, then the option that provides information is the correct answer. If, however, the client is expressing feelings, a therapeutic response is called for, and the test taker should select the option that addresses the patient's feelings.

29. 1. Asking the dietitian to consult with the client is a good intervention, but the nurse should assess the impact of the change in taste on the client.

2. The client did not complain of nausea. Antiemetic medication is used to prevent nausea associated with food odors and attempting to eat.

3. The nurse can recommend an over-the-counter supplement to increase nutrition, but the nurse should first assess the impact of the problem. Over-the-counter supplements are expensive, and the nurse should suggest the client try malts and milk shakes and fortified soups. Then, if the client does not like or gets tired of the taste, a family member can consume the food and it is not wasted.

4. Checking the client's weight change over a period of time is the first step in assessing the client's nutritional status and the impact of the taste changes on the client.

MAKING NURSING DECISIONS: The test taker should employ a systematic approach to problem-solving. The nursing process is a systematic approach, and assessment is the first step of the nursing process.

30. 1. A quality improvement project looks at the way tasks are performed and attempts to see whether the system can be improved. A medication delivery system in which it takes a long time for the nurse to receive a stat or "now" medication is an example of a system that needs improvement and should be addressed by a quality improvement committee.

2. Financial reimbursement of the staff is a management issue, not a quality improvement issue.

3. Collective bargaining is an administrative issue, not a quality improvement issue.

4. The number of medication errors committed by a nurse is a management-to-nurse issue and does not involve a systems issue, unless several nurses have committed the same error because the system is not functioning appropriately.

COMPREHENSIVE EXAMINATION

1. The elderly female client diagnosed with osteoporosis is prescribed the bisphospho-nate medication alendronate (Fosamax). Which intervention is priority when adminis-tering this medication?
   1. Administer the medication first thing in the morning.
   2. Ask the client whether she has a history of peptic ulcer disease.
   3. Encourage the client to walk daily for at least 30 minutes.
   4. Have the client remain upright for 30 minutes after administering.

2. The female nurse is discussing an upcoming surgical procedure with a 76-year-old male client diagnosed with cancer. Which action is an example of the ethical principle of fidelity?
   1. The nurse makes sure the client understands the procedure before signing the permit.
   2. The nurse refuses to disclose the client's personal information to the CNO.
   3. The nurse tells the client his diagnosis when the family did not want him to know.
   4. The nurse tells the client that she does not know the client's diagnosis.

3. The evening nurse in a long-term care facility is preparing to administer medications to a client diagnosed with atrial fibrillation. Which medication should the nurse ques-tion administering?

Client: Mr. A	Admit Number: 654321		Allergies: Penicillin
Date: Today	Height: 71 inches Weight: 77.27 kg 170 pounds		Diagnosis: Atrial Fibrillation
Medication	**0701–1500**	**1501–2300**	**2301–0700**
Warfarin (Coumadin) 5 mg PO daily INR: 3.4/today		1800	
Metoclopramide (Reglan) 5 mg P.O. TID	0900 DN 1300 DN	1800	
Docusate (Colace) PO BID	0900 DN	1800	
Atorvastatin (Lipitor) PO daily		1800	
Nurse's Name/ Initials	**Day Nurse RN/DN**	**Evening Nurse RN/EN**	

   1. Warfarin (Coumadin), an anticoagulant.
   2. Metoclopramide (Reglan), a gastric motility medication.
   3. Docusate (Colace), a stool softener.
   4. Atorvastatin (Lipitor), an antihyperlipidemic.

4. The nurse and the UAP enter the client's room and discover that the client is unresponsive. Which action, according to the American Heart Association (AHA) guidelines, should the nurse assign to the UAP first?
   1. Ask the UAP to check whether the client is asleep.
   2. Tell the UAP to administer two rescue breaths.
   3. Instruct the UAP to get the crash cart.
   4. Request the UAP to put the client in a recumbent position.

5. The elderly client on a medical unit has a do not resuscitate (DNR) order written. Which intervention should the nurse implement?
   1. Continue to care for the client's needs as usual.
   2. Place notification of the DNR inside the client's chart.
   3. Refer the client to a hospice organization.
   4. Limit visitors to two at a time, so as not to tire the client.

6. Which client laboratory data should the nurse report to the HCP immediately?
   1. The elevated amylase report on a client diagnosed with acute pancreatitis.
   2. The elevated WBC count on a client diagnosed with a septic leg wound.
   3. The urinalysis report showing many bacteria in a client receiving chemotherapy.
   4. The serum glucose level of 235 mg/dL on a client diagnosed with type 1 diabetes.

7. The elderly client frequently makes statements that are inappropriate for the situation and is not oriented to place, time, or date. The HCP has ordered a magnetic resonance imaging (MRI) scan of the client's brain. Which intervention should the nurse implement?
   1. Administer a mild sedative to prevent claustrophobia.
   2. Order a vest restraint for use by the client during the MRI.
   3. Make sure the client does not have a pacemaker.
   4. Ask a family member to stay with the client while the test is performed.

8. The elderly female client from an extended care facility is admitted to the hospital without family or friends present. Which resource(s) should the admission nurse utilize to obtain information about the client?
   1. The nurse should wait until a significant other can be contacted.
   2. The verbal report from the ambulance workers and stat lab work.
   3. The transfer form from the nursing home and old hospital records.
   4. The health-care provider's telephone orders about care needed.

9. The nurse administering medications to clients on a medical unit discovers that the wrong medication was administered to the elderly female client. The client had replied that she was Mrs. Smith when the nurse asked her name from the MAR. Which step in medication administration did the nurse violate when administering the medication?
   1. Asking the client to repeat her name.
   2. Verifying the client's arm band with the MAR.
   3. Checking the medication against the MAR.
   4. Documenting the medication on the MAR.

10. The elderly client becomes confused and wanders in the hallways. Which fall precaution intervention should the nurse implement first?
   1. Place a Posey vest restraint on the client.
   2. Move the client to a room near the station.
   3. Ask the HCP for an antipsychotic medication.
   4. Raise all four-side rails on the client's bed.

11. The admitting nurse is subpoenaed to give testimony in a case in which the client fell from the bed and fractured the left hip. The nurse initiated fall precautions on admission but was not on duty when the client fell. Which issue should the nurse be prepared to testify about the incident?
    1. What preceded the client's fall from the bed.
    2. The extent of injuries the client sustained.
    3. The client's mental status before the incident.
    4. The facility's policy covering falls prevention.

12. The RN, LPN, and UAP are caring for a group of clients on a surgical unit. Which nursing task should the nurse assign to the LPN?
    1. Insert an indwelling urinary catheter before surgery.
    2. Turn and reposition the client every 2 hours.
    3. Measure and record the urine in the bedside commode.
    4. Feed the client who gagged on the food during the last meal.

13. The charge nurse must notify a staff member to stay home because of low census. The unit currently has 35 clients who all have at least one IV and multiple IV medications. The unit is staffed with two RNs, three LPNs, and three UAPs. Which nurse should be notified to stay home?
    1. The least experienced RN.
    2. The most experienced LPN.
    3. The UAP who asked to be requested off.
    4. The UAP who was hired 4 weeks ago.

14. The charge nurse in a long-term care facility is reviewing the male resident's laboratory data and notes the following: H&H, 13/39; WBC count, 5.25 (10^3); and platelets, 39 (10^3). Which instructions should the nurse give to the UAP caring for the client?
    1. Place the client in reverse isolation immediately.
    2. Administer oxygen during strenuous activities.
    3. Do not shave the resident with a safety razor.
    4. Check the resident's temperature every 4 hours.

15. The charge nurse in an extended care facility notes an elderly male resident holding hands with an elderly female resident. Which intervention should the charge nurse implement?
    1. Do nothing, because this is a natural human need.
    2. Notify the family of the residents about the situation.
    3. Separate the residents for all activities.
    4. Call a care plan meeting with other staff members.

16. The Chief Nursing Officer (CNO) of an extended care facility is attending shift report with two charge nurses, and an argument about a resident's care ensues. Which action should the CNO implement first?
    1. Ask the two charge nurses to stop arguing and go to a private area.
    2. Listen to both sides of the argument and then implement a plan of care.
    3. Ask the family to join the discussion before deciding how to implement care.
    4. Tell the nurses to stop arguing and continue to give report.

17. Which action by the nurse is a violation of the Joint Commission's Patient Safety Goals?
    1. The surgery nurse calls a time-out when a discrepancy is noted on the surgical permit.
    2. The unit nurse asks the client for his or her date of birth before administering medications.
    3. The nurse educator gives the orientee the answers to the quiz covering the IV pumps.
    4. The admit nurse initiates the facility's fall prevention program on an elderly client.

18. The nurse on a medical unit has just received the evening shift report. Which client should the nurse assess first?
    1. The client diagnosed with a DVT who has a heparin drip infusion and a PTT of 92.
    2. The client diagnosed with pneumonia who has an oral temperature of 100.2°F.
    3. The client diagnosed with cystitis who complains of burning on urination.
    4. The client diagnosed with pancreatitis who complains of pain that is an "8."

19. The nurse is preparing to administer medications. Which medication should the nurse administer first?
    1. Digoxin (Lanoxin), a cardiac glycoside, due at 0900.
    2. Furosemide (Lasix), a loop diuretic, due at 0800.
    3. Propoxyphene (Darvon), an analgesic, due in 2 hours.
    4. Acetaminophen (Tylenol), an analgesic, due in 5 minutes.

20. The nurse is providing discharge instructions to a 68-year-old male client who had quadruple coronary bypass surgery. Which question should the nurse ask the client?
    1. "Are you sexually active?"
    2. "Can you still drive your car?"
    3. "Do you have pain medications at home?"
    4. "Do you know when to call your HCP?"

1. 1. Fosamax should be administered in the morning on an empty stomach to increase absorption, but it is not priority over the client's sitting up for 30 minutes. The client should main upright for at least 30 minutes to prevent regurgitation into the esophagus and esophageal erosion.
   2. The client with peptic ulcer disease may be more a risk for esophageal erosion, but the HCP should have assessed this prior to prescribing this medication for the client.
   3. The client with osteoporosis should be encouraged to walk to increase bone density, but this is not pertinent when administering the medication.
   4. **Fosamax should be administered on an empty stomach with a full glass of water to promote absorption of the medication. The client should remain upright for at least 30 minutes to prevent regurgitation into the esophagus and esophageal erosion.**

2. 1. This is an example of autonomy. The client needs all pertinent information prior to making an informed choice.
   2. **This is an example of fidelity. Fidelity is the duty to be faithful to commitments and involves keeping information confidential and maintaining privacy and trust.**
   3. This is an example of veracity, the duty to tell the truth.
   4. This is an example of nonmalfeasance, the duty to do no harm. This avoids telling a client facing surgery that he has cancer.

3. 1. **The client's international normalized ratio (INR) is 3.4. The therapeutic range is 2 to 3 for a client diagnosed with atrial fibrillation. This client is at risk for bleeding. The nurse should hold the medication and discuss the warfarin with the HCP.**
   2. Metoclopramide is used to stimulate gastric emptying. Nothing in the stem or the MAR indicates a problem with administering this medication. The nurse would administer this medication.
   3. Docusate is a stool softener. Nothing in the stem or the MAR indicates a problem with administering this medication. The nurse would administer this medication.
   4. Atorvastatin is a lipid-lowering medication. Nothing in the stem or the MAR indicates a problem with administering this medication. The nurse would administer this medication.

4. 1. The first step in cardiopulmonary resuscitation according to the AHA guidelines is to establish unresponsiveness by "shaking and shouting." If the client does not respond to being shaken, then the nurse can proceed to the next step, which is to "look, listen, and feel" for breaths. This is assessment and, according to AHA guidelines, the UAP could perform this function if alone. However, the nurse should assess the client before a UAP.
   2. Administering two rescue breaths comes after establishing unresponsiveness and lack of respiration.
   3. **The nurse can tell the UAP to get the crash cart while the nurse assesses the client. This is the best task to assign the UAP at this time.**
   4. The nurse should place the client in the recumbent position before attempting to perform chest compressions; the nurse should send the UAP for help and the crash cart.

5. 1. **The nurse should care for the client as if the DNR order was not on the chart. A DNR order does not mean the client no longer wishes treatment. It means the client does not want CPR or to be placed on a ventilator if the client's heart quits beating.**
   2. The information about the DNR status is already inside the chart. It may need to be placed on the outside of the chart and a special arm band or other notification made to other health-care personnel.
   3. The client has a DNR order, but this does not imply that there may be 6 months or less life expectancy for the client. (Hospice care may be requested for clients with less than a 6-month life expectancy.) An order for hospice must be written by the attending health-care provider before making this referral.
   4. The client should be allowed as many visitors as the hospital policy allows.

6. 1. An elevated amylase would be expected in a client diagnosed with acute pancreatitis. The nurse would not need to call the HCP immediately.
   2. An elevated WBC would be expected in a client diagnosed with a septic (infection) leg wound. The nurse would not need to call the HCP immediately.

3. The urinalysis report showing many bacteria is indicative of an infection. Clients receiving chemotherapy are at high risk of developing an infection. The nurse should notify the HCP immediately.

4. This blood glucose level is above normal range but would not be particularly abnormal for a client diagnosed with type 1 diabetes. The nurse would not need to call the HCP immediately.

7. 1. The client has not complained of claustrophobia. The client has some type of neurologic abnormality.

2. A vest restraint will not keep the client's head still during the MRI.

3. **The nurse should make sure that the client does not have any medical device implanted that could react with the magnetic field created by the MRI scanner. An implanted ECG device could prevent the client from having an MRI, depending on the age of the pacemaker and the material with which it was made.**

4. Family members are requested to stay outside of the area where the MRI is performed.

8. 1. The nurse needs as much information as possible in order to provide care for the client. The client may or may not have a significant other to be contacted. This is not the best way to try to get information on the client.

2. The ambulance workers will only be able to give a cursory report based on the limited information that was provided to them. This is not the best place to try to get information on the client.

3. **The nursing home should send a transfer form with the client that details current medications and diagnoses as well as hygiene needs. Previous hospital records will include a history and physical examination and a discharge summary. This is a good place to start to glean information regarding the client.**

4. The HCP orders may contain a current diagnosis but will not contain any information about the client's medical history. This is not the best place to try to get information on the client.

9. 1. The nurse asked the client her name, and the client replied that she was a different person.

2. **The step the nurse did not take was to verify the client's arm band against the MAR. Checking the identification band**

against the MAR would have prevented the error.

3. This is not the step that was overlooked.

4. This is not the step that was missed.

10. 1. The nurse should implement the least restrictive measures to ensure client safety. Restraining a client is one of the last measures implemented.

2. **Moving the client near the nursing station where the staff can closely observe the client is one of the first measures in most fall prevention policies.**

3. This is considered medical restraints and is one of the last measures taken to prevent falls.

4. Four side rails are considered a restraint. Research has shown that having four side rails up does not prevent falls and only gives the client farther to fall when the client climbs over the rails before falling to the floor.

11. 1. The nurse cannot testify to what preceded the client's fall because the nurse was not on duty at the time.

2. The nurse was not on duty to assess the client's injuries, so any information about the injuries received from the fall would have to be hearsay or obtained from the chart.

3. The nurse cannot testify to the client's mental status prior to the fall because the nurse was not on duty at the time.

4. **The nurse initiated a policy that is designed to prevent falls from occurring. This is all the nurse can testify to.**

12. 1. **The LPN is qualified to perform a sterile procedure, such as inserting an indwelling catheter before surgery. This is an appropriate assignment.**

2. Turing and repositioning a client can be delegated to a UAP.

3. Emptying a client's bedside commode and recording the amount of urine can be delegated to a UAP.

4. The nurse should feed the client who gagged during the last meal to assess the client's ability to swallow. This client is unstable and cannot be assigned/delegated.

13. 1. **The registered nurse, experienced or not, can be assigned nursing duties of assessment, planning, teaching, and other duties that cannot be delegated or assigned. The charge nurse only has two RNs for 35 clients. This nurse should not be requested to stay home.**

2. An experienced LPN will be needed by the unit to care for the many IV lines and medications.

3. **The UAP cannot administer medications or IVs and has requested to be allowed to stay home. This is the best staff member to request to stay home.**

4. This UAP may be less experienced on the floor but has not worked long enough to receive any paid time off, and this could greatly affect the UAP's pay.

14. 1. The resident's WBC count is within normal limits and indicates an ability to resist infection. The nurse should not place this resident in reverse isolation.

2. The resident's H&H is slightly lower than normal but not low enough to cause dyspnea during activity. The resident does not need oxygen.

3. **The resident's platelet count is very low and could cause the resident to bleed. The nurse should initiate bleeding precautions that include not using sharp blades to shave the resident and using soft bristle toothbrushes.**

4. The client is not at risk for developing an infection. The client does not need the temperature checked every 4 hours.

15. 1. **The charge nurse does not have a right to interfere with two consenting adults having a relationship. Doing nothing is the correct action for the charge nurse. If one of the residents involved is incapable of giving consent to a relationship, then the charge nurse might need to get involved.**

2. Two consenting adults have a right to form a bond. The family does not have a right to interfere with the expression of a basic human need, to form an intimate relationship with another human being.

3. The residents have the right to companionship. They should be allowed to participate in any activity that they wish, when they wish.

4. This is a normal situation, and no care plan meeting is needed.

16. 1. The argument should already be in a private area because the argument ensued during report. Report should always be held in a confidential area.

2. **The CNO should evaluate the concerns of each charge nurse and then make a decision as to a plan of care for the resident. The CNO is the next in**

command over the charge nurses in an extended care facility.

3. This argument does not involve the family. If, after listening to both sides, the CNO thinks there is a need for family member's input, then the CNO could contact the family, but a decision should be made until this can occur.

4. The nurses each have a concern over a resident. This situation should be resolved before continuing report.

17. 1. Calling a time-out when a discrepancy is noted on the surgical permit is an appropriate action to prevent an error during a surgical procedure.

2. The Joint Commission requires two identifiers be utilized prior to administering medications. Most hospitals use the client's date of birth for the second identifier. This is an appropriate action to prevent an error during a medication administration.

3. **A quiz during orientation is given to assess whether the new employee understands the information being taught. Giving the answers to the quiz completes the required documentation for the employee's files but does not ensure the new hire understands how to utilize the IV pump. This is a violation of the Patient Safety Goals.**

4. Initiating a fall prevention program for an elderly client to prevent falls is an appropriate action to attempt to ensure client safety.

18. 1. **The therapeutic PTT level should be $1\frac{1}{2}$ to 2 times the control. Most controls average 36 seconds, so the therapeutic levels of heparin would place the control between 54 and 72. With a PTT of 92, the client is at risk for bleeding, and the heparin drip should be held. The nurse should assess this client first.**

2. A client diagnosed with pneumonia would be expected to have a fever. This client can be seen after the client diagnosed with a DVT.

3. Cystitis is inflammation of the urinary bladder, and burning on urination is an expected symptom.

4. Pancreatitis is a very painful condition. Pain is a priority but not over potential for hemorrhage.

19. 1. Digoxin can be administered later because it is a routine medication.

2. Lasix can be administered within the 1-hour leeway (30 minutes before and after); it does not need to be administered first.

3. Darvon is not due yet; the nurse should assess the client and determine whether nonpharmacologic interventions to relieve pain can be implemented, but this medication cannot be administered for 2 hours.
4. Tylenol is administered for mild-to-moderate pain. By the time the nurse obtains the medication and performs all of the steps to administer a medication correctly, it will be time for the client to receive the Tylenol. This medication should be administered first.

20. 1. The nurse should be aware that sexual activity is important to most adults and should not decide that the client is not sexually active because of a client's age. The nurse should provide instructions regarding sexual activity before the client is discharged. This is the question that should be asked because many clients may be embarrassed to bring up the subject.
2. The client should not drive a motor vehicle until released to do so by the HCP. This is not an appropriate question at this time.
3. The client should be discharged with a prescription for oral pain medications to be taken as directed by the surgeon. The nurse should not encourage the client to use old medications the client may have at home. This is not an appropriate question.
4. The nurse is providing discharge instructions and should tell the client when to call the HCP. This is not an appropriate question.

Rehabilitation Nursing 7

"To be effective and organized, the nurse must continually prioritize what must be done."

—Ray A. Hargrove-Huttel

ABBREVIATION LIST

ABG	Arterial Blood Gas
ADA	Americans with Disabilities Act
ADLs	Activities of Daily Living
AP	Apical Pulse
BP	Blood Pressure
COPD	Chronic Obstructive Pulmonary Disease
CPM	Continuous Passive Motion
CVA	Cerebrovascular Accident (Brain Attack, Stroke)
DVT	Deep Vein Thrombosis
ED	Emergency Department
H&H	Hemoglobin and Hematocrit
HCP	Health-Care Provider
HIPAA	Health Insurance Portability and Accountability Act
INR	International Normalized Ratio
K+	Potassium
LPN	Licensed Practical Nurse
MAR	Medication Administration Record
NCSBN	National Council of State Boards of Nursing
NICU	Neonatal Intensive Care Unit
NSAID	Nonsteroidal Anti-inflammatory Drug
ORIF	Open Reduction and Internal Fixation
PO	Orally
PRN	As Needed
PT	Physical Therapist
RN	Registered Nurse
RF	Rheumatoid Factor
SCI	Spinal Cord Injury
THR	Total Hip Replacement
TKR	Total Knee Replacement
TPN	Total Parenteral Nutrition
UAP	Unlicensed Assistive Personnel
WBC	White Blood Cell

PRACTICE QUESTIONS

Setting Priorities When Caring for Clients

1. The rehabilitation nurse received the A.M. shift report on the following clients. Which client should the nurse assess first?
   1. The client with a C-6 SCI who has an elevated blood pressure and has a headache.
   2. The client diagnosed with a CVA who is crying and upset about being discharged home.
   3. The client who is 1 week postoperative for right THR who has a temperature of 100.4°F.
   4. The client who has full-thickness burns who needs to be medicated before being taken to whirlpool.

2. The nurse is working in an orthopedic rehabilitation department. Which client should the nurse assess first?
   1. The client who is 2 weeks postoperative ORIF of the right hip who is complaining of pain when ambulating.
   2. The client who is 10 days postoperative for left TKR who is refusing to use the continuous passive motion machine.
   3. The client who is 1 week postoperative for L3-4 laminectomy who is complaining of numbness and tingling of the feet.
   4. The client who is being admitted to the rehabilitation unit from the orthopedic surgical unit after a motor vehicle accident.

3. The client is 1 week postoperative for right below-the-knee amputation secondary to arterial occlusive disease. The rehabilitation nurse is unable to assess a pedal pulse in the left foot. Which intervention should the nurse implement first?
   1. Assess for paresthesia and paralysis.
   2. Utilize the Doppler device to auscultate the pulse.
   3. Place the client's leg in the dependent position.
   4. Wrap the client's left leg in a warm blanket.

4. The male client recovering from an acute deep vein thrombosis (DVT) is transferred to the rehabilitation unit. The client is complaining of bleeding when brushing his teeth. The nurse reviews the client's medication administration record (MAR). Which intervention should the nurse implement first?

Client's Name:	Account Number: 123456		Allergies: NKDA
Height: 72 inches	Weight: 240 pounds		
Date	**Medication**	**2301–0700**	**0701–1500**	**1501–2300**
	Levothyroxine (Synthroid) 1 tablet PO qd		0900 DN	
	Atenolol (Tenormin) 50 mg PO qd		0900 DN AP 72	
	Warfarin (Coumadin) 5 mg PO 1700			1700 DN
	Hydrocodone 5 mg/ 500 mg PO q 4–6 hours prn for pain			
Signature/Initials	Day Nurse RN DN			

   1. Prepare to administer AquaMephyton (vitamin K).
   2. Determine whether the client is using a soft bristle toothbrush.
   3. Check the client's apical pulse and blood pressure.
   4. Request the laboratory to draw a stat INR.

5. The nurse is preparing to administer medications to clients on the rehabilitation unit. Which medication should the nurse administer first?
   1. The NSAID to the client diagnosed with osteoarthritis.
   2. The antacid to the client complaining of heartburn.
   3. The stool softener to the client who is constipated.
   4. The antiplatelet to the client diagnosed with atherosclerosis.

6. The nurse is preparing to teach the male client how to irrigate his sigmoid colostomy. Which intervention should the nurse implement first?
   1. Demonstrate the procedure on a model.
   2. Provide the client with written instructions.
   3. Ask the client whether he has any questions.
   4. Show the client all of the equipment needed.

7. The rehabilitation nurse enters the room, and the client is beginning to have a tonic-clonic seizure. Which action should the nurse implement first?
   1. Identify the first area that began seizing.
   2. Note the time the client's seizure began.
   3. Pad the siding of the client's bed rails.
   4. Provide the client with privacy during the seizure.

8. The nurse on the rehabilitation unit is preparing to change a dressing on an 82-year-old client with a stage III pressure ulcer. Which intervention should the nurse implement first?
   1. Obtain the needed equipment to perform the procedure.
   2. Remove the client's old dressing with nonsterile gloves.
   3. Explain the procedure to the client in understandable terms.
   4. Check to determine whether the client has received pain medication.

9. Which client should the charge nurse on the rehabilitation unit assess first after receiving the A.M. shift report?
   1. The client diagnosed with an ORIF of the right hip who has a hemoglobin and hematocrit (H&H) of 8/24.
   2. The client diagnosed with rheumatoid arthritis who has a positive rheumatoid factor (RF).
   3. The client diagnosed with a stage IV pressure ulcer who has a white blood cell (WBC) count of 14,000.
   4. The client diagnosed with congestive heart failure who has a digoxin level of 1.8.

10. The client ambulating down the rehabilitation hallway unassisted fell to the floor. Which action should the nurse implement first?
    1. Complete an adverse occurrence report.
    2. Notify the clinical manager on the unit.
    3. Determine whether the client has any injuries.
    4. Ask why the client was in the hall alone.

Delegating and Assigning Nursing Tasks

11. The nurse and the unlicensed assistive personnel (UAP) are caring for clients on a rehabilitation unit. Which nursing task would be most appropriate for the nurse to delegate to the UAP?
    1. Flush the triple-lumen lines on a central venous catheter.
    2. Demonstrate for the client how to ambulate with a walker.
    3. Assist with bowel training by escorting the client to the bathroom.
    4. Feed the client diagnosed with a CVA who is dysphagic.

12. The UAP tells the rehabilitation nurse that the client with a right above-the-knee amputation has a large amount of bright red blood on the right leg residual limb. Which action should the nurse take?
    1. Assess the client's residual limb dressing.
    2. Tell the UAP to take the client's pulse and blood pressure.
    3. Remove the dressing to assess the incision.
    4. Request the UAP to reinforce the dressing.

13. Which action by the UAP would warrant immediate intervention by the rehabilitation nurse?
    1. The UAP tied the confused client to a chair with a sheet.
    2. The UAP escorted the client downstairs to smoke a cigarette.
    3. The UAP bought the client a carbonated beverage from the cafeteria.
    4. The UAP assisted the client to ambulate to the dayroom area.

14. The charge nurse, a licensed practical nurse (LPN), and two UAPs are caring for clients on a rehabilitation unit. The male client with type 2 diabetes mellitus is requesting someone cut his toenails. Which action would be most appropriate for the charge nurse to implement?
    1. Instruct the UAP to cut the toenails carefully straight across.
    2. Ask the LPN to cut the client's toenails before the end of the shift.
    3. Explain to the client that a podiatrist must cut the client's toenails.
    4. Cut the client's toenails after soaking in warm water for 20 minutes.

15. The nurse in the rehabilitation unit is caring for clients along with a UAP. Which action by the UAP warrants immediate intervention?
    1. The UAP assists a client 1 week postoperatively to eat a regular diet.
    2. The UAP calls for assistance when taking a client to the shower.
    3. The UAP is assisting the client who weighs 181 kg to the bedside commode.
    4. The UAP places the call light within reach of the client who is sitting in the chair.

16. The UAP on the rehabilitation unit is placing the client with a left above-the-knee amputation in the prone position. Which action should the nurse implement?
    1. Tell the UAP to place the client on the back.
    2. Praise the UAP for positioning the client prone.
    3. Report this action verbally to the charge nurse.
    4. Explain to the UAP that the client should not be placed on the stomach.

17. The UAP is applying elastic compression stockings to the client in the rehabilitation unit. Which action by the UAP indicates to the nurse the UAP understands the correct procedure for applying the elastic compression stockings?
    1. The UAP applied the stockings while the client is sitting in a chair.
    2. The UAP is unable to insert two fingers under the proximal end of the stocking.
    3. The UAP had the client elevate the legs prior to putting on the stockings.
    4. The UAP placed the toe opening of the elastic stocking on top of the client's foot.

18. The charge nurse on the acute care rehabilitation unit is making assignments for the shift. Which client should the charge nurse assign to the RN?
    1. The client diagnosed with a head injury who is refusing to go to therapy.
    2. The client diagnosed with an L-3 SCI who is being discharged home today.
    3. The client diagnosed with AIDS dementia who is confused and disoriented.
    4. The client diagnosed with a CAV who has new deficits in the visual fields.

19. The charge nurse on the busy 36-bed rehabilitation unit must send one staff member to the emergency department (ED). Which staff member would be the most appropriate person to send?
    1. The LPN who has worked on the rehabilitation unit for 3 years.
    2. The RN who has been employed on the rehabilitation unit for 8 years.
    3. The UAP who is completing the 4-week orientation to the rehabilitation
    4. The RN who transferred to the rehabilitation unit from the medical unit.

20. Which task should the rehabilitation nurse delegate to the UAP?
    1. Tell the UAP to show the client how to perform self-catheterization.
    2. Ask the UAP to place the newly confused client in the inclusion bed.
    3. Request the UAP to give the client 30 mL of Maalox, an antacid.
    4. Encourage the UAP to attend the multidisciplinary team meeting.

Managing Clients and Nursing Staff

21. The client with a C-5 SCI is complaining of a pounding headache, "9" on a pain scale of 1 to 10. Which intervention should the rehabilitation nurse implement first?
    1. Notify the health-care provider.
    2. Elevate the client's head of the bed.
    3. Assess for bladder distention.
    4. Take the client's blood pressure.

22. The elderly wife of a client with a total hip replacement who is being discharged home tells the nurse, "I am really worried about taking my husband home. I don't know how I will be able to take care of him." Which response would be most appropriate for the rehabilitation nurse?
    1. "We can arrange for a home health nurse to come visit your husband."
    2. "Have you thought about placing your husband in a nursing home?"
    3. "I will ask your husband's doctor to come and talk to you about your concerns."
    4. "I can see that you are worried but I am sure everything will be all right."

23. The male nurse who has been told by the female nurse on previous occasions not to talk to her about her body says, "You really look hot in that scrub suit. You have a great looking body." Which action should the female nurse take next?
    1. Document the comment in writing and file a formal grievance.
    2. Tell the male nurse this makes her feel very uncomfortable.
    3. Notify the clinical manager of the sexual harassment.
    4. Discuss the male nurse's behavior with the hospital lawyer.

24. The client who was admitted to the rehabilitation unit because of a debilitative state asks the nurse, "Why do I have to go to physical therapy every day?" Which statement is the nurse's best response?
    1. "The physical therapy will help you become more independent in caring for yourself."
    2. "You must have at least 3 hours of therapy a day to be able to stay in this rehab unit."
    3. "The multidisciplinary team determined that you should be in physical therapy daily."
    4. "The physical therapist will help you with exercises to improve your muscle strength."

25. The client diagnosed with a CVA is having trouble swallowing and has had two choking episodes. Which member of the multidisciplinary team should address this problem?
    1. The speech therapist.
    2. The registered dietitian.
    3. The occupational therapist.
    4. The rehabilitation physician.

26. The client with an L-4 SCI tells the nurse, "I was told I can't go back to my job because they do not have handicap accessible bathrooms or ramps." Which action by the rehabilitation nurse would be most helpful to the client?
    1. Discuss the situation with the multidisciplinary health-care team.
    2. Explain the Americans with Disability Act (ADA) to the client.
    3. Contact the client's employer via telephone and discuss the situation.
    4. Encourage the client to hire an attorney and sue the employer.

27. Which action by the female primary nurse would warrant immediate intervention by the charge nurse on the rehabilitation unit?
    1. The primary nurse tells the UAP to escort a client to the swimming pool.
    2. The primary nurse evaluates the client's plan of care with the family member.
    3. The primary nurse asks another nurse to administer an injection she prepared.
    4. The primary nurse requests another nurse to watch her clients for 30 minutes.

28. The client with a C-6 SCI tells the rehabilitation nurse, "I don't want to live like a vegetable. I can't feed myself or clean myself." Which statement is the nurse's best response?
    1. "I know this must be hard for you but you can have a life."
    2. "I can see you must feel helpless, I am here to listen."
    3. "Have you thought about killing yourself?"
    4. "You are in shock but in time things will get better."

29. The nurse on the rehabilitation unit is being sent to the neonatal intensive care unit (NICU) to work because the unit is short-staffed. The nurse has never worked in the NICU. Which response by the nurse supports the ethical principle of nonmalfeasance?
    1. The nurse requests not to be floated to the NICU.
    2. The nurse accepts the assignment to the NICU.
    3. The nurse asks why another nurse can't go to the NICU.
    4. The nurse talks another nurse into going to the NICU.

30. The client's husband is frustrated and tells the nurse, "Everyone is telling me something different as to when my wife is going to be able to go home. I don't know who to believe." Which statement is the rehabilitation nurse's best response?
    1. "I can see you are frustrated. Would you like to talk about how you feel?"
    2. "I will contact the case manager and have her talk to you as soon as possible."
    3. "Do not worry. Your wife won't go home until you and she are both ready."
    4. "Your wife's health-care provider should be able to give you that information."

Setting Priorities When Caring for Clients

1. 1. This client is exhibiting signs of autonomic dysreflexia, which requires immediate intervention. A distended bladder may be causing the signs/symptoms.
   2. This is a psychosocial need and should be addressed, but it is not priority over a physiologic need.
   3. This temperature is elevated and the client should be seen, but this is not priority over a client who is experiencing autonomic dysreflexia, which is a medical emergency.
   4. The client should be medicated prior to being taken to whirlpool, but this is not priority over a client experiencing autonomic dysreflexia, which is a medical emergency.

   MAKING NURSING DECISIONS: When deciding which client to assess first, the test taker should determine whether the signs/symptoms the client is exhibiting are normal or expected for the client situation. After eliminating the expected options, the test taker should determine which situation is more life threatening.

2. 1. The client having pain when ambulating after an ORIF of the hip is expected; this client would not need to be assessed first.
   2. The client should be ambulating and moving the left leg while in bed and would not need to be in the continuous passive motion (CPM) machine 10 days postoperatively.
   3. Numbness and tingling of the legs are signs of possible neurovascular compromise. This client should be assessed first.
   4. The client being transferred should be assessed but would be considered stable; therefore, this client would not be assessed before a client experiencing possible neurovascular compromise.

3. 1. An absent pulse is not uncommon in a client diagnosed with arterial occlusive disease. If the client can move the toes and denies tingling or numbness, then no further action should be taken.
   2. To identify the location of the pulse, the nurse should use a Doppler device to amplify the sound, but this is not the first

   intervention if the client is able to move the toes and denies numbness and tingling.
   3. Placing the client's leg in a dependent position will increase blood flow and may help the nurse palpate the pulse, but it is not the nurse's first intervention.
   4. Warming will dilate the arteries and may help the nurse to find the pedal pulse, but this is not the first intervention. (Cooling, in contrast, causes vasoconstriction and decreases the ability to palpate the pulse.)

4. 1. If the client's international normalized ratio (INR) is elevated, the antidote for the oral anticoagulant warfarin (Coumadin) is vitamin K, but this is not the nurse's first intervention.
   2. The client should be using a soft bristle toothbrush, but this is not the nurse's first intervention.
   3. The nurse can always check the client's vital signs, but it is not the first intervention when addressing the client's complaint of gums bleeding.
   4. The nurse should first check the client's INR to determine whether the bleeding is secondary to an elevated INR level—above 3.

5. 1. The NSAID is a routine medication and is not a priority medication.
   2. The client complaining of heartburn should receive the antacid first because the client is in pain. A client in pain should be the nurse's first priority.
   3. The client who is constipated needs the stool softener, but this is not priority over the client who is in pain.
   4. The antiplatelet is not priority over a client who is in pain.

6. 1. The nurse should demonstrate the procedure on a model, but the first intervention should be to assess, to determine whether the client has any questions.
   2. The nurse should provide the client with written instructions, but the first intervention should be to assess, to determine whether the client has any questions.
   3. The client cannot learn if he has any questions or concerns. Therefore, the first intervention is to ask the client whether he has any questions. The

nurse must allay any concerns or fears of the client before beginning to teach the client.

4. The nurse should show the client all the equipment, but the first intervention should be to assess, to determine whether the client has any questions.

7. 1. Identifying the first area that began seizing will provide information and clues as to the location of the seizure origin in the brain, but it is not the nurse's first intervention.
   2. **The nurse should first look at his or her watch and time the seizure. Assessment is the first intervention because there is no action the nurse can implement to stop or intervene with the seizure.**
   3. The client's bed rails should be padded, but this is not the first intervention when walking into a room where the client is beginning to have a seizure. The nurse should first assess the seizure and then pad the side rails if there is time. The seizure may be over by the time the nurse can pad the side rails.
   4. The client should be protected from onlookers, but the nurse should always assess and care for the client first.

8. 1. The nurse should obtain the needed equipment, but that is not the first intervention.
   2. The nurse should remove the old dressing with nonsterile gloves, but not before determining whether the client has been premedicated.
   3. The nurse should explain the procedure prior to performing the dressing change, but that is not the first intervention.
   4. **Dressing changes for a stage III pressure ulcer will be painful for the client, and the nurse should make sure the client has received pain medication at least 30 minutes prior to the procedure. This is showing client advocacy.**

9. 1. **The H&H are low, which requires the nurse to assess this client first. The nurse must take the client's vital signs, check the surgical dressing, and determine whether the client is symptomatic for hypovolemia.**
   2. The client with rheumatoid arthritis should have a positive rheumatoid factor (RF). The positive RF factor confirms the diagnosis of this disease process.
   3. A client with a stage IV pressure ulcer would frequently have an infection; therefore, the nurse would expect an elevated white blood cell (WBC) count.

4. The therapeutic level for digoxin is 0.8 to 2; therefore, this client would not need to be assessed first.

MAKING NURSING DECISIONS: The test taker must know normal laboratory data. See Appendix A for normal laboratory data.

10. 1. The nurse should complete a report documenting the client's fall, but this is not the first intervention.
    2. The nurse should notify the clinical manager, but this is not the nurse's first intervention.
    3. **The nurse must first determine whether the client has any injuries before taking any other action. This is the first intervention the nurse must implement prior to moving the client.**
    4. The nurse should determine why the client was ambulating alone, but it is not the priority nursing intervention. Determining whether the client has any injuries is the most important intervention.

Delegating and Assigning Nursing Tasks

11. 1. The triple-lumen lines should be flushed with 100 units/mL heparin solution, and this task should not be delegated to a UAP.
    2. This is teaching, and the nurse should not delegate teaching to the client.
    3. **The UAP can assist the client to the bathroom as part of the bowel training; the nurse is responsible for the training, but the nurse can delegate this task.**
    4. This client is unstable and at risk for choking; therefore, the nurse should not delegate this task.

MAKING NURSING DECISIONS: The nurse cannot delegate assessment, evaluation, teaching, administering medications, or an unstable client to a UAP.

12. 1. **Because the UAP is informing the nurse of pertinent information, the nurse should assess the client to determine which action to take.**
    2. The client may be hemorrhaging; therefore, the nurse cannot delegate assessing vital signs on an unstable client.
    3. The nurse should not remove the dressing. The nurse should reinforce the dressing and notify the HCP if bleeding does not stop or if the client is showing signs of hypovolemia. Reinforcing the dressing

would help decrease bleeding, but the nurse must assess first.

4. The client is potentially unstable; therefore, the nurse should not delegate any care to the UAP.

MAKING NURSING DECISIONS: Anytime the nurse receives information from another staff member about a client who may be experiencing a complication, the nurse must assess the client. The nurse should not make decisions about client's needs based on another staff member's information.

13. 1. Tying a client to a chair is a form of restraint, and the client cannot be restrained without an HCP order; therefore, the nurse should immediately free the client. This is a legal issue.
2. The UAP is not hired to smoke with the client and the nurse should talk to the UAP, but this does not warrant an immediate response. The client's being illegally restrained warrants immediate intervention.
3. The UAP's bringing a beverage to the client would not warrant immediate intervention.
4. The UAP can assist the client to ambulate.

14. 1. The client is diabetic, and the charge nurse should not delegate cutting the client's toenails to the UAP.
2. The LPN should not cut the client's toenails because the client is diabetic.
3. A podiatrist can cut the client's toenails, the nurse should make this referral.
4. The client is diabetic. This puts the client at risk for delayed healing if a cut on the foot occurs; therefore, this client is unstable and the nurse should not cut the toenails.

MAKING NURSING DECISIONS: When the test taker is deciding which option is the most appropriate task to delegate/assign, the test taker should choose the task that allows each member of the staff to function within his or her full scope of practice. Do not assign a task to a staff member that requires a higher level of expertise than the staff member has; similarly, do not assign a task to a staff member when it could be delegated/assigned to a staff member with a lower level of expertise.

15. 1. The UAP can assist a client to eat a regular meal; this would not warrant immediate action.
2. The UAP's request for assistance is appropriate because it is ensuring client safety. This action would not warrant immediate behavior.
3. The UAP is attempting to move a client who weighs 400 pounds to the bedside commode. The UAP should request assistance to ensure client safety as well as to protect the UAP's back. This is a dangerous situation and requires intervention by the nurse.
4. This action ensures client safety and does not require immediate intervention by the nurse.

16. 1. The client with a lower extremity amputation should be placed in the prone position to prevent contractures.
2. The nurse should praise the UAP for taking the initiative and placing the client in the prone position. The prone position will help prevent contractures of the residual limb, which helps when applying a prosthetic device.
3. This action is appropriate and should not be reported to the charge nurse. The nurse should first praise the UAP and then report this behavior to the charge nurse if wanting to reward the UAP for appropriate behavior.
4. The client with a lower extremity amputation presents one of the few times a client should be placed on the stomach, the prone position.

17. 1. Stockings should be applied after the legs have been elevated for a period of time when the amount of blood in the leg vein is at its lowest. Applying the stockings when the client is sitting in a chair indicates that the UAP does not understand the correct procedure for applying the elastic compression stockings.
2. The top of stocking should not be too tight. The UAP should be able to insert two to three fingers under the proximal end of the stocking. Not allowing this much space indicates the UAP does not understand the correct procedure for applying compression stockings.
3. Stockings should be applied after the legs have been elevated for a period of time when the amount of blood in the leg vein is at its lowest. Having the client elevate the legs before placing

the stockings on the legs indicates that the UAP understands the procedure for applying the elastic compression stockings.

4. The toe opening should be positioned on the bottom of the foot; therefore, this indicates the client does not understand the correct procedure for applying the elastic compression stockings.

18. 1. Someone must talk to this client, but the RN does not need to be assigned this client.

2. The multidisciplinary team has been preparing the client for discharge since admission to the rehabilitation unit; therefore, the charge nurse does not need to assign the RN this client.

3. The client with AIDS dementia would be confused and disoriented as a result of this diagnosis; therefore, the charge nurse would not need to assign the RN this client.

4. **New deficits in the visual fields in a client diagnosed with a CVA could indicate an expanding or a new problem. The RN should be assigned to this client.**

MAKE NURSING DECISIONS: When the nurse is deciding which client should be assigned to the RN, the most critical client or the client requiring more expert care should be assigned to the RN.

19. 1. The LPN should not be sent to the emergency department because the LPN's expertise is needed to care for the clients on the busy rehabilitation unit.

2. The RN has 8 years experience on the rehabilitation unit, and the charge nurse does not want to send a nurse who is a vital part of the rehabilitation team.

3. The UAP who is completing orientation should stay on the unit, and a UAP would not be able to do as much in the emergency department as a licensed nurse.

4. **The RN with medical unit experience would be the most appropriate nurse to send to the emergency department because this nurse has experience that would be helpful in the ED. The nurse is also an RN, who would be more helpful in the ED than a UAP or an LPN.**

20. 1. The UAP cannot teach the client; therefore, this task cannot be delegated.

2. The client is confused and should be assessed prior to being placed in an inclusion bed, which is used when a client wanders. The client should be assessed, and assessment cannot be delegated.

3. The UAP cannot administer medications; therefore, this task cannot be delegated.

4. **The UAP is a vital part of the health-care team and should be encouraged to attend the multidisciplinary team meeting and provide input into the client's care.**

Managing Clients and Nursing Staff

21. 1. This action will not address the client's pounding headache. The nurse should either assess the client or intervene prior to calling the HCP.

2. Elevating the head of the bed may help decrease the client's blood pressure by causing orthostatic hypotension, but the nurse must first determine whether the client's BP is elevated.

3. If the client's BP is elevated, this is probably autonomic dysreflexia, an acute emergency that occurs as a result of exaggerated autonomic responses to stimuli that are harmless in normal people and only occur after spinal shock has resolved in clients with an SCI above T-6. The most common cause of autonomic dysreflexia is a full bladder.

4. **The nurse must determine whether the client's blood pressure is elevated. If it is, then the client is probably experiencing autonomic dysreflexia, and the nurse should assess for bladder distention, the most common cause of autonomic dysreflexia.**

MAKING NURSING DECISIONS: If the test taker wants to select "notify the HCP" as the correct answer, the test taker must examine the other three options. If information in any of the other options is data the HCP would need to know in order to make a decision, then the test taker should eliminate the "notify the HCP" option.

22. 1. According to the National Council of State Boards of Nursing (NCSBN), management of care includes being knowledgeable about referrals. This client would benefit from a home health-care nurse to evaluate the

client's home and the wife's ability to care for the client.

2. The nurse should help the client care for her husband in the home. Placing him in a nursing home may be a possibility if she is unable to care for him, but the most appropriate response would be trying to help the wife care for her husband in the home.

3. The HCP can talk to the wife but will not be able to address her concerns of taking care of her husband when he is discharged home.

4. This is false reassurance and does not address the wife's concern about being able to care for her husband.

23. 1. This is a formal step in filing a grievance, but the nurse's next action should be to follow the chain of command and place an informal complaint with the clinical manager.

2. The female nurse has already told the male nurse this makes her feel uncomfortable; therefore, this action is not appropriate.

3. **If a direct request to the perpetrator does not stop the comments, then an informal complaint may be effective, especially if both parties realize a problem exists. The female nurse should utilize the chain of command and notify the clinical manager.**

4. The female nurse should follow the chain of command and notify the clinical manager as the next action.

MAKING NURSING DECISIONS: The nurse is responsible for knowing and complying with local, state, and federal standards of care.

24. 1. Assisting the client to become independent in self-care is the role of the occupational therapist.

2. The client must be able to be in therapy at least 3 hours a day, but the 3-hour period includes all types of therapy, not just physical therapy. This is a true statement, but it does not answer the client's question.

3. A multidisciplinary team decides which therapy the client should be receiving, but this does not answer the client's question.

4. **The physical therapist will assist in improving the circulation, strengthening muscles, and ambulating and transferring the client from a bed to a chair. This is the nurse's best response in explaining why the client goes to physical therapy daily.**

25. 1. **The speech therapist addresses swallowing problems as well as speech impediments. This is the most appropriate team member to address the problem.**

2. The registered dietitian addresses the client's nutritional status but does not help with swallowing difficulties.

3. The occupational therapist addresses the upper extremity activities of daily living, not choking difficulties.

4. The HCP can prescribe tests to determine why the client is having choking problems, but the speech therapist is the team member who can help the client with choking problems.

26. 1. The nurse can discuss this situation with the health-care team, but the most helpful intervention is to explain the rights of the disabled according to the ADA.

2. **The ADA was passed in 1990 and ensures that a client with a disability has a right to be employed. Employers must make "reasonable accommodations," such as equipment or access ramps to facilitate employment of a person with a disability.**

3. The nurse should not interfere and contact the client's employer. The nurse should empower clients to care independently for themselves.

4. This client might be able to do this, but the most helpful intervention is to contact the ADA. The employer is violating the 1990 Americans with Disability Act.

MAKING NURSING DECISIONS: The nurse is responsible for knowing and complying with local, state, and federal standards of care.

27. 1. The UAP can escort clients to the different rehabilitation therapies. This action would not warrant immediate intervention.

2. The family members/significant others are an integral part of the health-care team. This action would not warrant intervention by the charge nurse.

3. **The primary nurse cannot ask another nurse to administer medication that he or she prepared. The nurse preparing the injection must administer the medication. This action requires the charge nurse to intervene.**

4. Making sure someone watches the nurse's assigned clients is an appropriate action and would not require intervention by the charge nurse.

28. 1. This response does not address the client's fears and concerns.
    2. **This statement will allow the client to ventilate feelings of helplessness and fear. It is the nurse's best response.**
    3. The client is not verbalizing that he or she will kill himself or herself; therefore, this is not the nurse's best response.
    4. This is negating the client's feelings, and with a C-6 SCI things may not get much better; therefore, this is not the nurse's best response.

29. 1. **Nonmalfeasance is the duty to prevent or avoid doing harm. The nurse asking not to be assigned to the NICU because of lack of experience in caring for critically ill infants is supporting the ethical principle of nonmalfeasance.**
    2. The NICU is a very specialized unit requiring the nurse to be knowledgeable with equipment and caring for critically ill infants. Accepting the assignment may cause harm to one of the neonates.
    3. This is challenging the charge nurse's assignment, and this does not support the ethical principle of nonmalfeasance.
    4. This is blatantly violating the charge nurse's authority and does not support the ethical principle of nonmalfeasance.

30. 1. This is a therapeutic response that encourages the husband to ventilate feelings, but the client's husband needs specific information, not ventilate feelings.
    2. **According to the NCSBN, case management is content included in the management of care. The case manager is responsible for collaborating with and coordinating the services provided by all members of the health-care team, including the home health-care nurse who will be responsible for directing the client's care after discharge from the rehabilitation unit. This is the nurse's best response.**
    3. This is not addressing the husband's concern, and sometimes the client is discharged when the family and client are not ready in the client's opinion. This is false reassurance and is not the nurse's best response.
    4. In rehabilitation, the HCP is part of the team and is not the only team member to determine the discharge date. This is not the nurse's best response.

COMPREHENSIVE EXAMINATION

1. The client with an L-4 SCI tells the rehabilitation nurse, "I have no idea what I am going to do after I get discharged. How will I support my family? I will need to get a new job." Which statement would be the nurse's best response?
   1. "You should contact the American Spinal Cord Injury Association."
   2. "The state rehabilitation commission will help retrain you."
   3. "You should ask the social worker about applying for disability."
   4. "You are worried about how you will be able to support your family."

2. The client tells the rehabilitation nurse, "I do not like my doctor and I want another doctor." Which statement is the nurse's best response?
   1. "You should tell your doctor you are not happy with his care."
   2. "Can you tell me what you don't like about your doctor's care?"
   3. "I will notify my nursing supervisor and report your concern."
   4. "I am sorry you really must keep this doctor until you are discharged."

3. The rehabilitation nurse and the UAP are caring for a 74-year-old client who is 1 week postoperative bilateral femoral-popliteal bypass surgery. Which nursing task should be delegated to the UAP?
   1. Place the abductor pillow between the client's legs.
   2. Ensure the client stays on complete bed rest.
   3. Feed the client the evening meal.
   4. Elevate the client's foot of the bed.

4. The rehabilitation nurse tells the UAP to assist the client recovering from Guillain-Barré syndrome with A.M. care. Which action by the UAP warrants immediate intervention?
   1. The UAP closes the door and cubicle curtain.
   2. The UAP massages the client's back with lotion.
   3. The UAP checks the temperature of the bathing water.
   4. The UAP puts the side rails up when bathing the client.

5. The client diagnosed with a right-sided CVA, or brain attack, is admitted to the rehabilitation unit. Which interventions should be included in the nursing care plan? Select all that apply.
   1. Position the client to prevent shoulder adduction.
   2. Refer the client to occupational therapy daily.
   3. Encourage the client to move the affected side.
   4. Perform quadriceps exercises five times a day.
   5. Instruct the client to hold the fingers in a fist.

6. The overhead page has issued a Code Black indicating a tornado in the area. Which intervention should the charge nurse of the rehabilitation unit implement?
   1. Instruct the hospital staff to assist the clients and visitors to the cafeteria.
   2. Request the client and visitors to go into the bathroom in the client's room.
   3. Have the clients and visitors remain in the hallway with the doors closed.
   4. Tell the client and any visitors to remain in the client's room with the door open.

7. The 43-year-old client is diagnosed with an L-1 SCI. The client's wife tells the nurse, "My husband said we are supposed to talk to his case manager. What is a case manager?" Which statement is the nurse's best response?
   1. "A case manager discusses the cost and insurance issues concerning the rehabilitation."
   2. "The case manager is responsible for the medical treatment regimen for your husband."
   3. "The case manager is a member of the team who will assist your husband in finding another job."
   4. "The case manager is a nurse who will coordinate the rehabilitation team and keep you informed."

8. The 28-year-old male client who sustained an L-2 SCI is being discharged home to live with his wife and 3-year-old son. Which priority psychosocial intervention should the rehabilitation nurse discuss with the client?
   1. Ask the client whether he has any sexual concerns he needs to discuss.
   2. Determine whether the client's home is equipped for his wheelchair.
   3. Discuss the procedure for obtaining a specially equipped car.
   4. Explain the importance of getting psychological counseling.

9. The primary nurse overhears the UAP telling a family member of a client, "One of the clients at the rehabilitation unit will be going to prison because that person was charged with vehicular manslaughter because two people in a motor vehicle accident died." Which action should the primary nurse implement first?
   1. Apologize to the family member for the UAP's comments.
   2. Tell the UAP that the comment is a violation of HIPAA.
   3. Allow the UAP to complete the conversation then discuss the situation.
   4. Interrupt the conversation and tell the UAP to go to the nurse's station.

10. The clinical manager has verbally warned a female staff nurse about being late to work on two previous occasions. The nurse was 35 minutes late for today's shift. Which action should the charge nurse take?
    1. Ask the staff nurse why she was late again today.
    2. Notify the human resource department in writing.
    3. Initiate the hospital policy for unacceptable behavior.
    4. Do not allow the staff nurse to work on the unit today.

11. The charge nurse on the rehabilitation unit is making assignments for the day shift. Which assignment would be most appropriate for the LPN?
    1. Have the LPN administer the routine medications.
    2. Instruct the LPN to complete the admission assessment.
    3. Ask the LPN to teach the client about a high-fiber diet.
    4. Request the LPN to obtain the intake and output for the clients.

12. The charge nurse received laboratory data on clients in the rehabilitation unit. Which client warrants immediate intervention by the charge nurse?
    1. The client with COPD who has ABGs of pH, 7.35; PaO_2, 77; $PaCO_2$, 57; HCO_3, 24.
    2. The client diagnosed with bilateral TKR who has a WBC count of 10,400.
    3. The client on antibiotic therapy who has a serum potassium level of 3.3 mEq/L.
    4. The client receiving TPN who has a glucose level of 145 mg/dL.

13. The client in the rehabilitation unit tells the primary nurse, "I just finished completing my Living Will and I need you to witness my signature." Which action should the nurse take?
    1. Witness the client's Living Will using an ink pen.
    2. Explain that the nurse cannot witness this document.
    3. Tell the client the document does not need a witness's signature.
    4. Offer to have the hospital attorney to come notarize the form.

14. The rehabilitation nurse is preparing to ambulate the client in the hall. Which priority intervention should the nurse implement?
    1. Place rubber-soled shoes on the client.
    2. Put a gait belt around the client's waist.
    3. Explain the procedure to the client.
    4. Provide a clear path for client to walk.

15. The client in the rehabilitation unit tells the nurse, "I will not go to physical therapy again because it hurts so much when I do the exercises." Which statement supports the nurse is a client advocate?
    1. "You do not have to go to physical therapy if it causes you pain."
    2. "I will talk to the physical therapist (PT) about the exercises that cause you pain."
    3. "Let me check and see if you can receive pain medication before therapy."
    4. "I will discuss your concerns at the next multidisciplinary team meeting."

16. The rehabilitation nurse enters the client's room and the client is talking on the phone. The client asks the nurse to talk to his wife because she has some questions. Which action should the nurse take?
    1. Explain that HIPAA regulations prevent the nurse from talking to the wife.
    2. Tell the client it would be best for the nurse to talk to the wife in person.
    3. Request the client's wife to come to the weekly team meeting to ask questions.
    4. Honor the client's request and answer any questions the wife has on the phone.

17. The hospital will be implementing a new MAR for documenting medication administration. Which action should the clinical manager take first when implementing the new MAR?
    1. Discuss the new MAR with each nurse individually.
    2. Schedule meetings on all shifts to discuss the new MAR.
    3. Require the nurse to read a handout explaining the new MAR.
    4. Ask the nurses to watch a video explaining the new MAR.

18. Which action by the primary nurse requires immediate intervention by the charge nurse of the rehabilitation unit?
    1. The nurse is teaching the client how to use a glucometer.
    2. The nurse leaves the nurse's notes at the client's bedside.
    3. The nurse is discussing a client situation on the phone with the HCP.
    4. The nurse contacts the chaplain to come and talk to a client.

19. The nurse notices that the female UAP has multiple charge stickers stuck to her uniform top. Which action would be most appropriate for the rehabilitation nurse?
    1. Explain that if the charge stickers are lost, then the unit loses money.
    2. Notify central supply that the UAP is not following hospital procedure.
    3. Instruct the UAP to place the stickers on the appropriate client's charge card.
    4. Document the UAP's action in writing and file it in her employee file.

20. The UAP comes running up the hall and tells the rehabilitation nurse, "Mr. Smith is masturbating in his bed." Mr. Smith is a 28-year-old client who has been in the rehabilitation unit for 3 weeks. Which action should the nurse take first?
    1. Inform the client in private that this is inappropriate behavior.
    2. Tell the UAP to close the door and leave the client alone.
    3. Document the client's behavior in the nurse's notes.
    4. Notify the client's health-care provider about the behavior.

1. 1. The American Spinal Cord Injury Association is an appropriate referral for living with this condition, but it does not help find gainful employment after the injury.
   2. **The rehabilitation commission of each state will help evaluate and determine whether the client can receive training or education for another occupation after injury.**
   3. The client is not asking about disability. The client is concerned about employment. The nurse needs to refer the client to the appropriate agency.
   4. This does not address the client's concern about gainful employment. This is a therapeutic response that will allow the client to ventilate feelings, but the client is asking for information.

2. 1. The client is confiding in the nurse about a doctor, and the nurse should address the client's concern, not tell the client to talk to the doctor. Many clients do not feel comfortable talking to a doctor.
   2. **The nurse should determine what is concerning the client. It could be a misunderstanding or a real situation where the client's care is unsafe or inadequate.**
   3. After the nurse determines whether the client's concern warrants a new doctor, then the nurse should talk to the nursing supervisor and help the client get a second opinion. The nurse is the client's advocate.
   4. The choice of doctor is ultimately the client's, and the client has a right to another doctor.

3. 1. An abductor pillow is used for a client who has had a TKR, not a femoral-popliteal bypass.
   2. The client in the rehabilitation unit should be up and ambulating in the hall, not on complete bed rest.
   3. Just because the client is elderly does not mean the client must be fed. There is nothing in the stem of the question that would indicate the client could not feed himself or herself. The nurse should encourage independence as much as possible and delegate feeding the client to a UAP only when it is necessary.
   4. **After the surgery, the client's legs will be elevated to help decrease edema. The surgery has corrected the decreased blood supply to the lower legs.**

4. 1. Closing the door and cubicle curtain protects the client's privacy and would not warrant immediate intervention from the nurse.
   2. Providing a back massage is a wonderful action to take and would not warrant intervention by the nurse.
   3. Checking the temperature of the bath water prevents scalding the client with water that is too hot or making the client uncomfortable with water that is too cold. This action would not warrant immediate intervention.
   4. **The client is recovering from a potentially debilitating disease, and in the rehabilitation unit the client should be out of the bed as much as possible. Bathing the client in bed would warrant intervention by the nurse.**

5. 1, 2, 3, and 4 are correct.
   1. **Placing a small pillow under the shoulder will prevent the shoulder from adducting toward the chest and developing a contracture.**
   2. **The client should be referred to occupational therapy for assistance with performing activities of daily living (ADLs)**
   3. **The client should not ignore the paralyzed side, and the nurse must encourage the client to move it as much as possible; a written schedule may assist the client in exercising.**
   4. **These exercises should be done at least five times a day for 10 minutes to help strengthen the muscles used for walking.**
   5. The fingers should be positioned so that they are barely flexed, to prevent contracture.

6. 1. The procedure for tornados is to have all clients, staff, and visitors stay in the hallway and close the doors to all the rooms. This will help prevent any flying debris or glass from hurting anyone.
   2. This may be recommended for individuals in the home, but it is not the hospital protocol for tornados.
   3. **The procedure for tornados is to have all clients, staff, and visitors stay in the hallway and close the doors to all the rooms. This will help prevent any flying debris or glass from hurting anyone.**
   4. The client and visitors should be in the client's room with the door closed for a fire, but this is not the correct procedure for a tornado.

7. 1. The finance office is responsible for discussing the cost and insurance issues with the client.
   2. The physiatrist is a medical health-care provider who cares for clients in the rehabilitation area.
   3. The vocational counselor would assist the client with employment training if needed.
   4. **The case manager is responsible for coordinating the total rehabilitative plan, collaborating with and coordinating the services provided by all members of the health-care team including the home health-care nurse who will be responsible for directing the client's care after discharge from the rehabilitation unit.**

8. 1. **The rehabilitation nurse must recognize and address sexual issues in order to promote feelings of self-worth that are essential to total rehabilitation. The age of the client should not matter, but this client is young; therefore, this is priority.**
   2. This is not a psychosocial intervention, and the social worker or occupational therapist usually address the home situation.
   3. This is not necessarily a psychosocial intervention, but it should be addressed so the client can be independent. The social worker usually addresses transportation.
   4. The client may or may not need psychological counseling, but the priority psychosocial intervention of the rehabilitation nurse is to discuss the client's sexuality needs.

9. 1. The nurse could apologize for the UAP's comments, but this is not the first intervention.
   2. This is a violation of HIPPA and the nurse should tell this to the UAP, but it is not the first intervention.
   3. The nurse should not allow the conversation to continue. The UAP is violating confidentiality and is gossiping about another client.
   4. **The nurse should stop the conversation immediately, and asking the UAP to go to the nurse's station does not embarrass the UAP. This is a violation of HIPPA and is gossiping about another client on the unit.**

10. 1. After two verbal warnings, the clinical manager should document the behavior and start formal proceedings to correct the staff nurse's behavior.
   2. The human resource department would not need to be notified until the clinical manager has decided to terminate the staff nurse's employment.
   3. **Every hospital has a procedure for termination if the employee is not performing as expected. After two verbal warnings, the clinical manager should document the employee's actions in writing and implement the hospital policy for possible termination.**
   4. The clinical manager cannot allow the nurse to go home because this will affect the care of the clients during the shift. It would cause a hardship on the other staff members.

11. 1. **The LPN's scope of practice includes administering medications to clients; therefore, this assignment would be appropriate.**
   2. The LPN's scope of practice does not include assessment.
   3. The registered dietitian would be the most appropriate team member to teach diets.
   4. The UAP could obtain the intake and output; therefore this is not an appropriate assignment for an LPN.

12. 1. The client with COPD would be expected to have low oxygen and high CO_2 levels in the arterial blood; therefore, this laboratory data would not warrant intervention from the charge nurse.
   2. This WBC level is within normal limits; therefore, this client does not warrant immediate intervention from the charge nurse.
   3. **Antibiotic therapy can result in a superinfection that destroys the normal bacterial flora of the intestines and produces diarrhea. Diarrhea, in turn, causes an increased excretion of potassium, resulting in hypokalemia. This K^+ level is below normal, and the charge nurse should notify the health-care provider.**
   4. This glucose level is slightly elevated, and TPN is high in glucose; therefore, this laboratory result does not require immediate intervention.

13. 1. The nurse is an employee of the hospital and cannot witness documents for clients.
   2. **This is the correct action to take; the nurse is an employee of the hospital directly involved in providing care and cannot witness documents for clients.**

3. This is incorrect information; the document should be witnessed by individuals who are not family members or employees of the hospital providing direct care.
4. The Living Will must be witnessed by two individuals when the client is signing it, but it does not have to be notarized.

14. 1. The nurse should ensure the client has appropriate shoes when ambulating, but the priority is safety of the client, which means using a gait belt.
2. **The nurse's priority is to ensure the safety of the client, and placing a safety gait belt around the client's waist before ambulating the client helps to ensure safety. The gait belt provides a handle to hold onto the client securely during ambulation.**
3. The nurse should explain the procedure to the client, but it is not priority over ensuring safety for the client while walking in the hall.
4. The nurse should make sure there is a clear path to walk, but the priority intervention is to protect the client if he or she falls, and that can be prevented by placing a gait belt around the client's waist.

15. 1. Being a client advocate means the nurse will support the client's wishes, but in some situations the nurse must adhere to the medical regimen. Telling the client he or she does not have to attend therapy is detrimental to the client's recovery and is not being a client advocate.
2. Being a client advocate means the nurse will support the client's wishes, but in some situations the nurse must adhere to the medical regimen. Talking to the physical therapist will not help the client's recovery.
3. **Finding ways for the client to perform the exercises by the physical therapist is supporting the medical regimen. This action supports client advocacy. PTs cannot prescribe.**
4. Discussing the client concerns does not help the client's recovery; therefore, this statement does not support client advocacy.

16. 1. As long as the client gives permission, the nurse can discuss the client's condition with anyone.
2. The nurse can answer questions over the phone with the client's permission. It may

be difficult for the client's wife to come to the rehabilitation unit.
3. The client and wife are allowed and encouraged to come to the multidisciplinary team meeting, but the nurse should talk to the wife on the phone.
4. **The nurse can talk to anyone the client requests. This is not a violation of HIPAA as long as the client gives permission for the nurse to share information.**

17. 1. The clinical manager may need to discuss the MAR with some nurses individually, but it is not the clinical manager's first intervention.
2. **The first intervention should be to arrange meetings to explain the new MAR and allow nurses to ask questions to clarify the new policy.**
3. The clinical manager can provide a written handout explaining the new MAR, but the first intervention should be small discussion groups.
4. A video is an excellent tool for explaining new procedures, but the first intervention should be small discussion groups so that all questions can be answered.

18. 1. The nurse's scope of practice includes teaching the client how to use equipment.
2. **This is a violation of HIPAA. The client's right to confidentiality is being compromised because anyone could read the client's nurse's notes. The charge nurse should intervene.**
3. The nurse can discuss a client situation with the HCP; therefore, this action does not require intervention.
4. According to the NCSBN NCLEX-RN test plan, questions concerning referrals and consultation are included in the management of care area.

19. 1. The purpose of the charge stickers is to ensure the client is charged for all equipment used. If the stickers are not placed on the client's charge cards, then the client will not be charged, and the unit will lose money. The nurse should explain this to the UAP, but this is not the most appropriate intervention.
2. Central supply is responsible for charges, but the UAP is not in the chain of command of central supply personnel. The nurse should correct the UAP because the

nurse is responsible for supervising the UAP.

3. The most appropriate action for the nurse to take is to instruct the UAP to place the stickers on the appropriate client's charge card. The stickers should not be placed on the UAP's uniform top.

4. The nurse should first correct the UAP's behavior. The nurse should not document the behavior in writing unless there is a pattern of behavior.

20. 1. This behavior is very normal for a 28-year-old male client, and the UAP should allow the client privacy.

2. Closing the door and leaving the client alone should be the nurse's first actions. This allows the client privacy and is very normal behavior for a young man. The rehabilitation nurse must recognize and address sexual issues in order to promote feelings of self-worth, which are essential to total rehabilitation.

3. The nurse could document the client's behavior, but it is not the first intervention.

4. The HCP could be notified of the client's behavior, but it is not the nurse's first intervention.

Outpatient/Community Health Nursing

8

"Intuition will tell the thinking mind where to look next."

—Jonas Salk

ABBREVIATION LIST

ACE	Angiotensin-Converting Enzyme	**NCSBN**	National Council of State Boards of Nursing
AHA	American Heart Association		
BP	Blood Pressure	**NSAID**	Nonsteroidal Anti-Inflammatory Drug
D₅W	5% Dextrose in Water		
ECG	Electrocardiogram	**PPD**	Purified Protein Derivative
GERD	Gastroesophageal Reflux Disease	**PTT**	Partial Thromboplastin Time
HCP	Health-Care Provider	**PT**	Prothrombin Time
H&H	Hemoglobin and Hematocrit	**RN**	Registered Nurse
HIPAA	Health Insurance Portability and Accountability Act	**R/O**	Rule Out
		UAP	Unlicensed Assistive Personnel
INR	International Normalized Ratio	**UTI**	Urinary Tract Infection
IV	Intravenous	**WBC**	White Blood Cell
LPN	Licensed Practical Nurse		

PRACTICE QUESTIONS

Setting Priorities When Caring for Clients

1. The community health nurse is triaging victims at a bus accident. Which client would the nurse categorize as red, priority 1?
   1. The client with head trauma whose pupils are fixed and dilated.
   2. The client with compound fractures of the tibia and fibula.
   3. The client with a sprained right wrist with a 1-inch laceration.
   4. The client with a piece of metal embedded in the right eye.

2. The nurse is caring for clients in a family practice clinic. Which client should the nurse assess first?
   1. The client who is complaining of right lower abdominal pain.
   2. The client who is having burning and pain on urination.
   3. The client who has low back pain radiating down the right leg.
   4. The client who has a sore throat and had a fever last night.

3. The clinic nurse is reviewing the laboratory data of clients seen in the clinic the previous day. Which client requires immediate intervention by the nurse?
   1. The client whose white blood cell (WBC) count is 9.5 mm^3.
   2. The client whose cholesterol level is 230 mg/dL.
   3. The client whose calcium level is 10.4 mg/dL.
   4. The client whose international normalized ratio (INR) is 3.8.

4. Which child should the nurse in the pediatric clinic assess first?
   1. The 1-year-old male child who is crying and pulling at his ears.
   2. The 5-year-old female child who has a fever and red rash over her body.
   3. The 8-year-old male child who has neck stiffness and light hurts his eyes.
   4. The 15-year-old female adolescent whose mother thinks she may be pregnant.

5. The clinic nurse is caring for a client diagnosed with osteoarthritis. The client tells the nurse, "I am having problems getting in and out of my bathtub." Which intervention should the clinic nurse implement first?
   1. Determine whether the client has grab bars in the bathroom.
   2. Encourage the client to take a shower instead of a bath.
   3. Initiate a referral to a physical therapist for the client.
   4. Discuss whether the client takes nonsteroidal anti-inflammatory drugs (NSAIDs).

6. The employee health nurse has cared for six clients who have similar complaints. The clients have a fever, nausea, vomiting, and diarrhea. Which action should the nurse implement first after assessing the clients?
   1. Have another employee drive the clients home.
   2. Notify the public health department immediately.
   3. Send the clients to the emergency department.
   4. Obtain stool specimens from the clients.

7. The clinic nurse is scheduling a chest x-ray for a female client who may have pneumonia. Which question is most important for the nurse to ask the client?
   1. "Have you ever had a chest x-ray before?"
   2. "Can you can hold your breath for a minute?"
   3. "Do you or have you ever smoked cigarettes?"
   4. "Is there any chance you may be pregnant?"

8. The clinic nurse is returning phone messages from clients. Which phone message should the nurse return first?
   1. The client who called reporting being dizzy when getting up.
   2. The client who has been having abdominal cramping.
   3. The client who is complaining of nausea and vomiting.
   4. The client who has not had a bowel movement in 3 days.

9. The clinic nurse is caring for clients in a pediatric clinic. Which client should the nurse assess first?
   1. The 4-year-old child who fell and is complaining of left leg pain.
   2. The 3-year-old child who is drooling and does not want to swallow.
   3. The 8-year-old child who has complained of a headache for 2 days.
   4. The 10-year-old child who is thirsty all the time and has lost weight.

10. The community health nurse is triaging victims at the scene of a building collapse. Which intervention should the nurse implement first?
   1. Discuss the disaster situation with the media.
   2. Write the client's name clearly in the disaster log.
   3. Place disaster tags securely on the victims.
   4. Identify an area for family members to wait.

Delegating and Assigning Nursing Tasks

11. The nurse and an unlicensed assistive personnel (UAP) are working in a family practice clinic. Which task should the nurse delegate to the UAP?
    1. Give the client sample medications for a urinary tract infection (UTI).
    2. Show the client how to use a self-monitoring blood glucometer.
    3. Answer the telephone triage line and take messages from the client.
    4. Take the vital signs of a client scheduled for a physical examination.

12. The registered nurse (RN) is working in an outpatient clinic along with a licensed
practical nurse (LPN). Which client should the RN assign the LPN?
    1. The male client whose purified protein derivative (PPD) induration of the left
       inner arm is 14 mm.
    2. The client diagnosed with pneumonia whose pulse oximeter reading is 90%.
    3. The client diagnosed with arterial hypertension whose blood pressure
       (BP) is 148/94.
    4. The adolescent client whose pregnancy test came back positive.

13. Which task would be most appropriate for the clinic nurse to delegate to the unlicensed assistive personnel (UAP)?
    1. The client diagnosed with atrial fibrillation who needs an electrocardiogram.
    2. The client diagnosed with rule out (R/O) urinary tract infection who needs to give
       a urine specimen.
    3. The client diagnosed with gastroenteritis who needs an intravenous (IV) of D_5W
       125 mL/hour.
    4. The client diagnosed with a head injury who needs discharge teaching.

14. The unlicensed assistive personnel (UAP) tells the clinic nurse the male client in
room 1 is "really breathing hard and can't seem to catch his breath." Which action
should the nurse implement first?
    1. Tell the UAP to put 4 mL oxygen on the client.
    2. Ask the UAP whether the client is sitting up in a chair.
    3. Request the UAP to go with the nurse to the client's room.
    4. Instruct the UAP to take the client's vital signs.

15. The LPN informs the clinic nurse that the client diagnosed with atrial fibrillation
has an INR of 4.5. Which intervention should the nurse implement?
    1. Tell the LPN to notify the clinic health-care provider (HCP).
    2. Instruct the LPN to assess the client for abnormal bleeding.
    3. Obtain a stat electrocardiogram on the client.
    4. Take no action because this INR is within the normal range.

16. The nurse at a disaster site is triaging victims when a woman states, "I am a
certified nurse aide. Can I do anything to help?" Which action should the nurse
implement?
    1. Request the woman to please leave the area.
    2. Ask the woman to check the injured clients.
    3. Tell the woman to try and keep the victims calm.
    4. Instruct the woman to help the paramedics.

17. The clinic nurse hears the UAP tell the client, "You have gained over
15 pounds since your last visit." The scale is located in the office area. Which action
should the clinic nurse implement?
    1. Tell the UAP in front of the client to not comment on the weight.
    2. Ask the UAP to put the client in the room and take no action.
    3. Explain in private that this is an inappropriate comment and violates HIPAA.
    4. Report the UAP to the director of nurses of the clinic.

18. The clinic nurse is making assignments to the staff. Which assignment/delegation would be most appropriate?
    1. Request the LPN to escort the clients to the examination rooms.
    2. Ask the unlicensed assistive personnel (UAP) to prepare the room for the next client.
    3. Instruct the RN to administer the tetanus shot to the client.
    4. Tell the clinic secretary to call in a new prescription for a client.

19. The client tells the nurse that the female unlicensed assistive personnel (UAP) did not know how to take the blood pressure. Which action should the nurse take first?
    1. Discuss the client's comment with the UAP.
    2. Retake the BP and inform the client of the BP readings.
    3. Explain that the UAP knows how to take BP.
    4. Ask the UAP to demonstrate taking a BP.

20. Which task would be most appropriate for the clinic nurse to assign to an LPN?
    1. The intravenous push antiemetic to the client who is nauseated and vomiting.
    2. The subcutaneous epinephrine to a client who is having an asthma attack.
    3. The antacid to the client who is diagnosed with gastroesophageal reflux.
    4. The sublingual nitroglycerin to the client who is complaining of chest pain.

Managing Clients and Nursing Staff

21. The clinic RN manager is discussing osteoporosis with the clinic staff. Which activity is an example of a secondary nursing intervention when discussing osteoporosis?
    1. Obtain a bone density evaluation test on a female client older than 50.
    2. Perform a spinal screening examination on all female clients.
    3. Encourage the client to walk 30 minutes daily on a hard surface.
    4. Discuss risk factors for developing osteoporosis.

22. The clinic nurse is scheduling a 14-year-old client for a tonsillectomy. Which intervention should the clinic nurse implement?
    1. Obtain informed consent from the client.
    2. Send a throat culture to the laboratory.
    3. Discuss the need to cough and deep breathe.
    4. Request the laboratory to draw a PT and a PTT.

23. The female client calls the clinic nurse and reports being nauseated, vomiting, and having diarrhea for the last 6 hours. Which priority intervention should the nurse implement?
    1. Tell the client to not eat anything and to drink fluids.
    2. Ask the client what she has eaten in the last 24 hours.
    3. Request the client to bring a stool specimen to the clinic.
    4. Instruct the client to take an antidiarrheal medication.

24. The RN observes an LPN discussing a scheduled diagnostic test with a client in the waiting room of the outpatient clinic. Which action should the RN implement?
    1. Praise the LPN for talking to the client about the diagnostic test.
    2. Tell the LPN the RN needs to talk to her in the office area.
    3. Go to the waiting room and tell the LPN not to discuss this there.
    4. Inform the HCP that the LPN was talking to the client in the waiting room.

25. The charge nurse in a large outpatient clinic notices the staff is arguing and irritable with one other and the atmosphere has been very tense for the past week. Which action should the charge nurse implement?
    1. Wait for another week to see whether the situation resolves itself.
    2. Write a memo telling all staff members to stop arguing.
    3. Schedule a meeting with the staff to discuss the situation.
    4. Tell the staff to stop arguing or staff will be terminated.

26. The employee health nurse is obtaining a urine specimen for a pre-employment drug screen. Which intervention should the nurse implement?
    1. Obtain informed consent for the procedure.
    2. Maintain the chain of custody for the specimen.
    3. Allow the client to go to any bathroom in the clinic.
    4. Take and record the client's tympanic temperature.

27. The clinic nurse is assessing a client who is complaining of right leg calf pain. The right calf is edematous and warm to the touch. Which intervention should the nurse implement first?
    1. Notify the clinic HCP immediately.
    2. Ask the client how long the leg has been hurting.
    3. Complete a neurovascular assessment on the leg.
    4. Place the client's right leg in a dependent position.

28. The fire alarm starts going off in the family practice clinic. Which action should the nurse take first?
    1. Determine whether there is a fire in the clinic.
    2. Evacuate all the people from the clinic.
    3. Immediately call 911 and report the fire.
    4. Instruct clients to stay in the room and close the door.

29. The female unlicensed assistive personnel (UAP) tells the clinic nurse, "One of the medical interns asked me out on a date. I told him no but he keeps asking." Which statement is the nurse's best response?
    1. "I will talk to the intern and tell him to stop."
    2. "Did anyone hear the intern asking you out?"
    3. "He asks everyone out; that is just his way."
    4. "You should inform the clinic director of nurses."

30. The clinic nurse overhears another staff nurse telling the pharmaceutical representative, "If you bring us lunch from the best place in town, I will make sure you get to see the HCP." Which action should the clinic nurse take?
    1. Tell the representative the staff nurse's statement was inappropriate.
    2. Report this behavior to the clinic director of nurses immediately.
    3. Do not take any action and wait for the food to be delivered.
    4. Inform the HCP of the staff nurse and representative's behavior.

Setting Priorities When Caring for Clients

1. 1. This client should be categorized as black, priority 4, which means the injury is extensive and chances of survival are unlikely even with definitive care. Clients should receive comfort measures and be separated from other casualties but not abandoned.
   2. **This client should be categorized as red, priority 1, which means the injury is life threatening but survivable with minimal intervention. These clients can deteriorate rapidly without treatment.**
   3. This client should be categorized as green, priority 3, which means the injury is minor and treatment can be delayed hours to days. These clients should be moved away from the main triage area.
   4. The client should be categorized as a yellow, priority 2, which means the injury is significant and requires medical care but can wait hours without threat to life or limb. Clients in this category receive treatment only after immediate casualties are treated.

   MAKING NURSING DECISIONS: The nurse should remember the traffic light; red is first to be treated, yellow is treated next, green is treated last, and black is not treated until everyone else has been treated.

2. 1. **Right lower abdominal pain may indicate appendicitis, which requires surgery. This client needs a stat white blood cell count to obtain a definite diagnosis. This client should be assessed first. Right lower quadrant pain could indicate other conditions such as ectopic pregnancy, ovarian cyst, or exacerbation of Crohn's disease, which all should be assessed before UTI, back pain, or sore throat.**
   2. More than likely, this client has a urinary tract infection, which requires a midstream urinalysis. Because this is not life threatening, the client would not need to be assessed first.
   3. This client may have a bulging herniated disc and will need x-rays to confirm the herniated disc, but this is not potentially life

threatening. This client would not need to be assessed first.
   4. A sore throat is not life threatening; therefore, this client does not need to be assessed first.

   MAKING NURSING DECISIONS: When deciding which client to assess first, the test taker should determine whether the signs/symptoms the client is exhibiting are normal for the client situation. After eliminating the expected options, the test taker should determine which situation is more life threatening.

3. 1. The normal white blood cell count is 5.0 to 10.0 mm^3; therefore, this client does not require immediate intervention.
   2. The client's cholesterol level is elevated, but this would not require immediate intervention by the nurse. An elevated cholesterol level is not life threatening and can be discussed at the client's next appointment.
   3. The client's calcium level is within the normal range of 9.0 to 10.5 mg/dL; therefore, this client does not require an immediate intervention.
   4. **The therapeutic range for an INR is 2 to 3. This client is at risk for bleeding and requires immediate intervention by the nurse. The nurse should call the client and instruct the client to stop taking warfarin (Coumadin), an anticoagulant.**

   MAKING NURSING DECISIONS: The test taker must know normal laboratory data. See Appendix A for normal laboratory data.

4. 1. These are signs of otitis media (ear infection), which is not life threatening; therefore, this child does not need to be assessed first.
   2. These are signs/symptoms of rheumatic fever, which is not life threatening; therefore, this child does not need to be assessed first.
   3. **These are signs of bacterial meningitis, which can be potentially life threatening. This child should be isolated and be assessed first.**
   4. This adolescent does not need to be assessed first because possible pregnancy is not life threatening.

   MAKING NURSING DECISIONS: When deciding which client to assess first, the

test taker should determine whether the signs/symptoms the client is exhibiting are normal for the client situation. After eliminating the expected options, the test taker should determine which situation is more life threatening.

5. 1. **The first intervention is for the nurse to ensure the client is safe in the home. Assessing for grab bars in the bathroom is addressing the safety of the client.**
   2. Taking a shower in a stall shower may be safer than a getting in and out of a bathtub, but the nurse should first determine whether the client has grab bars and safety equipment even when taking a shower.
   3. According to the NCSBN NCLEX-RN test blueprint for management of care, the nurse must be knowledgeable of referrals. The physical therapist is able to help the client with transferring, ambulation, and other lower extremity difficulties and is an appropriate intervention, but it is not the nurse's first intervention. Safety is priority.
   4. NSAIDs are used to decrease the pain of osteoarthritis, but this intervention will not address safety issues for the client getting into and out of the bathtub.

   MAKING NURSING DECISIONS: The test taker should apply some systematic approach when answering a priority question. Maslow's Hierarchy of Needs should be used when determining which intervention to implement first. Safety is a priority.

6. 1. The employee health nurse should keep the clients at the clinic or send them to the emergency department. The clients should be kept together until the cause of their illnesses is determined. If it is determined that the clients are stable and not contagious, they should be driven home.
   2. **The employee health nurse should be aware that six clients with the same signs/symptoms indicate a potential deliberate or accidental dispersal of toxic or infectious agents. The nurse must notify the public health department so that an investigation of the cause can be instituted and appropriate action to contain the cause can be taken.**
   3. As long as the clients are stable, the nurse should keep the clients in the employee health clinic. The clients should not be exposed to clients and emergency department staff. If the clients must be transferred, decontamination procedures may need to be instituted.

4. The client may need to provide stool specimens, but this would be done at the emergency department. Employee health clinics do not have laboratory facilities to perform tests on stools.

7. 1. The nurse could ask this question because the radiologist may need to compare the previous chest x-ray with the current one, but this is not the most important question.
   2. The client will have to hold her breath when the chest x-ray is taken, but this is not the most important question.
   3. Smoking or a history of smoking is pertinent to the diagnosis of pneumonia, but it is not the most important question.
   4. **This is the most important question because if the client is pregnant, the x-rays can harm the fetus.**

   MAKING NURSING DECISIONS: The test taker should realize that for any female client of childbearing age, the most important questions or concerns will probably address the chance of pregnancy. Most medications and many diagnostic tests and treatments can harm the fetus.

8. 1. **This client should be called first so that the nurse can determine whether the dizziness when getting up is the result of medication or some other reason. Orthostatic hypotension can be life threatening; therefore, this client may need to be assessed immediately.**
   2. Abdominal cramping is not life threatening, and this client's call can be returned after the call to the client who is possibly experiencing orthostatic hypotension is completed.
   3. Nausea and vomiting are not life threatening. The nurse needs to talk to the client but not before returning the call from the client who is possibly experiencing orthostatic hypotension.
   4. This client is constipated, which is not priority over a client possibly experiencing orthostatic hypotension.

   MAKING NURSING DECISIONS: The test taker should apply some systematic approach when answering priority questions. All of the clients are experiencing physiologic problems, the first priority according to Maslow's Hierarch of Needs. Once that is established, then the test taker should determine which physiologic problem is most life threatening—in this case, dizziness when standing because of its possible cause, hypotension, which can be life threatening.

9. 1. This child needs an x-ray to rule out a fractured left leg, but this is not life threatening.
   2. **Drooling and not wanting to swallow are the cardinal signs of epiglottitis, which is potentially life threatening. This child should be assessed first. The nurse should not attempt to visualize the throat area and should allow the HCP to do this in case an emergency tracheostomy is required.**
   3. A child usually does not complain of a headache and this child should be assessed, but it is not life threatening.
   4. This client may have type 1 diabetes mellitus and should be assessed, but this is not life threatening at this time.

10. 1. A spokesperson should address the media away from the victim care area as soon as possible. This could be a nurse in some situations, but it is not the priority intervention when triaging victims.
    2. The disaster tag number and the client's name should be recorded in the disaster log book, but it is not the priority intervention. The disaster tag must be attached to the client prior to logging the client into the disaster log book.
    3. **Client tracking is a critical component of casualty management. Disaster tags, which include name, address, age, location, description of injuries, and treatments or medications administered, must be securely attached to the client.**
    4. Family and friends arriving at the disaster must be cared for by the disaster workers, but it is not the first intervention for the nurse who is triaging disaster victims.

Delegating and Assigning Nursing Tasks

11. 1. The nurse should not delegate medication administration, including giving the client boxes of sample medications, to a UAP.
    2. Showing the client how to use a glucometer is teaching the client, and the nurse cannot delegate teaching.
    3. The UAP should not talk to clients who are requesting health-care advice. The UAP is not trained to assess and ask pertinent questions.
    4. **The UAP is trained to take vital signs on a client who is stable. This task could safely be delegated by the nurse.**

MAKING NURSING DECISIONS: The nurse cannot delegate assessment, evaluation, teaching, administration of medications, or care of an unstable client to a UAP.

12. 1. An induration greater than 10 mm is positive for tuberculosis. This client needs to be assessed and followed up to rule out tuberculosis. This client should not be assigned to an LPN.
    2. A pulse oximeter reading less than 93% is life threatening; therefore, this client should not be assigned to an LPN.
    3. **This blood pressure is high, but not life threatening; therefore, the LPN could be assigned this client.**
    4. The adolescent client who is pregnant will need teaching; therefore, this client should not be assigned to an LPN.

MAKING NURSING DECISIONS: The nurse should assign the LPN the client who has the lowest level of need but for whom the task still remains in the LPN's scope of practice. The nurse cannot assign assessing, teaching, evaluating, or an unstable client to an LPN.

13. 1. The UAP may or may not be able to perform an ECG, but the stem asks which task is most appropriately delegated to a UAP. The nurse should delegate the task that requires the least amount of education, which, in this case, is collecting a urine specimen.
    2. **The UAP can request the client to urinate into a specimen cup. This is the task that requires the least amount of expertise and therefore is the most appropriate task to assign the UAP.**
    3. The UAP cannot start an intravenous line. This is an invasive procedure.
    4. The client with a head injury must be taught and must understand the signs/symptoms that require a visit to the emergency department. This task, which involves teaching, should not be delegated to a UAP.

MAKING NURSING DECISIONS: The nurse cannot delegate assessment, evaluation, teaching, administering medications, or an unstable client to a UAP.

14. 1. The UAP cannot administer oxygen to a client. Oxygen is considered a medication.

2. The nurse should not depend on the UAP to care for the client who is experiencing a potentially life-threatening condition.
3. This is the first intervention because the nurse must assess the client. Asking the UAP to accompany the nurse will allow the nurse to stay with the client while the UAP obtains any needed equipment.
4. The nurse should immediately assess the client. The UAP does not have the knowledge or skills to care for the client experiencing shortness of breath.

MAKING NURSING DECISIONS: Any time the nurse receives information from another staff member about a client who may be experiencing a new problem, complication, or life-threatening problem, the nurse must assess the client. The nurse should not make decisions about client needs based on another staff member's information.

15. 1. The LPN can contact the HCP and give pertinent information. The INR is high (therapeutic is 2 to 3), and the HCP should be informed.
2. The RN cannot assign assessment to an LPN.
3. The INR is elevated, but this will not affect the client's atrial fibrillation. The client is at risk for abnormal bleeding, not a life-threatening dysrhythmia.
4. The normal INR is 2 to 3; therefore, some action should be implemented.

16. 1. In a disaster, the nurse should utilize as many individuals as possible to help control the situation; therefore, this is an inappropriate intervention.
2. The unlicensed assistive personnel cannot assess clients; therefore, this is not an appropriate action.
3. Unlicensed assistive personnel have the ability to keep the victims calm; therefore, this is an appropriate action. This action is not critical to the safety of the victims.
4. The paramedics do not need civilians assisting them as they stabilize and transport the victims. This is not an appropriate action.

17. 1. The clinic nurse should not correct the UAP in front of the client. This is embarrassing to the UAP and makes the client uncomfortable.

2. The clinic nurse must correct the UAP's behavior. The client's weight gain should not be announced in the office area so that all staff, clients, and visitors can hear. This is a violation of confidentiality.
3. The clinic nurse should correct the UAP's behavior, but it should be done in private and with an explanation as to why the action is inappropriate. This is a violation of confidentiality because the scale is located in the office area and any client or visitor passing by, as well as other staff members, can hear the comment.
4. The clinic nurse should handle this situation. If the UAP's behavior shows a pattern of behavior, then it should be reported to the director of nurses.

MAKING NURSING DECISIONS: In any business, including a health-care facility, argument or discussion of confidential information should not occur among staff of any level where the customers—in this case, the clinic clients—can hear it or see it.

18. 1. The UAP could escort the clients to the room so that the LPN could be assigned tasks that are within the LPN's scope of practice.
2. The UAP can make sure the room is clear of the previous client's gown and equipment used with the previous client. The UAP can also make sure there are gowns, tongue blades, and additional equipment in the examination room.
3. The LPN can administer medication; therefore, it would be more appropriate to assign this task to the LPN, so that the RN could be assigned tasks that are beyond the scope of practice of an LPN and within the RN scope of practice.
4. The clinic secretary is unlicensed personnel and does not have the authority to call in a new prescription for a client.

MAKING NURSING DECISIONS: When the test taker is deciding which option is the most appropriate task to delegate/assign, the test taker should choose the task that requires each member of the staff to function within his or her full scope of practice. Do not assign a task to a staff member that requires a higher level of expertise than the staff member has, and do not assign a task to a staff member when the task could be delegated/assigned to a staff member with a lower level of expertise.

19. 1. The nurse should discuss the client's comment, but it is not the nurse's first intervention.
    2. **The nurse should first take the client's BP correctly and address the client's concern.**
    3. If the nurse's BP reading and the UAP's BP reading are close to the same, the nurse could reassure the client that the UAP does know how to take BP readings. However, this is not the nurse's first intervention.
    4. This is an appropriate action, but it is not the first intervention. The nurse is responsible for making sure the UAP has the ability to perform any delegated tasks correctly.

20. 1. Intravenous push medications cannot be assigned to an LPN. It is the most dangerous route for administering medication, and only an RN (or HCP) can perform this task.
    2. The client who is having an asthma attack is not stable; therefore, this client should not be assigned to the LPN.
    3. **GERD is not a life-threatening disease process, and an antacid is an oral medication that the LPN can administer. Therefore, this task would be the most appropriate to assign the LPN.**
    4. The client may be having a myocardial infarction; therefore, this client is unstable and should not be assigned to an LPN.

    MAKING NURSING DECISIONS: The test taker must determine which option absolutely is included within the LPN's scope of practice. LPNs are not routinely taught how to administer intravenous push medications. The test taker must also determine which client is the most stable, which makes this an "except" question. Three clients are either unstable or have potentially life-threatening conditions and should not be assigned to an LPN.

Managing Clients and Nursing Staff

21. 1. A secondary nursing intervention includes screening for early detection. The bone density evaluation will determine the density of the bone and is diagnostic for osteoporosis.
    2. Spinal screening examinations are performed on adolescents to detect scoliosis. This is a secondary nursing intervention, but not to detect osteoporosis.

    3. Teaching the client is a primary nursing intervention. This is an appropriate intervention to help prevent osteoporosis, but it is not a secondary intervention.
    4. Discussing risk factors is an appropriate intervention, but it is not a secondary nursing intervention.

22. 1. The parent/guardian must sign the consent for surgery because the client is under the age of 18.
    2. The client has already been diagnosed with tonsillitis; therefore, a throat culture is not needed prior to surgery.
    3. The client should not cough after this surgery because it could cause bleeding from the incision site.
    4. **A PT/PTT will assess the client for any bleeding tendencies. This is priority before this surgery because bleeding is a life-threatening complication.**

23. 1. This may be an appropriate intervention, but the nurse should first assess the client's food intake to determine whether the symptoms may be caused by food poisoning or by a viral infection.
    2. **This is the priority intervention because the nurse should first attempt to determine the cause of the signs/symptoms—which will then guide further instructions.**
    3. This may be an appropriate intervention, but the nurse should first assess the client's food intake to determine whether this may be food poisoning or a viral infection.
    4. This may be an appropriate intervention, but the nurse should first assess the client's food intake to determine whether this may be food poisoning or a viral infection.

24. 1. This is a breach of confidentiality. The LPN should not discuss the client's health problem in the waiting room area where everyone can hear.
    2. **The RN should remove the LPN from the situation without embarrassing the LPN. Asking the LPN to come to the office area is the appropriate action for the RN to take. The LPN's action is a violation of HIPAA.**
    3. The RN should not correct the LPN's behavior in front of the client. This is embarrassing to both the LPN and the client.
    4. The RN does not have to report this to the HCP. The RN can talk to the LPN concerning this breach of confidentiality.

The nurse is responsible for knowing and complying with local, state, and federal standards of care. The LPN's discussion of a confidential matter in a public area is a violation of HIPAA.

25. 1. The charge nurse must address this situation because it has been going on for more than a week.
    2. Writing a memo does not find out what is causing the tense atmosphere.
    3. **The charge nurse should call a meeting and attempt to determine what is causing the staff's behavior and the tense atmosphere. The charge nurse could then problem-solve, with the goal being to have a more relaxed atmosphere in which to work.**
    4. This is threatening, which is not an appropriate way to resolve a staff problem.

MAKING NURSING DECISIONS: In any business, including a health-care facility, arguing should not occur among staff of any level where the customers—in this case, the clients—can hear it or see it. The nurse should address the situation directly with the staff.

26. 1. Obtaining a urine sample is not an invasive procedure and does not require informed consent.
    2. **The urine specimen must adhere to a chain of custody so that the client cannot dispute the results.**
    3. The bathroom for drug testing should not have access to any water via a sink so that the client cannot dilute the urine specimen.
    4. The tympanic temperature is taken in the client's ear and is not required for a urine drug sample.

27. 1. **The nurse should realize the client probably has a deep vein thrombosis, which is a medical emergency. The HCP should be notified immediately so the client can be started on IV heparin and admitted to the hospital.**
    2. This data may be needed, but the nurse should notify the HCP based on the signs/symptoms alone.
    3. A neurovascular assessment should be completed, but not before notifying the HCP. The signs/symptoms alone indicate a potentially life-threatening condition.
    4. The client's leg should be elevated, not placed hanging over the side of the bed, which would be appropriate for an arterial occlusion.

MAKING NURSING DECISIONS: The test taker needs to read all of the options carefully before choosing the option that says, "Notify the HCP." If any of the options will provide information the HCP needs to know in order to make a decision, the test taker should choose that option. If, however, the HCP does not need any additional information to make a decision and the nurse suspects the condition is serious or life threatening, the priority intervention is to call the HCP.

28. 1. **The nurse should first determine whether there is a fire or whether someone accidentally or on purpose pulled the fire alarm. Because this is a clinic, not a hospital, the nurse should keep calm and determine the situation before taking action.**
    2. The nurse should not evacuate clients, visitors, and staff unless there is a real fire.
    3. The nurse should assess the situation before contacting the fire department.
    4. This is an appropriate intervention, but this is not the first intervention. The nurse should first assess to determine whether there is a fire.

MAKING NURSING DECISIONS: The nurse must be knowledgeable of emergency preparedness. Employees receive this information in employee orientation and are responsible for implementing procedures correctly. The NCSBN NCLEX-RN blueprint includes questions on safe and effective care environment.

29. 1. The clinic nurse should allow the director to address sexual harassment allegations. This is a matter that should be handled legally.
    2. This is an appropriate question to ask when investigating sexual harassment allegations, but the clinic nurse should allow the director of nurses to pursue this situation.
    3. The clinic nurse is responsible for taking the appropriate action when sexual allegations are reported. This is not taking the allegations seriously and could result in disciplinary action against the nurse.
    4. **This is the most appropriate response because sexual harassment allegations are a legal matter. The clinic nurse implemented the correct action by making sure the UAP reported the allegation to the director of nurses.**

MAKING NURSING DECISIONS: The nurse is responsible for knowing and complying with local, state, and federal standards of care.

30. 1. The clinic nurse should not discuss the staff nurses' statement with the pharmaceutical representative because the staff member's behavior is unethical and could have repercussions. The clinic nurse should notify the director of nurses.
    2. This behavior is unethical and is making promises that the staff nurse may or may not be able to keep. Because this situation includes the HCP, an outside representative, and the staff nurse, this situation should be reported to the director of nurses for further action.
    3. This behavior must be reported. This is bribing the pharmaceutical representative and using a meeting with the HCP as the reward.
    4. The clinic nurse should maintain the chain of command and report this to the nursing supervisor, not to the HCP.

COMPREHENSIVE EXAMINATION

1. The clinic nurse is evaluating vital signs for clients being seen in the outpatient clinic. Which client would warrant intervention?
   1. The 10-month-old infant who has a pulse rate of 140.
   2. The 3-year-old toddler who has a respiratory rate of 28.
   3. The 24-week gestational woman who has a BP of 142/96.
   4. The 42-year-old client who has a temperature of 100.2°F.

2. The nurse accidentally sticks herself with a needle she used to administer an intradermal injection for a PPD. Which action should the nurse implement?
   1. Take no action because this is an injection under the skin.
   2. Immediately wash the area with soap and water.
   3. Ask the client whether he or she has AIDS or hepatitis.
   4. Place an antibiotic ointment and Band-Aid on the site.

3. The client diagnosed with arterial hypertension and has been taking a calcium channel blocker, a loop diuretic, and an ACE inhibitor for 3 years. Which statement by the client would warrant intervention by the nurse?
   1. "I have to go to the bathroom a lot during the morning."
   2. "I get up very slowly when I have been sitting for a while."
   3. "I do not salt my food when I am cooking it but I add it at the table."
   4. "I drink grapefruit juice every morning with my breakfast."

4. The director of nurses in the clinic is counseling a unlicensed assistive personnel (UAP) in the clinic who returned late from her lunch break seven times in the last 2 weeks. Which conflict resolution utilizes the win-lose strategy?
   1. The UAP explains she is checking on her ill mother during lunch, and the nurse allows her to take a longer lunch break if she comes in early.
   2. The director of nurses offers the UAP a transfer to the emergency weekend clinic so that she will be off during the week.
   3. The director of nurses terminates the UAP explaining that all staff must be on time so that the clinic runs smoothly.
   4. The UAP is placed on 1-month probation, and any further occurrences will result in being terminated from this position.

5. The clinic nurse has told the female unlicensed assistive personnel (UAP) twice to change the sharps container in the examination room, but it has not been changed. Which action should the nurse implement first?
   1. Tell the UAP to change it immediately.
   2. Ask her why the sharps container has not been changed.
   3. Change the sharps container as per clinic policy.
   4. Document the situation and place a copy in the employee file.

6. The clinic nurse is making assignments for the large family practice clinic. Which task should be assigned to the staff nurse who is 4 months pregnant?
   1. Have the staff nurse answer the telephone calls from clients.
   2. Instruct the staff nurse to work in the radiology department.
   3. Tell the staff nurse to work in the front desk triage area.
   4. Assign the staff nurse to work in the oncology clinic.

7. Which task would be most appropriate for the clinic nurse to delegate to the unlicensed assistive personnel (UAP)?
   1. Request the UAP to ride in the ambulance with a client.
   2. Ask the UAP to escort the client in a wheelchair to the car.
   3. Instruct the UAP to show the client how to use crutches.
   4. Tell the UAP to call the pharmacy to refill a prescription.

8. The employee health nurse is caring for an employee who fell off a ladder and is complaining of low back pain radiating down both legs. Which action should the nurse implement first?
   1. Refer the client to an HCP for further evaluation.
   2. Complete the workers' compensation documentation.
   3. Investigate the cause of the fall off the ladder.
   4. Notify the employee's supervisor of the incident.

9. The clinic nurse is reviewing laboratory results for clients seen in the clinic. Which client warrants intervention from the nurse?
   1. The client who has a hemoglobin of 9 g/dL and a hematocrit of 29%.
   2. The client who has a WBC count of 9.0 mm^3.
   3. The client who has a serum potassium level of 4.8 mEq/L.
   4. The client who has a serum sodium level of 137 mEq/L.

10. The Hispanic female client is complaining of nausea, vomiting, and diarrhea. The Hispanic husband answers questions even though the nurse directly asks the client. Which action should the nurse take?
    1. Ask the husband to allow his wife to answer the questions.
    2. Request the husband to leave the examination room.
    3. Continue to allow the husband to answer the wife's questions.
    4. Do not ask any further questions until the client starts answering.

11. The clinic nurse walks into the examination room, and the client is lying on the table and is not breathing. Which interventions should the nurse implement? Rank in order of performance.
    1. Open the client's airway.
    2. Check the client's carotid pulse.
    3. Assess for rise and fall of the chest.
    4. Perform compressions at a 30:2 rate.
    5. Pinch the nose and give two breaths.

12. The client had an allergic reaction to penicillin, an antibiotic, and was admitted to the hospital 2 weeks ago. The client is being seen at the clinic for a follow-up visit. Which priority intervention should the nurse implement?
    1. Recommend the client wears a medic alert bracelet.
    2. Encourage the client to tell the pharmacy about the allergy.
    3. Tell the client not to be around any person taking penicillin.
    4. Allow the client to ventilate feelings about the hospitalization.

13. Which action would be most appropriate for the clinic nurse who suspects another staff nurse of stealing narcotics from the clinic?
    1. Confront the staff nurse with the suspicion.
    2. Call the State Board of Nurse Examiners.
    3. Notify the director of nurses immediately.
    4. Report the suspicion to the clinic's HCP.

14. The employee health nurse is caring for a male employee who reports tripping and is complaining of right knee pain. There is no visible injury, and the client has a normal neurovascular assessment. Which intervention should the nurse implement?
    1. Request the employee to return to work.
    2. Obtain a urine specimen for a drug screen.
    3. Send the client to the emergency department.
    4. Place a sequential compression device on the leg.

15. The community health nurse is triaging victims at the site of a disaster. Which client should the nurse categorize as black, priority 4?
    1. The client who is alert and has a sucking chest wound.
    2. The client who cannot stop crying and can't answer questions.
    3. The client whose abdomen is hard and tender to the touch.
    4. The client who has full thickness burns over 60% of the body.

16. The client comes to the clinic reporting pain and burning on urination. Which action should the nurse implement first?
    1. Assess and document the client's vital signs.
    2. Determine whether the client has seen any blood in the urine.
    3. Request the client give a midstream urine specimen.
    4. Ask the client whether she wipes front to back after a bowel movement.

17. The nurse is working at the emergency health clinic in a disaster shelter. Which intervention is priority when initially assessing the client?
    1. Find out how long the client will be in the shelter.
    2. Determine whether the client has his or her routine medications.
    3. Document the client's health history in writing.
    4. Assess the client's vital signs, height, and weight.

18. The wife of a client calls the clinic and tells the nurse her husband is having chest pain but won't go to the hospital. Which action should the nurse implement first?
    1. Instruct the wife to call 911 immediately.
    2. Tell the wife to have the client chew an aspirin.
    3. Ask the wife what the client had to eat recently.
    4. Request the husband talk to the clinic nurse.

19. The HCP orders an intravenous pyelogram for the 27-year-old male client diagnosed with R/O renal calculi. The client is diagnosed with schizophrenia and is delusional. Which action should the clinic nurse implement?
    1. Ask the client whether he is allergic to yeast.
    2. Request him to sign a permit for the procedure.
    3. Obtain informed consent from his significant other.
    4. Discuss the local hospital's day surgery procedure.

20. The clinic nurse administered 200,000 units of intramuscular penicillin to a client. Which priority intervention should the nurse implement?
    1. Place a Band-Aid over the intramuscular injection site.
    2. Tell the client to put a warm compress over the injection site.
    3. Document the medication injection in the client's chart.
    4. Inform the client to stay in the waiting room for 30 minutes.

1. 1. The normal pulse rate for a 1- to 11-month old is 100 to 150. This client would not warrant immediate intervention.
   2. The normal respiratory rate for a toddler is 20 to 30. This client would not warrant immediate intervention.
   3. **A 24-week gestation woman with a BP of 142/96 would warrant intervention because the average systolic BP should be between 90 and 140 mm Hg and the diastolic BP should be between 60 and 85 mm Hg. This BP could indicate pregnancy-induced hypertension.**
   4. This is an elevated temperature, but it would not warrant intervention from the nurse. This is not a potentially life-threatening temperature.

2. 1. A dirty needle stick is a dirty needle stick and should be treated according to hospital policy. It does not matter which route was used.
   2. **The nurse should wash the area with soap and water and attempt to squeeze the area to make it bleed.**
   3. The nurse should not ask this question directly to the client. The nurse could ask whether the client would agree to have blood drawn for testing, but not directly ask whether the client has AIDS or hepatitis.
   4. The puncture site would not require antibiotic ointment unless it is infected, which it wouldn't be immediately after the incident.

3. 1. If the client takes the loop diuretic in the morning, then going to the bathroom a lot in the morning would not warrant intervention.
   2. Rising from a sitting position slowly helps prevent orthostatic hypotension, which is a potential side effect of all the medications. This statement would not warrant intervention.
   3. This statement indicates the client is adhering to a low-sodium diet, as he should be. No intervention is warranted.
   4. **Grapefruit juice can cause calcium channel blockers to rise to toxic levels. Grapefruit juice inhibits cytochrome P450-3A4 found in the liver and intestinal wall. This statement warrants intervention by the nurse.**

4. 1. This is a win-win strategy which focuses on goals (to have adequate staff) and attempts to meet the needs of both parties. The director of nurses keeps an experienced nurse, and the UAP keeps her position. Both parties win.
   2. This is a possible win-win strategy in which both parties win. The UAP keeps her job, and the director of nurses can hire a UAP who will be able to work the assigned hours.
   3. This is a win-lose strategy in which during the conflict one party (the director of nurses) exerts dominance and the other party (UAP) must submit and loses.
   4. This is negotiation in which the conflicting parties give and take on the issues. The UAP gets one more chance, and the director of nurse's authority is still intact.

5. 1. A full sharps container is a violation of Occupational Health and Safety Administration (OSHA) regulations, and because the UAP has not done it after being asked twice, a third request is not necessary.
   2. The nurse should discuss why the sharps container has not been changed, but it is not the first intervention.
   3. **A full sharps container is a violation of Occupational Health and Safety Administration (OSHA) regulations and may result in a $25,000 fine. The nurse should first take care of this situation immediately and then discuss it with the UAP. This is modeling appropriate behavior.**
   4. The situation should be documented because the UAP was told twice, but documentation is not the first intervention.

6. 1. **This would be the most appropriate assignment because the nurse would not be exposed to any contagious diseases or dangerous radiologic procedures.**
   2. The pregnant nurse should not be exposed to x-rays, which could endanger the fetus.
   3. Working in the front desk triage area would allow the pregnant nurse to be exposed to any type of contagious or infectious disease. This is not an appropriate assignment.
   4. The oncology clinic will have clients receiving chemotherapeutic agents that may endanger the fetus; this would not be the most appropriate assignment. Even if the

nurse is not administering the medication, the most appropriate assignment is to assign the nurse to an area that poses no danger to the fetus.

7. 1. If the client must be transferred from the clinic to the hospital, then the client is unstable and therefore should not be assigned to a UAP.
   2. **The client is stable because he or she is being sent home; therefore, the UAP could safely complete this task.**
   3. Showing the client how to walk with crutches is teaching, and the nurse cannot delegate teaching to the UAP.
   4. The UAP should not be calling a pharmacy because this is not within the scope of practice of unlicensed personnel. The HCP is responsible for delegating this task.

8. 1. **The nurse should first care for the client and refer the client to an HCP for possible x-rays, pain medication, and further treatment. The employee health nurse's responsibility is to ensure the employee is safe to work, and this client is not.**
   2. This information should be completed because any injury on the job must be covered by workers' compensation insurance so that all costs will be covered for the client. Documentation is never priority over caring for the client.
   3. The employee health nurse should determine whether there are unsafe areas in the workplace or whether the employee was negligent, but this is not the nurse's first intervention.
   4. The employee's supervisor does need to be notified, but this is not the nurse's first intervention. The safety of the client is always first.

9. 1. **The normal hemoglobin is 12 to 15 g/dL, and normal hematocrit is 39% to 45%. This client's H&H is low. The nurse should contact the client and make an immediate appointment.**
   2. The normal WBC count is 4.0 to 10.0 mm³. This client's WBC count is within normal range and does not warrant intervention from the clinic nurse.
   3. The normal serum potassium level is 3.5 to 5.5 mEq/L. This client's level is within normal range and does not warrant intervention from the clinic nurse.
   4. The normal serum sodium level is 135 to 145 mEq/L. This client's level is within the normal range, and the client does not warrant intervention from the clinic nurse.

10. 1. In the Hispanic culture, the husband often speaks for the wife and family, and requesting the husband not to speak may be insulting. This action may cause the wife to leave as well.
    2. In the Hispanic culture, the husband often is the spokesman and makes decisions for the wife and family. Asking the husband to leave the room may cause the client to leave as well.
    3. **This behavior may be cultural, and the nurse should continue to allow the husband to answer the questions, while the nurse looks at the client. The nurse must be respectful of the client's culture. The nurse can, however, ask whether the client agrees with the husband's answers.**
    4. This is disrespectful to the client's culture. Many times the nurse must honor the client's culture while caring for the client.

11. The correct order is 1, 3, 5, 2, 4.
    1. The nurse should open the client's airway to ensure a patent airway.
    3. After opening the airway, the nurse should check and determine whether or not the client is breathing.
    5. The nurse should then administer two breaths while the client's nose is pinched.
    2. The nurse then must determine whether the client's heart is pumping by checking the carotid pulse.
    4. The American Heart Association recommends 30 compressions followed by two breaths.

12. 1. **This is the nurse's priority intervention because any emergency personnel who may come into contact with the client should be aware of the client's allergy. A penicillin allergy can kill the client.**
    2. The client's pharmacy can be made aware of the allergy, but this is helpful only when the client is having prescriptions filled.
    3. Unless the client has an allergy to penicillin dust, which is rare, coming into contact with another person taking penicillin will not cause the client to have an allergic reaction.
    4. Therapeutic communication allows the client to ventilate feelings, which is an appropriate intervention, but it is not priority over teaching the client how to prevent a potentially life-threatening reaction.

13. 1. The clinic nurse should not confront the staff nurse without objective data that supports the allegation.
2. The State Board of Nurse Examiners cannot do anything to the nurse until the nurse has been convicted of the crime. Many states have programs to help addicted nurses, but some states may revoke the nurse's license to practice nursing.
3. **The clinic nurse should report the suspicions so that appropriate actions can be taken, such as a urine drug screen for the nurse, watching the nurse for the behavior, and possibly notifying the police department.**
4. The nurse should follow the chain of command, which does not include the HCP.

14. 1. If a client is complaining of pain, the nurse should not ask the client to return to work. If nothing else, the client should be allowed to stay in the clinic until the pain subsides.
2. **The employee must submit to a urine drug screen anytime there is an injury. This is standard practice by many employers to help determine whether the employee was under the influence during the time of the accident. Workers' compensation will not be responsible if the employee is under the influence of alcohol or drugs.**
3. Because there are no visible injuries and the neurovascular assessment is normal, a referral to the emergency department is not warranted. The employee health nurse could send the employee home with further instructions. None of the complaints warrants the employee's needing an x-ray.
4. A sequential compression device is used to help prevent deep vein thrombosis for clients on bed rest. This is not an appropriate intervention.

15. 1. An alert client with a sucking chest wound should be categorized as red, priority 1, which means the injury is life threatening but survivable with minimal intervention. These clients can deteriorate rapidly without treatment.
2. A client who cannot stop crying and cannot answer questions should be categorized as green, priority 3, which means the injury is minor and treatment can be delayed hours to days. These clients should be moved away from the main triage area. Clients with behavioral and psychological problems are included in this category.
3. A client whose abdomen is hard and tender should be categorized as a yellow, priority 2, which means the injury is significant and requires medical care but can wait hours without threat to life or limb. Clients in this category receive treatment only after immediate casualties are treated.
4. **This client should be categorized as black, priority 4, which means the injury is extensive and chances of survival are unlikely even with definitive care. Clients should receive comfort measures and be separated from other casualties, but not abandoned.**

16. 1. Any client seen in the clinic should have the vital signs taken, but given the signs/symptoms of the client, the nurse should first obtain a urinalysis. The laboratory test can be completed before the client is seen by the HCP.
2. The nurse should determine whether there has been blood in the urine, but it is not the nurse's first intervention. The HCP needs a urinalysis to confirm the probable diagnosis.
3. **The client is verbalizing the classic signs/symptoms of a urinary tract infection, but it must be confirmed with a urinalysis. The nurse should first obtain the specimen so that the results will be available by the time the HCP sees the client.**
4. The nurse should always teach the client and asking this question is appropriate, but it is not the clinic nurse's first intervention.

17. 1. The nurse may need to know how long the client will be in the shelter, but this is not priority during the initial assessment of the client.
2. **During a disaster, the priority is to determine whether the client has routine medications that can be taken while in the shelter. If clients do not have life-sustaining medications, then obtaining the medications becomes priority. Remember, psychiatric medications are life sustaining.**
3. The client's health history is important, but no matter what the history is, if the client does not have life-sustaining medications, the client will end up in the hospital.
4. The client should be assessed, but unless the client has a specific complaint in this

situation, assessment of vital signs, height, and weight is not priority.

18. 1. The wife should call 911, but the American Heart Association recommends chewing a baby aspirin at the onset of chest pain.
    2. **The AHA recommends the client having chest pain chew an aspirin to help decrease platelet aggregation. This is the first intervention the clinic nurse should tell the wife to do.**
    3. This question could be asked to determine whether the pain is secondary to a gallbladder attack or gastric irritation, but this is not the first intervention.
    4. The clinic nurse could possibly talk to the client while the wife is getting an aspirin, but this is not the first intervention.

19. 1. The nurse should ask whether the client is allergic to iodine, such as shellfish.
    2. An incompetent client cannot sign the consent form. Because the client is diagnosed with schizophrenia, asking him to sign a permit form is not an appropriate intervention.
    3. **An incompetent client is an individual who is not autonomous and cannot give or withhold consent—for example, individuals who are cognitively**
impaired, mentally ill, neurologically incapacitated, or under the influence of mind-altering drugs. **This client is diagnosed with schizophrenia, a mental illness; therefore, the client's significant other must sign for the procedure.**
    4. This procedure is performed in the radiology department, not in a day surgery department.

20. 1. The nurse can or cannot place a Band-Aid over the injection site. This is not a priority intervention.
    2. Warm compresses will help increase the absorption of the medication, but this is not the priority nursing intervention.
    3. The medication injection must be documented in the client's chart in a clinic, just as it must be in an acute care area, but documentation is not priority over a possible life-threatening allergic reaction.
    4. **The client is at risk for having an allergic reaction to the penicillin, which is a life-threatening complication. Therefore, the client must stay in the waiting room for at least 30 minutes so the nurse can determine whether an allergic reaction is occurring.**

Home Health Nursing

9

"If something comes to life in others because of you, then you have made an approach to immortality."

—Norman Cousins

ABBREVIATION LIST

AIDS	Acquired Immunodeficiency Syndrome	**HIPAA**	Health Insurance Portability and Accountability Act
BP	Blood Pressure	**NAHC**	National Association for Home Care
CHF	Congestive Heart Failure	**NCSBN**	National Council State Board of Nursing
CVA	Cerebrovascular Accident		
COPD	Chronic Obstructive Pulmonary Disease	**NPO**	Nothing per (by) Os (Mouth)
DNR	Do Not Resuscitate	**ROM**	Range of Motion
DVT	Deep Vein Thrombosis	**SCI**	Spinal Cord Injury
HCP	Health-Care Provider	**UAP**	Unlicensed Assistive Personnel
HH	Home Health		

PRACTICE QUESTIONS

Setting Priorities When Caring for Clients

1. The home health (HH) nurse enters the home of an 80-year-old female client who had a cerebrovascular accident (CVA), or "brain attack," 2 months ago. The client is complaining of a severe headache. Which intervention should the nurse implement first?
   1. Determine what medication the client has taken.
   2. Assess the client's pain on a 1-to-10 pain scale.
   3. Ask whether the client has any acetaminophen (Tylenol).
   4. Tell the client to sit down, and take her blood pressure.

2. The HH nurse received phone messages from the agency secretary. Which client should the nurse phone first?
   1. The client diagnosed with hypertension who is reporting a BP of 148/92.
   2. The client diagnosed with cystic fibrosis who has a pulse oximeter reading of 93%.
   3. The client diagnosed with congestive heart failure who has edematous feet.
   4. The client diagnosed with chronic atrial fibrillation who is having chest pain.

3. The HH director of nurses is orienting new HH nurses to the agency. Which information should the director tell the new HH nurse is priority to be successful in HH nursing?
   1. Discuss the importance of the weekly team conference meetings.
   2. Discuss the need for clients to have an Advance Directive.
   3. Explain that the greatest challenge is motivating the client to learn.
   4. Explain how to coordinate the client's care with other disciplines.

4. The HH nurse is scheduling visits for the day. Which client should the nurse visit first?
   1. The client with an L-4 SCI who is complaining of a severe, pounding headache.
   2. The client with chronic leukemia who is depressed and does not want to live.
   3. The client with chronic obstructive pulmonary disease who is short of breath.
   4. The client with type 2 diabetes mellitus who has numbness in the legs.

5. The HH nurse is visiting a client diagnosed with end-stage congestive heart failure. The nurse finds the client lying in bed, short of breath, unable to talk, and with buccal cyanosis. Which intervention would the HH nurse implement first?
   1. Assist client to a sitting position.
   2. Assess the client's vital signs.
   3. Call 911 for the paramedics.
   4. Auscultate the client's lung sounds.

6. The HH nurse is visiting a 92-year-old client with an out-of-hospital do not resuscitate (DNR) order who has stopped breathing and has no pulse or blood pressure. The client's family is at the bedside. Which action should the HH nurse implement first?
   1. Contact the agency's chaplain.
   2. Pronounce the client's death.
   3. Ask the family to leave the bedside.
   4. Call the client's funeral home.

7. The male HH nurse is planning his visits for the day. Which client should the nurse visit first?
   1. The client diagnosed with AIDS who has developed Kaposi's sarcoma.
   2. The client diagnosed with dementia who is having difficulty dressing himself.
   3. The client diagnosed with a venous stasis ulcer who is complaining of pain.
   4. The client diagnosed with Parkinson's disease who is hallucinating.

8. The HH nurse in the office is notified that the female client on warfarin (Coumadin), an oral anticoagulant, has an international normalized ratio (INR) of 3.8. Which action should the HH nurse implement first?
   1. Document the result of the INR in the client's chart.
   2. Contact the client and ask whether she has any abnormal bleeding.
   3. Notify the client's health-care provider of the INR results.
   4. Schedule an appointment with the client to draw another INR.

9. The HH nurse received laboratory results on the following clients. Which client should the HH nurse contact first?
   1. The client who has an INR of 2.8.
   2. The client who has a serum potassium level of 3.8 mEq/L.
   3. The client who has a serum digoxin level of 2.6 mg/dL.
   4. The client who has a glycosylated hemoglobin of 6%.

10. The HH nurse is caring for a 22-year-old female client who sustained an L-5 spinal cord injury 2 months ago. The client says, "I will never be happy again. I can't walk, I can't drive, and I had to quit college." Which intervention should the nurse implement first?
    1. Allow the client to ventilate her feelings of powerlessness.
    2. Refer the client to the home health-care agency social worker.
    3. Recommend contacting the American Spinal Cord Association.
    4. Ask the client whether she has any friends who come and visit.

Delegating and Assigning Nursing Tasks

11. Which action by the HH aide indicates to the HH nurse that the aide understands the correct procedure for applying compression stockings to the client recovering from a pulmonary embolus?
    1. The HH aide instructs the client to sit in the chair when applying the stockings.
    2. The HH aide cannot insert one finger under the proximal end of the stocking.
    3. The HH aide ensures the toe opening is placed on the top side of the feet.
    4. The HH aide checked to make sure the toes were warm after putting the stockings on.

12. The female HH aide calls the office and reports pain after feeling a pulling in her back when she was transferring the client from the bed to the wheelchair. Which priority action should the HH nurse tell the HH aide?
    1. Explain how to perform isometric exercises.
    2. Instruct her to go to the local emergency room.
    3. Tell her to complete an occurrence report.
    4. Recommend that she apply an ice pack to the back.

13. The female client with osteoarthritis is 6 weeks postoperative for open reduction and internal fixation of the right hip. The HH aide tells the HH nurse the client will not get in the shower in the morning because she hurts all over. Which action would be most appropriate by the HH nurse?
    1. Tell the HH aide to allow the client to stay in bed until the pain goes away.
    2. Instruct the HH aide to get the client up to a chair and give her a bath.
    3. Explain to the HH aide to the client should get up and take a warm shower.
    4. Arrange an appointment for the client to visit her health-care provider.

14. The HH nurse is discussing the care of a client with the female HH aide. Which task can the HH nurse delegate to the HH aide?
    1. Instruct her to assist the client with a shower.
    2. Ask her to prepare the breakfast meal for the client.
    3. Request her to take the client to an HCP's appointment.
    4. Tell her to show the client how to use a glucometer.

15. The HH care agency director is teaching a class to the HH aides concerning safety in HH nursing. Which statement by the HH aide indicates the director needs to re-teach safety information?
    1. "It is all right to call the agency if I am afraid of going into the home."
    2. "I should wear my uniform and name tag when I go into the home."
    3. "I must take my cellular phone when visiting the client's home."
    4. "It is all right if I don't wear gloves when touching bodily fluids."

16. The HH care agency director is making assignments. Which client should be assigned to the most experienced HH nurse?
    1. The client who is recovering from Guillain-Barré syndrome who reports being tired all the time.
    2. The client who has multiple stage 3 and 4 pressure ulcers on the sacral area.
    3. The client who is 2 weeks postoperative for laryngectomy secondary to laryngeal cancer.
    4. The client who is being discharged from service within the next week.

17. The HH nurse is visiting the client diagnosed with end-stage chronic obstructive pulmonary disease (COPD) while the HH aide is providing care. Which action by the HH aide would warrant intervention by the nurse?
    1. The HH aide keeps the bedroom at a warm temperature.
    2. The HH aide maintains the client's oxygen rate at 2 L/min.
    3. The HH aide helps the client sit in the orthopneic position.
    4. The HH aide allows the client to sleep in the recliner.

18. Which task would be most appropriate for the HH nurse to delegate to a female HH aide?
    1. Instruct her to change the client's subclavian dressing.
    2. Ask her to reinsert the client's Foley catheter.
    3. Request her to demonstrate ambulation with a walker.
    4. Tell her to get the client up in a chair three times a day.

19. In the local restaurant, the HH nurse overhears one of the HH aides talking to her friend about a client. The HH aide is telling her friend how nice the client is and how beautiful the home is. Which action should the HH nurse take?
    1. Do not approach the HH aide in the restaurant.
    2. Ask the HH aide not to discuss anything about the client.
    3. Contact the HH care agency and report the behavior.
    4. Tell the client the HH aide was violating her confidentiality.

20. The 92-year-old client has a hospital bed in the home and is on strict bed rest. The HH aide cares for the client in the morning 5 days a week. Which statement by the HH aide warrants intervention by the HH nurse?
    1. "I do not give her a lot of fluids so she won't wet the bed."
    2. "I perform passive range of motion exercises every morning."
    3. "I put her on her side so that there will be no pressure on her butt."
    4. "I do not pull her across the sheets when I am moving her in bed."

Managing Clients and Nursing Staff

21. The HH aide calls the HH nurse to report the client has a reddened area on the sacral area. Which intervention should the nurse implement first?
    1. Notify the client's health-care provider.
    2. Visit the client to assess the reddened area.
    3. Document the finding in the client's chart.
    4. Refer the client to the wound care nurse.

22. The 32-year-old male client with a traumatic right above-the-elbow amputation tells the HH he is worried about supporting his family and finding employment since he can't be a mechanic anymore. Which intervention should the nurse implement?
    1. Contact the HH agency's occupational therapist.
    2. Refer the client to the state rehabilitation commission.
    3. Ask the HH agency's social worker about disability.
    4. Suggest he talk to his wife about his concerns.

23. The HH nurse is completing the admission assessment for an obese client diagnosed with a myocardial infarction with comorbid type 1 diabetes and arterial hypertension. Which priority intervention should the nurse implement?
    1. Encourage the client to walk 30 minutes a day.
    2. Request HH registered dietitian to talk to the client.
    3. Refer the client to a cardiac rehabilitation unit.
    4. Discuss the need to lose 1 to 2 pounds a week.

24. The HH director of nurses hears an HH nurse and the occupational therapist loudly disagreeing about the care of a newly admitted client while they are sitting in an area that is accessible to anyone coming into the office. Which action should the director of nurses implement first?
    1. Ask the staff members to move the argument to another room.
    2. Request both individuals to come into the director's office.
    3. Call the secretary with instructions for the staff to quit arguing.
    4. Tell the staff members that arguing is not allowed in the office.

25. The HH nurse is visiting a 62-year-old client diagnosed with type 2 diabetes mellitus. The client shows the nurse an area on his right leg that is reddened, inflamed, and has multiple ant bites. Which priority intervention should the nurse implement?
    1. Clean the area with warm soap and water.
    2. Apply warm moist packs to the right leg.
    3. Elevate the right foot on two pillows.
    4. Have the client see the HCP today.

26. The HH nurse is visiting a female client diagnosed with colon cancer who has had a sigmoid colostomy. The client is crying and tells the nurse that she was told the cancer has spread and she will die very soon. Which intervention should the nurse implement?
    1. Discuss the possibility of being placed on hospice services.
    2. Contact the client's oncologist to discuss the client's prognosis.
    3. Ask the client whether she has planned her funeral services.
    4. Recommend the client get a second opinion concerning her prognosis.

27. The female client diagnosed with diverticulosis called the HH care agency and told the nurse "I am having really bad pain in my left lower stomach and I think I have a fever." Which action should the HH nurse take?
    1. Recommend the client take an antacid and lie flat in the bed.
    2. Instruct one of the HH nurses to visit the client immediately.
    3. Tell the client to have someone drive them to the emergency room.
    4. Ask the client what she has had to eat in the last 8 hours.

28. The HH nurse is admitting a female client diagnosed with myasthenia gravis. The client tells the nurse, "Even with my medication I get exhausted when I do anything." Which intervention should the nurse implement?
    1. Talk to the client's husband about helping around the house more.
    2. Contact the HH occupational therapist to discuss the client's concern.
    3. Allow the client to verbalize her feelings of being exhausted.
    4. Recommend the client make an appointment with her HCP.

29. The HH nurse notes the 88-year-old female client is unable to cook for herself and mainly eats frozen foods and sandwiches. Which intervention should the nurse implement?
    1. Discuss the situation with the client's family.
    2. Refer the client to the HH occupational therapist.
    3. Request the HH aide to cook all the client's meals.
    4. Contact the community Meals on Wheels.

30. Which legal intervention should the nurse implement on the initial visit when admitting a client to the home health-care agency?
    1. Discuss the professional boundary crossing policy with the client.
    2. Provide the client with a copy of the NAHC Bill of Rights.
    3. Tell the client how many visits the client will have while on service.
    4. Explain that the client must be homebound to be eligible for home health care.

1. 1. The nurse should determine what medication the client has taken, but the nurse should first attempt to determine whether the headache is secondary to high blood pressure.
   2. No matter what number the client identifies on the pain scale in the home setting, the nurse must attempt to determine the cause. One way to try to determine the cause or to eliminate a possible cause is to take the client's blood pressure.
   3. If the client's blood pressure is not elevated, the client could take the non-narcotic analgesic acetaminophen (Tylenol), but if the client's blood pressure is elevated, the Tylenol will not help.
   4. **The number 1 risk factor for a CVA is arterial hypertension. Because the client has a history of a CVA and is complaining of a severe headache, which is a symptom of hypertension, the nurse should first take the client's blood pressure. If it is elevated, the client needs to be taken to the emergency department. In the home setting, asking about the pain scale would not affect the care the nurse provides.**

2. 1. This blood pressure—148/92—is elevated, but it would not be life threatening for someone diagnosed with hypertension; therefore, the nurse would not contact this client first.
   2. A pulse oximeter reading of 93% is low but still within normal limits, and a client with cystic fibrosis, a chronic respiratory condition, would be expected to have a chronically low oxygen level. This client would not need to be contacted first.
   3. The client with CHF would be expected to have edematous feet; this client would not need to be contacted first.
   4. **The client with chronic atrial fibrillation is at risk for pulmonary emboli, a potentially life-threatening complication. Chest pain is a common symptom of pulmonary embolism. The nurse should contact this client first.**

   MAKING NURSING DECISIONS: When deciding which client to assess first, the test taker should determine whether the signs/symptoms the client is exhibiting are normal or expected for the client situation. After eliminating the expected option, the test taker should determine which situation is more life-threatening.

3. 1. Weekly conferences are an important part of the HH team, but this is not the most important information to tell the new HH nurse.
   2. All clients should have an Advance Directive, but it is not mandated by law, and clients can decide not to have one. This is not vital for a nurse to be successful in HH nursing.
   3. **According to the NCSBN NCLEX-RN test blueprint, staff education is part of the management of care. The HH director of nursing should impress on the new HH nurse the importance of motivating a client to learn about any health issues the client has and how to deal with them because the client is responsible for his or her own health. Discovering what motivates the client to want to learn and focusing on what is most important can tax the ingenuity of even the most dedicated HH nurse.**
   4. Coordinating the client's care is an important part of the HH nurse's responsibility, but it is not vital.

4. 1. A severe, pounding headache would be priority for a client with a T-6 or above spinal cord injury (SCI) because it could be autonomic dysreflexia, but not in a client with a lower-level lesion.
   2. **As in the acute care setting, at times the client with a psychosocial need is priority over a client with physiologic problems that are expected with the disease process. This client should be visited first.**
   3. The nurse would expect a client with COPD to be short of breath, so this client would not need to be visited first.
   4. The nurse would expect a client with type 2 diabetes mellitus to have signs/symptoms of diabetic neuropathy, such as numbness in the legs. This client does not need to be visited first.

5. 1. The nurse's first intervention is to assist the client to a sitting position to decrease the workload of the heart by decreasing venous return and maximizing lung expansion. This will, it is hoped, help relieve the client's respiratory distress.
   2. The nurse should assess the client's vital signs, but the first intervention is to help the client breathe.
   3. The nurse should contact the paramedics if the client does not get better after being placed in a sitting position, but this is not the nurse's first intervention.
   4. The nurse should auscultate the client's lungs, but the first intervention is to help the client breathe more easily.

   MAKING NURSING DECISIONS: The nurse should remember that if a client is in distress and the nurse can do something to relieve the distress, that should be done first, before assessment. The test taker should select an option that directly helps the client's condition.

6. 1. The HH nurse can contact the agency's chaplain to provide spiritual support for the client's family, but the first intervention is to pronounce the client's death.
   2. Nurses in home health have been given the authority to pronounce death for client's who are on service and death is imminent. This action should be implemented first.
   3. The family should be able to stay at the bedside, but if for some reason they need to leave, the nurse's asking them to leave is not the first intervention. The nurse can assess the apical pulse with the family at the bedside.
   4. The client's funeral home needs to be contacted, but it is not the nurse's first action, and often the family will call the funeral home.

7. 1. A client with AIDS would be expected to have Kaposi's sarcoma; therefore, this client would not need to be visited first.
   2. A client with dementia would be expected to have difficulty dressing; therefore, this client would not need to be visited first.
   3. A client with a venous stasis ulcer would be expected to have pain; therefore, this client would not need to be visited before the client who is hallucinating.
   4. Hallucinations are not an expected symptom of Parkinson's disease; therefore, this client should be seen first.

Hallucinations are sometimes an adverse effect of anti-parkinsonian medication.

MAKING NURSING DECISIONS: When deciding which client to assess first, the test taker should determine whether the signs/symptoms the client is exhibiting are normal or expected for the client situation. After eliminating the expected options, the test taker should determine which situation is more dangerous for the client.

8. 1. The nurse should document the results in the client's chart, but this is not the nurse's first intervention.
   2. The therapeutic value for INR is 2 to 3; levels higher than that increase the risk of bleeding. The nurse should first contact the client and determine whether she has any abnormal bleeding and then instruct the client to not take any more Coumadin.
   3. The nurse should notify the client's HCP, but the nurse should first determine whether the client has any abnormal bleeding so that can be reported to the HCP.
   4. The client will need to have another INR drawn, but it is not the nurse's first intervention.

   MAKING NURSING DECISIONS: Any time the nurse receives information from another source about a client who may be experiencing a complication, the nurse must assess the client. In this scenario, the nurse assesses by talking to the client on the phone. The nurse should not make decisions about client needs unless the nurse talks to the client.

9. 1. The therapeutic range for INR is 2 to 3; therefore; this client would not need to be contacted first.
   2. The client's serum potassium level is within the normal range—3.5 to 5.5 mEq/L. Therefore, this client would not need to be contacted first.
   3. The client's digoxin level is higher than the therapeutic level for digoxin, which is 0.8 to 2 mg/dL. This client should be contacted first to assess for signs/symptoms of digoxin toxicity.
   4. The glycosylated hemoglobin, which is the average of blood glucose levels over 3 months, should not be more than 8%. This client, with a level of 6%, does not need to be contacted.

   MAKING NURSING DECISIONS: The test taker must know normal laboratory data. See Appendix A for normal laboratory data.

10. 1. Therapeutic communication addresses the client's feelings and attempts to allow the client to verbalize feelings. The client is still grieving over her loss, and the nurse should let her vent feelings.
    2. The social worker may be able to help the client with driving and going back to college, but this is not the nurse's first intervention.
    3. The American Spinal Cord Association is an excellent resource for clients with spinal cord injuries, but the client is still grieving, and the nurse should allow the client to express her feelings.
    4. Attempting to help identify a support system for the client is an appropriate intervention, but the first intervention is to allow the client to vent her feelings.

Delegating and Assigning Nursing Tasks

11. 1. Stockings should be applied after the legs have been elevated for a period of time when the amount of blood in the leg vein is at its lowest. Applying the stockings when the client is sitting in a chair indicates the HH aide does not understand the correct procedure for applying compression stockings.
    2. If a finger cannot be inserted under the proximal end of the stocking, the compression hose is too tight, and the HH worker does not understand the correct procedure for applying the stockings.
    3. The toe opening should be placed on the plantar side of the foot. Placing the toe opening on the top side of the foot indicates the HH aide does not understand the correct procedure for applying compression stockings.
    4. Warm toes mean the stockings are not too tight and there is good circulation. Checking that the toes are warm indicates the HH aide understands the correct procedure for applying the compression stockings.

12. 1. Isometric exercises such as weight lifting increase muscle mass. The HH nurse should not instruct the HH aide to do this type of exercises.
    2. The HH aide may go to the emergency department, but the HH nurse should address the aide's back pain. Many times, the person with back pain does not need to be seen in the emergency room.

3. An occurrence report explaining the situation is important documentation and should be completed. It provides the staff member with the required documentation to begin a workers' compensation case for payment of medical bills. However, the HH nurse on the phone should help decrease the HH aide's pain, not worry about paperwork.
4. The HH aide is in pain, and applying ice to the back will help decrease pain and inflammation. The HH nurse should be concerned about a co-worker's pain. Remember ice for acute pain and heat for chronic pain.

13. 1. Allowing the client to stay in bed is inappropriate because a client with osteoarthritis should be encouraged to move, which will decrease the pain.
    2. A bath at the bedside does not require as much movement from the client as getting up and walking to the shower. This is not an appropriate action for a client with osteoarthritis.
    3. Movement and warm or hot water will help decrease the pain; the worse thing the client can do is not to move. The HH aide should encourage the client to get up and take a warm shower or bath.
    4. Osteoarthritis is a chronic condition, and the HCP could not do anything to keep the client from "hurting all over."

14. 1. The HH aide's responsibility is to care for the client's personal needs, which include assisting with A.M. care.
    2. The HH aide is not responsible for cooking the client's meals.
    3. The HH aide is not responsible for taking the client to appointments. This also presents an insurance problem with the client in the HH aide's car.
    4. Even in the home, the HH nurse should not delegate teaching.

    MAKING NURSING DECISIONS: The nurse cannot delegate assessment, evaluation, teaching, medications, or care of an unstable client to a UAP.

15. 1. If the HH aide is fearful for any reason, the HH aide should not go into the home and should notify the agency. The employee's safety is important. This statement does not require re-teaching.
    2. For safety purposes, the HH aide should be clearly identified when entering the client's neighborhood and home. This statement does not require re-teaching.

3. The HH aide should be able to contact the HH nurse or agency about any potential or actual concerns. This is for the safety of the client as well as the employee. This statement does not require re-teaching.
4. According to the **NCSBN NCLEX-RN** test blueprint, staff education is a component of the management of care. Standard precautions apply in the home as in the hospital. If the HH aide has the potential to touch the client's bodily fluids, then the aide should wear gloves and wash his or her hands. The statement indicates the HH aide needs re-teaching.

16. 1. The client diagnosed with Guillain-Barré syndrome would have been on bed rest for days to weeks and would be in a debilitated state; therefore, reports of being tired all the time would be expected. This client would not require the most experienced nurse.
2. **The client with pressure ulcers requires meticulous nursing care and experience with wounds. The most experienced nurse should be assigned this client.**
3. The client with a laryngectomy has received teaching prior to and after the procedure and would not require extensive teaching or nursing care; therefore, this client would not require the most experienced nurse.
4. Discharge teaching starts on admission into the home health-care agency; therefore, most of the teaching would have been completed, and this client would not need the most experienced nurse.

17. 1. **The client with end-stage COPD usually prefers a cool climate, with fans to help ease breathing. A warm area would increase the effort the client would need to breathe. This action would warrant intervention by the nurse.**
2. The client with end-stage COPD should be maintained on a low oxygen rate, such as 2 L/min to prevent depression of the hypoxic drive. High levels of oxygen will depress the client's ability to breathe. This action would not warrant intervention by the nurse.
3. The client will usually sit in the orthopneic position, usually slumped over a bedside table, to help ease breathing. This is called the three-point stance. This action

would not warrant intervention by the nurse.
4. The client in end-stage COPD has great difficulty breathing; therefore; sleeping in a recliner is sometimes the only way the client can sleep. This action would not warrant intervention by the nurse.

18. 1. The HH aide cannot perform sterile dressing changes.
2. The HH aide cannot perform sterile procedures.
3. The HH aide cannot teach the client.
4. **The HH aide can transfer the client from the bed to the chair three times a day.**

MAKING NURSING DECISIONS: The nurse cannot delegate assessment, evaluation, teaching, medications, or an unstable client to a UAP.

19. 1. The HH aide is violating HIPAA, and the HH nurse should take action immediately.
2. **The HH nurse should first ask the HH aide not to discuss the client with a friend. Discussing any information about a client is a violation of HIPAA.**
3. The HH nurse should address the HH aide in the restaurant. The HH nurse could tell the HH agency, but the HH nurse must stop the conversation in the restaurant immediately.
4. The HH nurse should not tell the client about the breach of confidentiality.

20. 1. **This statement warrants intervention because fluids will help prevent dehydration and renal calculi. The nurse should explain the client needs to increase fluids.**
2. ROM exercises help prevent deep vein thrombosis (DVT). This statement does not require intervention by the HH nurse.
3. Keeping the client off the buttocks is an appropriate intervention for a client on strict bed rest. This comment does not require intervention by the HH nurse.
4. Pulling the client across the sheets will cause skin breakdown. Because the HH aide is not doing this, no intervention by the HH nurse is needed.

Managing Clients and Nursing Staff

21. 1. The client's HCP may need to be notified, but it is not the nurse's first intervention.

2. The nurse must first assess the reddened area to determine the stage of the pressure ulcer and what treatment should be recommended.
3. The reddened area should be documented in the chart, but this is not the first intervention.
4. The client may or may not need to be referred to a wound care nurse, but it is not the nurse's first intervention. If the reddened area is stage 1 or 2, the wound care nurse probably would not be notified.

MAKING NURSING DECISIONS: Anytime the nurse receives information about a client that must be confirmed, this client becomes a priority to assess.

22. 1. The occupational therapist assists the client with activities of daily living, not with employment concerns.
2. **The NCSBN NCLEX-RN test blueprint lists referrals under management of care. After a client has been injured and is unable to return to previous employment because of the injury, the rehabilitation commission of each state will help evaluate the client and determine whether the client is eligible to receive training or education for another occupation.**
3. The client is not asking about disability but rather about employment. The nurse needs to refer the client to the appropriate agency.
4. The client should discuss his concerns with his wife, but the nurse should refer the client to an agency that can address his concerns about employment.

23. 1. The client should be encouraged to exercise, but it should be in a supervised setting such as a cardiac rehabilitation unit because the client has diabetes and hypertension.
2. The client should adhere to a low-fat, low-cholesterol, carbohydrate-counting diet, but this is not the priority intervention. The client needs to be in a supervised setting, and diet teaching is included in cardiac rehabilitation.
3. **The NCSBN NCLEX-RN test blueprint lists referrals under management of care. Cardiac rehabilitation includes progressive exercise, diet teaching, and classes on modifying risk factors. This supervised setting would be the priority intervention for this client when the client is discharged from HH.**
4. The client should lose weight slowly, but the priority intervention for this client

would be a referral to a supervised setting where the client can lose weight slowly and safely.

24. 1. Moving the staff members to another room will just allow the argument to continue. This is not the director's first intervention.
2. **The director should intervene and listen to both staff members' concerns and attempt to help resolve the disagreement. This is the director's first intervention.**
3. The director should not ask another staff member to intervene in the argument. The director should address the professional staff about the unprofessional behavior.
4. The director should not act unprofessionally and correct the staff in front of everyone in the office. This should be done in private.

MAKING NURSING DECISIONS: In any business, arguments should not occur among staff of any level where the customers or other staff can hear or see it.

25. 1. This is an appropriate intervention, but the priority intervention is to have the client see the HCP today.
2. Warm moist packs cause dilatation, which is needed, but it is not the priority intervention because the client needs medical treatment.
3. Elevating the foot above the heart will decrease edema, but it is not the priority intervention because the client needs medical treatment.
4. **The priority intervention for the HH nurse is to make sure the client sees an HCP today. The client with type 2 diabetes is a risk for delayed wound healing and must be placed on antibiotics. The HH nurse's responsibility is to assess clients in the home and make sure those clients who have a condition that needs immediate medical attention receive it.**

26. 1. Hospice is a service for clients who have less than 6 months to live. If the client has been told she will die "very soon," then this is probably less than 6 months. If the client does not die within the 6 months, she will not automatically be discharged from hospice. Each client is assessed individually for the need to remain on hospice. If the client does not want any heroic measures and wants to

die at home, then hospice will provide these services. This intervention would be appropriate for the HH nurse.

2. The HH nurse is not responsible for discussing the client's prognosis. The oncologist would have to write a letter stating the client had less than 6 months to live to be placed on hospice services. The client should discuss this with the oncologist, not the HH nurse.

3. Because the client is crying and upset, it would be more appropriate for the nurse to discuss a plan for living and hospice services than to discuss what is going to happen after she dies. At some point this should be done, but this is not an appropriate time.

4. The client does have a right to a second opinion, but the nurse should not tell the client this unless the client is questioning the diagnosis.

27. 1. The client is having signs/symptoms of diverticulitis, which can be potentially life threatening; therefore, the client should get medical assistance immediately.

2. The client needs to be seen by a medical doctor to be prescribed antibiotics; therefore, there is no reason for an HH nurse to visit the client.

3. **The HH nurse must have knowledge of disease processes. The client is verbalizing signs of acute diverticulitis, which requires the client to be NPO and prescribed antibiotics. The client needs to receive immediate medical attention.**

4. The client is verbalizing signs/symptoms of acute diverticulitis, which requires medical attention. It does not matter what the client has had to eat.

28. 1. The client has a chronic illness. The nurse should empower the client to deal with her disease process, not put more responsibility on her husband.

2. **The occupational therapist could assist the client in identifying ways to save energy when performing activities of daily living. Myasthenia gravis is a neurological condition that causes skeletal muscle weakness.**

3. The HH nurse should realize that exhaustion is a symptom of her disease process and should utilize any member of the home health-care team who could help the client. Allowing the client to verbalize her feelings about exhaustion is

an appropriate therapeutic intervention, but this client needs specific advice on how to handle her exhaustion.

4. If the client is taking her medication, she does not need to be referred to her HCP. Myasthenia gravis is a chronic illness, and muscle weakness is the primary symptom.

29. 1. The nurse should not make the client dependent on family members to prepare meals. If the family were willing to do this, they would probably already be doing it.

2. The occupational therapist would teach the client how to cook, but this client is 88 years old and needs meals provided. Therefore, providing meals through Meals on Wheels is the most appropriate intervention.

3. The HH aide's duties do not include cooking all three meals for the client.

4. **Meals on Wheels delivers a hot, nutritionally balanced meal once a day on week days, usually at noon for older people who do not have assistance in the home for food preparation. This intervention would be most helpful to the client.**

30. 1. HH care agency employees are responsible for knowing and adhering to the professional boundary crossing standards. The nurse should not discuss this with the client.

2. **Home health-care agencies are required by law to address the concepts in the National Association for Home Care (NAHC) Bill of Rights with all home health clients on the initial visit. The agencies may also make additions to the NAHC's original bill of rights.**

3. The nurse should discuss this with the client, but it is not a legal intervention.

4. This is a true statement, but it is not a legal intervention. If the client is not homebound, he or she is not eligible for home health care.

MAKING NURSING DECISIONS: The nurse is responsible for knowing and complying with local, state, and federal laws and standards of care.

COMPREHENSIVE EXAMINATION

1. The HH nurse enters the yard of a client and is bitten on the leg by the client's dog. Which intervention should the nurse implement first?
   1. Clean the dog bite with soap and water and apply antibiotic ointment.
   2. Obtain the phone number and contact the client's veterinarian.
   3. Contact the HH care agency and complete an occurrence report.
   4. Ask the client whether the dog has had all the required vaccinations.

2. The HH nurse is visiting a client diagnosed with arterial occlusive disease. Which statement by the client would warrant immediate intervention by the nurse?
   1. "My legs start to hurt when I walk to check my mail."
   2. "My legs were so cold I had to put a heating pad on them."
   3. "I hang my legs off the side of my bed when I sleep."
   4. "I noticed that the hair on my feet and up my leg is gone."

3. The HH nurse has completed a home assessment on the client and finds out there are no smoke detectors in the home. The client tells the nurse they just cannot afford them. Which action should the nurse implement first?
   1. Purchase at least one smoke detector for the client's home.
   2. Notify the HH care agency social worker to discuss the situation.
   3. Ask the client whether a family member could buy a smoke detector.
   4. Contact the local fire department to see whether they have smoke detectors.

4. The HH nurse is admitting a 72-year-old female client and notes multiple bruises on the face, arms, and legs along with possible cigarette burns on her upper arms. The client states she fell on the ashtray and doesn't want to talk about it. Which intervention is priority?
   1. Document the objective findings in the client's chart.
   2. Tell her she must talk about the situation with the nurse.
   3. Report the situation to the Adult Protective Services.
   4. Take photographs of the bruises and cigarette burns.

5. The client who sustained a severe head injury was referred to the HH care agency. The client's wife is concerned about what to do if he has a seizure as he did in the hospital. Which statement indicates the wife understands the most important action to take if her husband has a seizure?
   1. "I should check to see if my husband urinates on himself."
   2. "I will move all the furniture out of his way."
   3. "I will call 911 as soon as the seizure begins."
   4. "I will make sure he rests after the seizure is over."

6. The HH nurse is admitting a client diagnosed with a DVT. Which statement by the client warrants immediate intervention by the nurse?
   1. "I take baby aspirin every day at breakfast."
   2. "I have ordered me a medic alert bracelet."
   3. "I eat spinach and greens at least twice a week."
   4. "I got a new recliner so I can elevate my legs."

7. The HH nurse is preparing for the initial visit to a client diagnosed with congestive heart failure. Which intervention should the nurse implement first?
   1. Prepare all the needed equipment for the visit.
   2. Call the client to arrange a time for the visit.
   3. Review the client's referral form/pertinent data.
   4. Make the necessary referrals for the client.

8. Which information should the experienced HH nurse discuss when orienting a new nurse to HH nursing?
   1. If the client or family is hostile or obnoxious, call the police.
   2. Carry the HH care agency identification in a purse or wallet.
   3. Visits can be scheduled at night with permission from the agency.
   4. Inform the agency of the times of the client's scheduled visits.

9. The client with a sigmoid colostomy has an excoriated area around the stoma that has not improved for more than 2 weeks. Which intervention is most appropriate for the HH nurse to implement?
   1. Refer the client to the wound care nurse.
   2. Notify the client's health-care provider.
   3. Continue to monitor the stoma site.
   4. Place Karaya paste over the excoriated area.

10. The HH nurse is admitting a female client diagnosed with end-stage renal disease who refuses to be placed on hemodialysis. The client is ready to die but verbalizes having so many regrets in her life. Which intervention would be most appropriate for the nurse?
    1. Contact the agency chaplain to come talk to the client.
    2. Call her church pastor and discuss the client's concerns.
    3. Ask the client whether she would like to pray with the nurse.
    4. Determine whether the client has an Advance Directive.

11. The HH agency director of nursing is making assignments for the nurses. Which client should be assigned to the HH nurse new to HH nursing?
    1. The client diagnosed with AIDS who is dyspneic and confused.
    2. The client who does not have the money to get prescriptions filled.
    3. The client with full-thickness burns on the arm who needs a dressing change.
    4. The client complaining of pain who is diagnosed with diabetic neuropathy.

12. The HH nurse along with an HH aide is caring for a client who is 3 week postoperative for open reduction and internal fixation of a right hip fracture. Which task would be appropriate for the nurse to delegate to the aide?
    1. Instruct the HH aide to palpate the right pedal pulse.
    2. Ask the HH aide to change the right hip dressing.
    3. Tell the HH aide to elevate the right leg on two pillows.
    4. Request the HH aide to mop the client's bedroom floor.

13. The HH nurse tells the director of the HH care agency that the nurses are upset and arguing over how the clients are being assigned by the assistant director. Which statement indicates a democratic leadership style?
    1. "My assistant makes the assignments and I support how she does it."
    2. "As long as there are no complaints from the clients I will not interfere."
    3. "I appreciate you telling me about the situation and I will handle it."
    4. "I will schedule a meeting and we will all sit down and discuss the situation."

14. The HH aide tells the HH nurse that the grandson of the client she is caring for asked her out on a date. Which statement is the HH nurse's best response?
    1. "I am so excited for you; he seems like a very nice young man."
    2. "You should not go out with him as long as she is a client of our agency."
    3. "I think you should tell the director of the HH care agency about this date."
    4. "You should never date someone you meet while taking care of a client."

15. The HH nurse's primary responsibility is teaching the client diagnosed with congestive heart failure. Which teaching interventions should the nurse discuss with the client? Select all that apply.
    1. Notify the HCP if the client gains more than 2 lbs in one day.
    2. Keep the head of the bed elevated when sleeping.
    3. Take the loop diuretic once a day before going to sleep.
    4. Teach the client which foods are high in sodium and should be avoided.
    5. Perform isotonic exercises at least once a day.

16. The client tells the HH nurse, "My oncologist told me they can't do anything else for my cancer. I do not want my children to know, but I had to tell someone. You won't tell them, will you?" Which statement is the nurse's best response?
    1. "Since you told me about the prognosis, I must talk to your children."
    2. "I don't think it is a good idea not to tell your children; they should know."
    3. "I will not say anything to your children, but I will contact the HH doctor."
    4. "You are concerned I might talk to your children about your prognosis."

17. The male client with peripheral vascular disease tells the female HH nurse, "I know my foot is really bad. My doctor told me I don't have any choice and I must have an amputation, but I don't want one." Which action supports the HH nurse's being a client advocate?
    1. Support the medical treatment, and recommend he have the amputation.
    2. Recommend the client talk to his wife and children about his decision.
    3. Explain that he has a right to a second opinion if he doesn't want an amputation.
    4. Tell the client she will go with him to discuss his decision with the doctor.

18. The multidisciplinary team is meeting to discuss a client with right-sided weakness who has developed a pressure ulcer over the sacral area that is not healing. Which priority intervention should the client's HH nurse recommend?
    1. Recommend the client get a hospital bed with a trapeze bar.
    2. Recommend an HH aide provide care 7 days a week for the client.
    3. Recommend the client's being transferred to a skilled nursing unit.
    4. Recommend a referral to the HH care agency wound care nurse.

19. The HH aide tells the HH nurse that the client is having problems getting out of the bed to the chair and is now having problems getting into the shower. Which intervention should the nurse implement?
    1. Ask the HH aide whether the bathroom has grab bars.
    2. Assess the client's ability to transfer in the home.
    3. Instruct the HH aide to give the client a bed bath.
    4. Contact the agency physical therapist about the situation.

20. The female HH nurse finds that the client is not at home at the scheduled time. The neighbor told the nurse the client went to the mall to do some shopping. Which intervention is most appropriate?
    1. Tell the neighbor to inform the client she was at the home.
    2. Notify the agency that the client should be discharged from service.
    3. Leave a note on the client's door that the HH nurse was there.
    4. Reschedule the visit when it is convenient for the client.

1. 1. The nurse should first take care of the bite and then determine whether the dog is up to date on the required vaccinations. The nurse should be concerned about the possibility of rabies.
   2. If the dog is not up to date on the required vaccinations, then the veterinarian should be notified to quarantine the dog to check for rabies.
   3. The nurse should complete an occurrence report and document the dog bite. If the nurse must pay for anything concerning the dog bite, it should be covered by workers' compensation.
   4. Beside an infection of the dog bite, the worst complication would be the nurse's contracting rabies. If the dog is up to date on the required vaccinations, then this should not be a concern.

2. 1. This would not warrant immediate intervention because intermittent claudication, pain when walking, is the hallmark sign of arterial occlusive disease.
   2. **This comment warrants immediate intervention because the client's legs have decreased sensation secondary to the arterial occlusive disease, and a heating pad could burn the client's legs without the client's realizing it. The client should not use a heating pad to keep the legs warm.**
   3. Hanging the legs off the bed helps increase the arterial blood supply to the legs, which, in turn, helps decrease the leg pain. This comment would not warrant immediate intervention by the nurse.
   4. Hair growth requires oxygen, and the client has decreased oxygen to the legs; therefore, decreased hair growth would be expected and not require immediate intervention.

3. 1. The nurse cannot purchase supplies for the client. This is professional boundary crossing.
   2. The social worker does assist with financial concerns and referrals for the client, but purchasing smoke detectors is not within the social worker's scope of practice.
   3. The nurse should not encourage the client to be dependent on family members for purchasing supplies for the client's home. This may be a possibility when all other avenues have been pursued.
   4. **The nurse should contact the fire department. Many fire departments will** supply and install smoke detectors for people who cannot afford them. The nurse should investigate this option first because it is the most immediate response to the safety need.

4. 1. The nurse should document the objective findings in the chart, but this is not the priority intervention.
   2. The nurse cannot force the client to talk about the situation.
   3. **The bruises and burns should make the nurse suspect elder abuse, and the nurse is mandated by law to report this to Adult Protective Services.**
   4. The nurse should let Adult Protective Services take pictures of the suspected abuse because there is a legal chain of custody that must be followed if the case goes to court.

5. 1. The wife should check to determine whether the client is incontinent of urine, but the client's safety is priority.
   2. **The most important action the wife can take if her husband has a seizure is to make sure he does not get injured during the seizure. Moving all the furniture out of the way will help ensure the client's safety.**
   3. Seizures are not life threatening. If the wife calls 911, the ambulance will probably arrive after the client's seizure has ended. Seizures lasting longer than 4 to 5 minutes warrant calling 911.
   4. The client should be allowed to rest after the seizure when he is in the postictal state, but it is not the most important action to take. Safety of the client during the seizure is priority.

6. 1. **Aspirin, an antiplatelet agent, puts the client at risk for bleeding. The client diagnosed with deep vein thrombosis will be on warfarin (Coumadin), an anticoagulant, which puts the client at risk for bleeding; therefore, this comment requires immediate intervention by the nurse.**
   2. The client should wear a medic alert bracelet to notify any emergency HCP of the client's condition and medication. This statement would not warrant immediate intervention.
   3. Most books recommend not eating green leafy vegetables that are high in vitamin K, because is it the antidote to Coumadin toxicity. The client would have to eat green

leafy vegetables more than twice a week to counteract the Coumadin; therefore, this comment would not warrant immediate intervention as much as the client's taking daily aspirin.

4. Elevating the client's legs would not warrant intervention by the nurse.

7. 1. The nurse should prepare the needed equipment, but it is not the nurse's first intervention.

2. The nurse should call and arrange a time convenient for the visit, but the nurse should first review the client referral so the nurse is aware of the need for the visit.

3. **The nurse should review the client's referral form and other pertinent data concerning the client's condition first before taking any further steps. The nurse may need to contact the referring agency if the information is unclear or if important information is missing.**

4. The nurse will not know which referrals will be needed until after the first visit.

8. 1. If the client or family is intoxicated, hostile, or obnoxious, the nurse should leave and reschedule the visit. There is no need to call the police unless the nurse thinks he or she will be hurt.

2. The HH nurse should wear the agency identification on the shirt or blouse; it should be visible to anyone talking to the nurse.

3. To be eligible for HH visits, the client must be homebound, and all visits should be done in the daylight hours as a safety precaution.

4. **The agency should be informed of the schedule so the nurse can be located if the nurse does not return when expected.**

9. 1. **According to the NCSBN NCLEX-RN test blueprint under management of care, the nurse should be knowledgeable of referrals. The wound care nurse is trained to care for clients with colostomy and is knowledgeable in treating complications.**

2. The most appropriate intervention is to refer the client to a member of the multidisciplinary team who has expertise in the area in which the client is having the problem. In this case, the wound care nurse has the expertise to care for the stoma site.

3. After 2 weeks, the nurse should obtain further assistance in treating the stoma site.

4. Karaya paste will not be effective in treating the excoriated area; therefore, this is not an appropriate intervention.

10. 1. **The NCSBN NCLEX-RN test blueprint includes referrals under management of care. The client is in spiritual distress, and the chaplain is the member of the team who addresses spiritual needs.**

2. The nurse should not discuss the client's concerns with the client's pastor. The nurse should contact the agency chaplain, and then, if needed, the agency chaplain could talk to the client's pastor.

3. This is crossing professional boundaries. The nurse should not impose his or her religious beliefs on the client. If the client asks the nurse to pray, then the nurse could—but the nurse should not ask the client to pray.

4. The client is verbalizing thoughts about dying, not asking questions about Living Wills. This would not be an appropriate intervention.

11. 1. Dyspnea and confusion are not expected with a client diagnosed with AIDS; therefore, this client would warrant a more experienced nurse to assess the reason for the complications.

2. The client with financial problems should be assigned to a social worker, not to a nurse.

3. A full-thickness (third-degree) burn is the most serious burn and requires excellent assessment skills to determine whether complications are occurring. This client should be assigned to a more experienced nurse.

4. **The client diagnosed with diabetic neuropathy would be expected to have pain; therefore, this client could be assigned to a nurse new to home health nursing. The client is not exhibiting a complication or an unexpected sign/symptom.**

12. 1. The nurse cannot delegate assessment to the HH aide.

2. The HH aide cannot assess the incisional wound, and the wound should be assessed. The nurse cannot delegate assessment.

3. **The HH aide can place the right leg on two pillows. This task does not require assessment, teaching, or evaluating, and the client is stable.**

4. Mopping the floor is not part of the HH aide's responsibility. This is not an appropriate task to delegate.

13. 1. This statement does not allow the nurses to have any input into the assignments; therefore, this is the statement of an autocratic manager. These managers use an authoritarian approach to direct the activities of others.
   2. Laissez-faire managers maintain a permissive climate with little direction or control. Allowing the assistant to have total control is laissez-faire management. Supporting the assistant in front of the nurse is an appropriate action, but it does not address the needs of the field nurses.
   3. This statement does not support a democratic leadership style. It is more autocratic: the director is going to take care of the problem.
   4. **Democratic managers are people oriented and emphasizes efficient group functioning. The environment is open, and communication flows both ways. Meetings to discuss concerns illustrate a democratic leadership style.**

14. 1. This is professional boundary crossing. Even though the grandson is not the client, he is related to the client. The HH aide should not go out with him.
   2. **This statement protects the HH aide. This is professional boundary crossing. The employee should not date any relatives of the client because this may pose a conflict of interest. The HH aide should wait until the client is no longer on service.**
   3. The nurse's best response is to tell the HH aide the facts about dating relatives of clients. The director would tell the HH aide the same information.
   4. The HH aide could date the grandson when the client is no longer on service. So this statement is not the nurse's best response.

15. 1, 2, 4, and 5 are correct.
   1. **A 2-lb weight gain indicates the client is retaining fluid and should contact the HCP. This is an appropriate teaching intervention.**
   2. **Keeping the head of the bed elevated will help the client breathe easier; therefore, this is an appropriate teaching intervention.**
   3. The loop diuretic should be taken in the morning to prevent nocturia. This is not an appropriate teaching intervention.
   4. **Sodium retains water. Telling the client to avoid eating foods high in sodium is an appropriate teaching intervention.**

5. **Isotonic exercise, such as walking or swimming, helps tone the muscles, and discussing this with the client is an appropriate teaching intervention.**

16. 1. If the nurse talks to the children, then the nurse has violated HIPAA and the client's right to confidentiality.
   2. The client has a right to decide whether she wants her children to know her prognosis. The nurse should not try to talk the client into changing her mind.
   3. **The nurse cannot say anything to the children but should discuss the client with the HCP to determine a plan of care.**
   4. This is a therapeutic response used to prompt the client to verbalize feelings, which may be appropriate. However, in this case, the client is asking a direct question, and the nurse should answer the question directly.

17. 1. The HH nurse should be a client advocate and support the client's wishes, not support the HCP's recommendation even if it is best for the client.
   2. Recommending the client talk to his family may be an appropriate action, but it does not support the HH nurse's being a client advocate.
   3. The client does have a right to a second opinion, but this action is not supporting the client's decision not to have an amputation and thus is not client advocacy.
   4. **This action is being the client's advocate. Offering to go talk to the HCP about the amputation and making sure the HCP hears the client's opinion is being a client advocate. Another discussion may change the client's decision, but either way, client advocacy is supporting the client's decision.**

18. 1. The client may benefit from a hospital bed, but this is not the priority intervention to address the client's nonhealing pressure ulcer.
   2. HH care agencies do not provide care 7 days a week. Even if the client could have an HH aide 7 days a week, it is not the priority intervention to address the client's nonhealing pressure ulcer.
   3. The client does not need to be transferred to a skilled nursing unit. The wound care nurse should attempt to heal the pressure ulcer in the home first.

4. The wound care nurse's primary role is to address nonhealing pressure ulcers. This referral is the priority intervention.

19. 1. Grab bars address safety issues, but the client is having transfer difficulty, which requires the help of the physical therapist.
2. In most situations, the nurse should assess the client prior to taking action, but the HH aide has the ability and knowledge to determine if the client is having problems getting out of the bed and into the shower. The nurse should allow the physical therapist to assess the client's transfer ability.
3. The goal of HH nursing is to keep the client as independent as possible, and having the client receive a bed bath is increasing the client's dependency on the HH aide.
4. **The NCSBN NCLEX-RN test blueprint includes referral under management of care. The physical therapist is the member of the health-care team who is responsible for helping the client with mobility issues.**

20. 1. It is not the neighbor's responsibility to tell the client the nurse was at the client's home.
2. **One of the requirements for home health-care eligibility is the client must be homebound. If the client is well enough to go to the mall to shop, then the client does not need to be receiving home health-care services.**
3. This is not the nurse's most appropriate intervention; the nurse should follow policy and report the client is at the mall.
4. The nurse should not reschedule the visit because the client should no longer be eligible for home health-care services.

Mental Health Setting

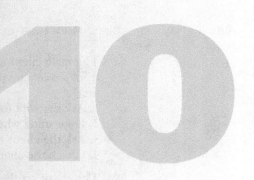

"All the kindness which a man puts out into the world works on the heart and thoughts of mankind."

—Albert Schweitzer

ABBREVIATION LIST

AMA	Against Medical Advice	**MHW**	Mental Health Worker (unlicensed assistive personnel)
ECT	Electroconvulsive Therapy		
ED	Emergency Department	**OTC**	Over-the-Counter
HCP	Health-Care Provider	**prn**	As Needed
HIPAA	Health Insurance Portability and Accountability Act	**RN**	Registered Nurse
		SANE	Sexual Assault Nurse Examiner
IM	Intramuscular	**UAP**	Unlicensed Assistive Personnel
LPN	Licensed Practical Nurse	**WBC**	White Blood Cell

PRACTICE QUESTIONS

Setting Priorities When Caring for Clients

1. The nurse in the outpatient psychiatric unit is returning phone calls. Which client should the psychiatric nurse call first?
   1. The female client diagnosed with histrionic personality who needs to talk to the nurse about something very important.
   2. The male client diagnosed with schizophrenia who is hearing voices telling him to hurt his mother.
   3. The male client diagnosed with major depression whose wife called and said he was talking about killing himself.
   4. The client diagnosed with bipolar disorder who is manic and has not slept for the last 2 days.

2. The nurse is caring for children in a psychiatric unit. Which client requires immediate intervention by the psychiatric nurse?
   1. The 10-year-old child diagnosed with oppositional defiant disorder who refuses to follow the directions of the mental health worker (MHW).
   2. The 5-year-old child diagnosed with pervasive developmental disorder who refuses to talk to the nurse and will not make eye contact.
   3. The 7-year-old child diagnosed with conduct disorder who is throwing furniture against the wall in the day room.
   4. The 8-year-old mentally retarded child who is sitting on the playground and eating dirt and sand.

3. The male client diagnosed with major depression is returning to the psychiatric unit from a weekend pass with his family. Which intervention should the nurse implement first?
   1. Ask the wife for her opinion of how the visit went.
   2. Determine whether the client took his medication.
   3. Ask the client for his opinion of how the visit went.
   4. Check the client for sharps or dangerous objects.

4. The client on the psychiatric unit is yelling at other clients, throwing furniture, and threatening the staff members. The charge nurse determines the client is at imminent risk for harming the staff/clients and instructs the staff to place the client in seclusion. Which intervention should the charge nurse implement first?
   1. Document the client's behavior in the nurse's notes.
   2. Instruct the MHWs to clean up the day room area.
   3. Obtain a restraint/seclusion order from the HCP.
   4. Ensure that none of the other clients were injured.

5. A woman comes to the emergency department (ED) and tells the triage nurse she was raped by two men. The woman is crying, disheveled, and has bruises on her face. Which action should the triage nurse implement first?
   1. Ask the client whether she wants the police department notified.
   2. Notify a Sexual Assault Nurse Examiner (SANE) to see the client.
   3. Request an ED nurse to take the client to a room and assess for injuries.
   4. Assist the client to complete the emergency department admission form.

6. The nurse is working in an outpatient mental health clinic and returning phone calls. Which client should the psychiatric nurse call first?
   1. The client diagnosed with agoraphobia who is calling to cancel the clinic appointment.
   2. The client diagnosed with a somatoform disorder who has numbness in both legs.
   3. The client diagnosed with hypochondriasis who is afraid she may have breast cancer.
   4. The client diagnosed with post-traumatic stress disorder who is threatening his wife.

7. The psychiatric nurse is working in an outpatient mental health clinic. Which client should the nurse intervene with first?
   1. The client who had a baby 2 months ago and who is sitting alone and looks dejected.
   2. The client whose wife just died and who wants to go to heaven to be with her.
   3. The client whose mother brought her to the clinic because the mother thinks the client is anorexic.
   4. The client who is rocking compulsively back and forth in a chair by the window.

8. The emergency department nurse is assessing a female client who has a laceration on the forehead and a black eye. The nurse asks the man who is with the client to please leave the room. The man refuses to leave the room. Which action should the nurse take first?
   1. Tell the man the client needs to go to the x-ray department.
   2. Notify hospital security and have the man removed from the room.
   3. Explain that the man must leave the room while the nurse checks the client.
   4. Give the client a brochure with information about a woman's shelter.

9. The charge nurse received laboratory data for clients in the psychiatric unit. Which client data warrants notifying the psychiatric health-care provider?
   1. The client on lithium (Eskalith) whose serum lithium level is 1.0 mEq/L.
   2. The client on clozapine (Clozaril) whose white blood cell count is 13,000.
   3. The client on alprazolam (Xanax) whose potassium level is 3.7 mEq/L.
   4. The client on quetiapine (Seroquel) whose glucose level is 128 mg/dL.

10. The client diagnosed with a panic attack disorder in the busy day room of a psychiatric unit becomes anxious, starts to hyperventilate and tremble, and is diaphoretic. Which intervention should the nurse implement first?
    1. Administer the benzodiazepine alprazolam (Xanax).
    2. Discuss what caused the client to have a panic attack.
    3. Escort the client from the day room to a quiet area.
    4. Instruct unlicensed assistive personnel (UAP) to take the client's vital signs.

Delegating and Assigning Nursing Tasks

11. The clinical manager assigned the psychiatric nurse a client diagnosed with major depression who attempted suicide and is being discharged tomorrow. Which discharge instruction by the psychiatric nurse would warrant intervention by the clinical manager?
    1. The nurse provides the client with phone numbers to call if needing assistance.
    2. The nurse makes the client a follow-up appointment in the psychiatric clinic.
    3. The nurse gives the client a prescription for a 1-month supply of antidepressants.
    4. The nurse tells the client not to take any over-the-counter medications.

12. The charge nurse is caring for clients in an acute care psychiatric unit. Which client would be most appropriate for the charge nurse to assign to the licensed practical nurse (LPN)?
    1. The client diagnosed with dementia who is confused and disoriented.
    2. The client diagnosed with schizophrenia who is experiencing tardive dyskinesia.
    3. The client diagnosed with bipolar disorder who has a lithium level of 2.0 mEq/L.
    4. The client diagnosed with chronic alcoholism who is experiencing delirium tremens.

13. Which task would be inappropriate for the psychiatric charge nurse to delegate to the MHW?
    1. Instruct the MHW to escort the client to the multidisciplinary team meeting.
    2. Ask the MHW to stay in the day room and watch the clients.
    3. Tell the MHW to take care of the client on a 1-to-1 suicide watch.
    4. Request the MHW to draw blood for a serum carbamazepine (Tegretol) level.

14. The male client in the psychiatric unit asks the MHW to mail a letter to his family for him. Which action would warrant intervention by the psychiatric nurse?
    1. The MHW tells the client to place the letter in the mailbox.
    2. The MHW informs the client he cannot send mail to his family.
    3. The MHW takes the letter and places it in the unit mailbox.
    4. The MHW reports the client mailed a letter at the team meeting.

15. The male client admitted to the medical unit after a motor vehicle accident admits using heroin. The UAP tells the nurse the client is really agitated, anxious, and has slurred speech. Which intervention should the nurse implement first?
    1. Assess the client for heroin withdrawal.
    2. Ask the UAP to take the client's vital signs.
    3. Notify the client's health-care provider.
    4. Administer chlordiazepoxide (Librium), an antianxiety medication.

16. Which task would be most appropriate for the psychiatric nurse to delegate to the MHW?
    1. Request the MHW to take the client with lithium toxicity to the emergency room.
    2. Have the MHW sit with a client diagnosed with bulimia for 1 hour after the meal.
    3. Encourage the MHW to teach the client how to express his or her anger in a positive way.
    4. Ask the MHW to sit with the client while the client talks to his mother on the telephone.

17. The psychiatric charge nurse is making shift assignments for the admission unit. The staff includes one registered nurse (RN), two LPNs, four MHWs, and a unit secretary. Which assignment would be most appropriate to assign to the LPN?
    1. Update the client's individualized care plans.
    2. Stay in the lobby area and watch the clients.
    3. Administer routine medications to the clients.
    4. Transcribe the admission orders for a client.

18. The MHW has tried to calm down the client on the psychiatric unit who is angry and attempting to fight with another client. The nurse observes the MHW "taking down" the client to the floor. Which intervention should the nurse implement?
    1. Assist the MHW with the "take down" of the client.
    2. Call the hospital security to come and assist the MHW.
    3. Document the client "take down" in the nurse's notes.
    4. Remove the other clients from the day room area.

19. The MHW reports to the psychiatric nurse that two clients were kissing each other while watching the movie in the lobby area. Which action should the nurse implement?
    1. Tell the MHW to tell the clients not to kiss each other again.
    2. Discuss the inappropriate behavior at the weekly team meeting.
    3. Transfer one of the clients to another psychiatric unit.
    4. Talk to the clients about kissing each other in the lobby area.

20. The nurse is caring for clients in the psychiatric unit. Which task would be most appropriate for the nurse to delegate to the MHW?
    1. Instruct the MHW to walk with the client who is agitated and anxious.
    2. Ask the MHW to clean up the floor where the client has urinated.
    3. Tell the MHW to phone the HCP to obtain a prn medication order.
    4. Request the MHW to explain seizures precautions to another staff member.

Managing Clients and Nursing Staff

21. The nurse on the substance abuse unit is administering medications. Which client would the nurse question administering the medication?
    1. The client admitted for alcohol detoxification who is receiving lorazepam (Ativan) and has an apical pulse of 110.
    2. The client admitted for heroin addiction who is receiving methadone (Methadose) and has a respiratory rate of 22.
    3. The client admitted for opioid withdrawal who is receiving clonidine (Catapres) and has a blood pressure (BP) of 88/60.
    4. The client diagnosed with Wernicke-Korsakoff syndrome receiving intravenous thiamine (vitamin B_1) who has an oral temperature of 96.8°F.

22. The psychiatric nurse overhears an MHW telling a client diagnosed with schizophrenia, "You cannot use the phone while you are here on the unit." Which action should the psychiatric nurse take?
    1. Praise the MHW for providing correct information to the client.
    2. Tell the MHW this is not correct information in front of the client.
    3. Explain to the MHW that the client does not lose any rights.
    4. Discuss this situation at the weekly multidisciplinary team meeting.

23. The client diagnosed with bipolar disorder is admitted to the psychiatric unit in an acute manic state. The nurse needs to complete the admission assessment, but the client is restless, very energetic, and agitated. Which intervention should the nurse implement?
    1. In a very firm voice, ask the client to sit down.
    2. Administer lithium (Eskalith), an antimania medication.
    3. Ask questions while walking and pacing with the client.
    4. Do not complete the admission assessment at this time.

24. The client in the psychiatric setting tells the nurse, "There were so many people at the team meeting; I am not sure what the psychiatric social worker is suppose to do for me." Which statement is the psychiatric nurse's best response?
    1. "The social worker evaluates the effectiveness of the client's medication."
    2. "This person provides activities that promote constructive use of leisure time."
    3. "The social worker will assist you in keeping your job or help you find a new one."
    4. "This person works with your family and community and makes referrals if needed."

25. The male client diagnosed with paranoid schizophrenia is yelling, talking to himself, and blocking the view of the television. The other clients in the day room are becoming angry. Which action should the nurse take first?
    1. Obtain a restraint order from the HCP.
    2. Escort the other clients from the day room.
    3. Administering an intramuscular (IM) antipsychotic medication.
    4. Approach the client calmly along with two MHWs.

26. A young child, Joey, was admitted to the pediatric unit with a fractured jaw, bruises, and multiple cigarette burns to the arms. The mother reported the father hurt the child. A man comes to the nurse's station saying, "I am Joey's father, can you tell me how he is doing?" Which statement is the nurse's best response?
    1. "Your son has a fractured jaw and some bruises but he is doing fine."
    2. "I am sorry I cannot give you any information about your son."
    3. "You should go talk to your wife about your son's condition."
    4. "The social worker can discuss your son's condition with you."

27. During an interview, the female client tells the psychiatric nurse in a mental health clinic, "Sometimes I feel like life is not worth living. I am going to kill myself." Which interventions should the nurse implement? Select all that apply.
    1. Make a no-suicide contract with the client.
    2. Place the client on a 1-to-1 supervision.
    3. Ask the client whether she has a plan.
    4. Commit the client to the psychiatric unit.
    5. Assess the client's support system.

28. The psychiatric nurse is caring for clients on a closed unit. Which client would warrant immediate intervention by the nurse?
    1. The client who refuses to attend the anger management class.
    2. The client who is requesting to go outside to smoke a cigarette.
    3. The client who is nauseated and has vomited twice.
    4. The client who has her menses and has abdominal cramping.

29. The clinical manager wants to reward the staff on the psychiatric unit for having no tardies or absences for 1 month. Which action would be most appropriate for the clinical manager?
    1. Provide pizza, drinks, and dessert for all the shifts.
    2. Post a thank you note on the board in the employee lounge.
    3. Individually acknowledge this accomplishment with the staff.
    4. Place official documentation in each staff's employee file.

30. The nurse is working in an outpatient psychiatric clinic. The male client tells the nurse, "I am going to kill my wife if she files for divorce. I know I can't live without her." Which action should the nurse implement?
    1. Take no action because this is confidential information.
    2. Document the statement in the client's nurse's notes.
    3. Inform the client's psychiatric health-care provider (HCP) of the comment.
    4. Encourage the client to talk to his wife about the divorce.

Setting Priorities When Caring for Clients

1. 1. The client with a histrionic personality has excessive emotionality and seeks attention. Her saying "something important" must be understood within this context and would not warrant the psychiatric nurse's calling this client first.
   2. **The nurse should contact this client first because the client realizes the voices are telling him to hurt his mother. The nurse should inform this client to come to the clinic immediately, and he should be admitted to a psychiatric unit.**
   3. Because the wife called the clinic, the client is being watched and should be safe from killing himself. The nurse should call this client immediately but not before a client who made the phone call and who may be by himself and hearing voices.
   4. The nurse should expect the client who is manic not to be sleeping; therefore, this is expected behavior. The nurse should call this client immediately but not before the client who is hearing voices telling him to hurt his mother.

2. 1. Oppositional defiant disorder consists of a pattern of uncooperative, defiant, and hostile behavior toward authority figures. Not following the MHW's directions would be expected behavior in a child diagnosed with this disorder and would not require immediate intervention by the nurse.
   2. Refusal to talk and/or make eye contact is a sign of autism, the best known of the pervasive developmental disorders; therefore, this client would not require immediate intervention by the nurse.
   3. **The child with conduct disorder is aggressive to people and animals, bullies, threatens, destroys property, and sets fires. The child's throwing furniture could endanger the child or other clients. This behavior warrants immediate intervention.**
   4. Eating dirt and sand is pica, or the ingestion of non-nutritive substances such as paint, hair, cloth, leaves, sand, clay, or soil. It is commonly seen in mentally retarded children, but it is not life threatening unless a medical complication such as a bowel obstruction, infection, or a toxic condition (e.g., lead poisoning) occurs. This behavior would not require immediate intervention.

MAKING NURSING DECISIONS: When deciding which client to assess first, the test taker should determine whether the signs/symptoms the client is exhibiting are normal for the client's situation. After eliminating the expected options, the test taker should determine which situation is more life threatening.

3. 1. The nurse should discuss how the visit went, but it is not the first intervention.
   2. The nurse should make sure the client took his medications during the weekend pass, but it is not the first intervention.
   3. The client should discuss how the visit went, but it is not the first intervention.
   4. **The nurse's first intervention should be to ensure the client's safety by checking to make sure the client has no sharps or dangerous objects that he could use to hurt himself because he is diagnosed with major depression.**

4. 1. The nurse must document the client's behavior that prompted the need for seclusion, but it is not the first intervention.
   2. The day room area should be cleaned up, but it is not the nurse's first intervention.
   3. **The use of restraints and seclusion requires a HCP's order every 24 hours. The nurse must obtain this order first after placing the client in the seclusion room. The nurse can place the client in seclusion for the safety of the client/staff/other clients, but the nurse must then immediately obtain a HCP's order.**
   4. The charge nurse should make sure the other clients are not injured, but the first intervention is to keep the client who is acting out safe and legally put into seclusion.

5. 1. The client may or may not want the police notified, but this is not the triage nurse's first intervention. The triage nurse should first care for the client.

2. The SANE nurse is a nurse who is specialized in caring for clients who have been raped. The SANE nurse is able to spend time with the client, is knowledgeable of legal issues, and would be an appropriate intervention, but it is not the triage nurse's first intervention.
3. The triage nurse's first intervention is to address the client's physiologic needs, which means to assess for any type of trauma or injury.
4. The client can complete the admission form while in the room; the triage nurse's first intervention should be to care for the client, not paperwork.

MAKE NURSING DECISIONS: When the question asks which intervention to implement first, the test taker should determine whether any of the options concern the physiologic needs of the client and then apply Maslow's Hierarchy of Needs to find the correct answer. Remember, physiologic needs take priority over all other needs.

6. 1. The client with agoraphobia is afraid to leave the house; therefore, canceling a clinic appointment would be expected of this client. The nurse would not need to return this client's phone call first.
2. The client with a somatoform disorder has physical symptoms without a physiologic cause; therefore, complaining of numbness in the legs is expected behavior. The nurse would not need to return this client's phone call first.
3. The client with hypochondriasis is preoccupied with the fear that one has or will get a serious disease; fearing breast cancer is then expected behavior. The nurse would not need to return this client's phone call first.
4. Post-traumatic stress disorder is an illness that occurs to someone who has experienced a traumatic event. The client feels a numbing of general responsiveness but has outbursts of anger. The nurse should return this call first and assess the situation to determine whether the client should be seen in the clinic.

MAKING NURSING DECISIONS: When deciding which client to assess first, the test taker should determine whether the signs/symptoms the client is exhibiting are normal or expected for the client situation. After eliminating the expected options, the test taker should determine which situation is more life threatening.

7. 1. The client who is depressed would be expected to look dejected; therefore, the nurse would not need to assess this client first.
2. This client who says he wants to go to heaven to be with his wife may be suicidal and should be assessed first to see whether he has a plan.
3. This client needs to be assessed for anorexia but not before a client who may be suicidal.
4. The nurse should not interrupt a client who is acting compulsively. The nurse should wait until the client finishes the behavior before talking to the client.

8. 1. The nurse needs to remove the man from the room so that the nurse can talk to the client and discuss probable abuse. Taking the client to the x-ray department may not rouse suspicion in the man and may allow the client to discuss the situation.
2. This may be needed, but it is not the first intervention. This action may cause the man to get angrier in the emergency room department, or it may cause more problems for the woman if she goes home with him.
3. The nurse could demand the man leave the room, but this action may cause the man's anger to escalate; therefore, the first intervention is to remove the client from the room.
4. The nurse should not allow the man to see the nurse discussing a woman's shelter with the client or providing a client with a brochure. This could cause further anger in the man, especially if the woman goes home with the man.

9. 1. The therapeutic serum level for lithium is 0.6 to 1.5 mEq/L. Because the client's 1.0 mEq/L level is within normal limits, the charge nurse would not need to notify the psychiatric HCP.
2. The WBC count is elevated, which may indicate that the client is experiencing agranulocytosis, a life-threatening complication of clozapine. This laboratory data would warrant notifying the psychiatric health-care provider.
3. The client's serum potassium level is within normal limits; therefore, this laboratory data does not warrant notifying the psychiatric health-care provider.
4. This glucose level is slightly elevated but would not warrant notifying the psychiatric health-care provider.

10. 1. This is an appropriate medication for an anxiety attack, but it will take at least 15 to 30 minutes for the medication to treat the physiologic signs/symptoms. Therefore, this is not the first intervention.
2. The nurse should discuss the panic attack and what prompted it, but it is not the nurse's first intervention.
3. The first intervention is to remove the client from the busy day room to a quiet area to help decrease the anxiety attack.
4. The client's vital signs should be taken, but this is not the nurse's first intervention.

Delegating and Assigning Nursing Tasks

11. 1. Providing phone numbers for the client and family is an intervention that the nurse should discuss with the client and would not warrant intervention by the clinical manager.
2. Follow-up appointments are important for the client after being discharged from a psychiatric facility; therefore, this instruction would not warrant intervention by the clinical manager.
3. The client should be given a 7-day supply of antidepressants because safety of the client is priority. As antidepressant medications become more effective, the client is at a higher risk for suicide; therefore, the nurse should ensure that the client cannot take an overdose of medication. This instruction warrants intervention by the clinical manager.
4. The client should not take any OTC medications without talking to the HCP or pharmacist. This instruction would not warrant intervention by the clinical manager.

12. 1. The client diagnosed with dementia would be expected to have confusion and disorientation; therefore, the LPN could be assigned this client. This client is not experiencing any potentially life-threatening complication of dementia.
2. The client is experiencing tardive dyskinesia, a potentially life-threatening complication of antipsychotic medication. An experienced RN should be assigned to this client.

3. The therapeutic serum level for lithium is 0.6 to 1.5 mEq/L. The client's level is toxic, and an experienced RN should care for the client.
4. This client is experiencing a potentially life-threatening complication of alcohol withdrawal. An experienced RN should be assigned to this client.

MAKING NURSING DECISIONS: The test taker must determine which client is the most stable, which makes this an "except" question. Three clients are either unstable or have potentially life-threatening conditions.

13. 1. Clients are allowed, encouraged, and expected to participate in the multidisciplinary team meeting. This is an appropriate task to delegate to the MHW.
2. One of the MHW's primary responsibilities is to watch clients in the day room area. This is an appropriate task to delegate.
3. The MHW can remain with a client who is on 1-to-1 suicide watch. This is an appropriate nursing task to delegate.
4. The MHW does not draw blood, and this would be an inappropriate task to delegate. The laboratory technician draws the client's blood work.

14. 1. Telling the client to place the letter in the mailbox is empowering the client to take responsibility. This action would not warrant intervention by the nurse.
2. The nurse should explain to the MHW that mental health clients retain all of the civil rights afforded to all persons, except the right to leave the hospital in the case of involuntary commitments. The client has the right to mail and receive letters.
3. Mailing the client's letter is an appropriate action to take; therefore, this would not warrant intervention by the nurse.
4. Reporting the client mailed a letter to his family at the team meeting may or may not be pertinent to the client's care, but this action would not warrant intervention by the nurse.

15. 1. Whenever the nurse is given information that indicates a complication or is potentially life threatening, the nurse must first assess the client.
2. The client is unstable; therefore, the nurse should not instruct the UAP to take the client's vital signs.
3. The nurse should not notify the healthcare provider before assessing the client.

4. Librium is a medication used for alcohol withdrawal, not for heroin withdrawal.

MAKING NURSING DECISIONS: If the test taker wants to select "notify the HCP" as the correct answer, the test taker must examine the other three options. If information in any of the other options is data the HCP would need to make a decision, then the test taker should eliminate the "notify the HCP" option.

16. 1. The client with lithium toxicity is unstable, and the nurse should not delegate this task to an MHW.
    2. **Having someone stay with the client after a meal will prevent the client from inducing vomiting and could be delegated to an MHW. The client diagnosed with bulimia needs someone there to prevent vomiting, which is a sign of this mental health problem.**
    3. The nurse should not delegate teaching. Helping the client with anger management would be the responsibility of the nurse or possibly the therapy department.
    4. The client has a right to talk to his mother on the phone without someone listening.

17. 1. The RN should be assigned to update the individualized care plans.
    2. The MHW should be assigned to watch the clients in the day area.
    3. **The LPN's scope of practice allows the administration of medication. This is an appropriate assignment.**
    4. The LPN can transcribe HCP's orders, but the unit secretary can also transcribe orders, which the RN/LPN can co-sign. This would not be the most appropriate assignment for the LPN.

18. 1. All psychiatric staff members are taught how to "take down" a client physically if the client is a danger to himself or herself or to others. The nurse should assist the MHW in subduing the client so that no one is injured.
    2. The psychiatric staff members are trained to deal with clients who are angry and aggressive; there is no need to contact hospital security.
    3. The nurse can document the occurrence, but because the nurse observed the "take down," the nurse should assist the MHW. The psychiatric staff members have to be able to depend on each other no matter what the situation.

4. The nurse can have other staff members remove clients from the day room area; the psychiatric nurse should help the MHW with the "take down."

19. 1. The nurse should address the behavior with the clients and not delegate this task to the MHW. This inappropriate behavior needs further investigation to determine whether it is consensual or under duress.
    2. The inappropriate behavior should be addressed immediately with both clients.
    3. If the behavior does not stop, one of the clients may need to be transferred to another unit, but this is not the appropriate action at this time.
    4. **The nurse needs to talk to the clients to determine whether the kissing was consensual or under duress. Either way, the behavior is inappropriate, and the clients should be told there is no kissing or sexual activity allowed between clients while they are hospitalized on the psychiatric unit.**

20. 1. **The MHW could walk with the client who is agitated. This may help decrease the client's agitation and anxiety.**
    2. The nurse should not assign a task that is the responsibility of another staff member. The housekeeping or custodial department should be assigned to clean the floor.
    3. The MHW cannot take or transcribe phone orders from a HCP. This must be done by a licensed nurse.
    4. The nurse cannot delegate teaching to an MHW. The nurse should explain seizure precautions to staff members.

MAKING NURSING DECISIONS: The nurse cannot delegate assessment, evaluation, teaching, administering medications, or the care of an unstable client to UAP.

Managing Clients and Nursing Staff

21. 1. Lorazepam is used to prevent delirium tremens, and an elevated pulse would not warrant questioning administering this medication.
    2. Methadone is prescribed to prevent withdrawal symptoms from heroin addiction, and an increased respiratory rate would not warrant questioning administering this medication.

3. Clonidine is administered primarily to treat hypertension but is also used to reduce the symptoms of withdrawal from opioids, nicotine, and alcohol. The nurse would question administering this medication because of the client's low blood pressure, no matter why it is being prescribed.
4. Thiamine is used to diminish Wernicke-Korsakoff encephalopathy, which is characterized by confusion, memory loss, and loss of cranial nerve function resulting from chronic alcohol abuse. The nurse would not question giving this medication to a client with Wernicke-Korsakoff syndrome, and a subnormal temperature would not warrant questioning administering this medication.

22. 1. This is not correct information; therefore; the nurse should not praise the MHW.
2. The psychiatric nurse should not correct the MHW in front of the client because it will compromise the MHW's authority with the client.
3. **The nurse should explain to the MHW that the mental health client retains all of the civil rights afforded to all persons, except the right to leave the hospital in the case of involuntary commitments. The client may have phone calls restricted if that is included in the care plan—for example, if the client is calling and threatening the president.**
4. This situation does not need to be discussed at the weekly team meeting. The psychiatric nurse can discuss this on a one-to-one basis with the MHW.

23. 1. The client has a chemical imbalance in the brain, and a firm voice will not be effective in getting the client to sit down. The client cannot sit still.
2. This is the medication of choice, but it takes up to 3 weeks to become therapeutic; therefore, this intervention would not help the nurse complete the admission assessment.
3. **Walking or pacing with the client will allow the client to work off energy and may decrease restlessness and agitation. The nurse should implement this intervention to obtain information for the admission assessment.**
4. The nurse must obtain an admission assessment; therefore, the nurse should walk and pace with the client while attempting to obtain the priority admission assessment.

24. 1. Evaluating the effectiveness of a client's medication is primarily the role of the psychiatric nurse, psychologist, and psychiatrist, not the social worker.
2. The recreational therapist helps the client to balance work and play in his or her life and provides activities that promote constructive use of leisure or unstructured time.
3. The vocational therapist helps the client with job-seeking or job-retention skills as well as with the pursuit of further education if needed and desired.
4. **According to the NSCBN referrals area content on the NCLEX-RN test blueprint, the psychiatric social worker may conduct therapy and often has the primary responsibility for working with families, for community support, and for referrals.**

25. 1. The first intervention should be to talk to the client and remove him from the day room to the least restrictive environment. Restraining the client is the most restrictive environment.
2. The nurse should first attempt to talk to the client and remove the client from the day room area, not try to remove all the other clients.
3. The client will probably need a prn medication to calm the behavior, but it is not the nurse's first intervention. An intramuscular medication takes at least 30 minutes to become effective.
4. **The first intervention is to approach the client calmly and attempt to remove him from the day room. Staff members should not approach the agitated client alone but should be accompanied by other personnel.**

26. 1. This child has been abused, and until Child Protective Services have been notified, the nurse should not share any information with the child's father.
2. **The Health Insurance Portability and Accountability Act (HIPAA) considers parents the "personal representative" of the minor child with the right to information. However, there are exceptions to this rule, including when the provider reasonably believes that the minor may be a victim of abuse or neglect by the parents/guardians. This statement is the nurse's best response.**
3. Because the mother is accusing the father of the abuse, this is not an appropriate response.

4. The social worker must adhere to HIPAA regulations; therefore; referring the father to the social worker will not help the father find out how is son is doing.

MAKING NURSING DECISIONS: The nurse is responsible for knowing and complying with local, state, and federal standards of care.

27. 1, 3, and 5 are correct.
    1. A no-suicide contract is one of the first interventions the nurse implements with the client. It states that if the client feels suicidal, he or she will talk to someone and will not take action on the thoughts.
    2. This is the most stringent form of supervision in which one staff person per shift is assigned to be no greater than one arm's length away from the client. This would be implemented in an inpatient psychiatric unit, not an outpatient clinic.
    3. The nurse should ask the client whether she has a plan. The more the specific the plan is, the more seriously the statement should be taken.
    4. The nurse cannot commit to a psychiatric unit every client with thoughts of killing himself or herself. The nurse must assess the lethality, the absolute possibility, and the available support systems prior to committing a client to the psychiatric unit. After the nurse requests an emergency commitment, the client must be evaluated by a psychiatrist.
    5. The nurse should assess the client's support system and the type of help each person or group can give the client such as hotlines, church groups, and self-help groups, as well as family members.

28. 1. This client should be instructed to go to the anger management class, but this does not warrant immediate intervention.
    2. The MHW could escort the client outside to smoke, but this does not warrant immediate intervention by the nurse.
    3. This client who is nauseated and has vomited has a physiologic problem that should be assessed by the nurse immediately. This client warrants immediate intervention.
    4. A client who has her menses, or "period," may experience abdominal cramping and would need to be assessed but not before the client who has vomited twice.

29. 1. Because the clinical manager wants to reward the unit for no absences or tardies, the manager must reward all shifts, so providing a thank you meal to all shifts would be most appropriate. This allows all the staff members to celebrate the unit accomplishment.
    2. A thank you note is a nice action, but knowing the clinical manager took the time to arrange for the meal means a lot to staff members. The meal could encourage the staff to try and do the same the next month.
    3. Individually telling the staff "job well done" is a possible action to take, but for the clinical manager to take the time to arrange for the meal on all shifts is above and beyond just saying thank you to each individual staff member.
    4. Having no absences or tardies for 1 month for an individual employee is the expected behavior. The fact the entire unit had no absences/tardies is what is being acknowledged.

30. 1. The nurse must take action to protect the wife.
    2. The statement can be documented, but this is not the appropriate action for the nurse to implement.
    3. Mental health clinicians have a duty to warn identifiable third parties of threats made by a person even if these threats were discussed during a therapy session (Tarasoff v. Regents of the University of California, 1976). The nurse should notify the client's psychiatric HCP so that the wife can be notified of the threat.
    4. The nurse should not encourage this behavior because it could cause serious harm to the wife.

COMPREHENSIVE EXAMINATION

1. The client diagnosed with bipolar disorder and who is prescribed lithium, an antimania medication, is admitted to the psychiatric unit in an acute manic state. Which intervention should the nurse implement first?
   1. Have the laboratory draw a stat serum lithium level.
   2. Evaluate what behavior prompted the psychiatric admission.
   3. Assess and treat the client's physiologic needs.
   4. Administer a stat dose of lithium to the client.

2. The psychiatric unit staff is upset about the new female charge nurse who just sits in her office all day. One of the staff members informs the clinical manager about the situation. Which statement by the clinical manager indicates a laissez-faire leadership style?
   1. "I will schedule a meeting to discuss the concerns of the charge nurse."
   2. "I hired the new charge nurse and she is doing what I told her to do."
   3. "You and the staff really should take care of this situation on your own."
   4. "I will talk to the charge nurse about your concerns and get back to you."

3. The MHW reports that one of the nurses threatened to force-feed the male client diagnosed with schizophrenia if the client did not eat the lunch tray. Which action should the charge nurse take first?
   1. Tell the MHW that this intervention is part of the client's care plan.
   2. Request the nurse to come to the office and discuss the MHW's allegation.
   3. Ask the client what happened between him and the nurse during lunch.
   4. Ask the MHW to write down the situation to submit to the head nurse.

4. The client diagnosed with paranoid schizophrenia is imminently aggressive and is dangerous to self, the other clients, and the psychiatric staff members. The client is placed in a seclusion room. Which interventions should the psychiatric nurse implement? Select all that apply.
   1. Assess the client every 2 hours for side effects of medication.
   2. Tell the client what behavior will prompt the release from seclusion.
   3. Do not notify the client's family of the initiation of seclusion.
   4. Explain that the client will be in the seclusion room for 24 hours.
   5. Instruct the MHW to check the client every 10 to 15 minutes.

5. The psychiatric nurse overhears an MHW arguing with a client diagnosed with paranoid schizophrenia. Which action should the nurse implement?
   1. Ask the MHW to go to the nurse's station.
   2. Tell the MHW to quit arguing with the client.
   3. Notify the clinical manager of the psychiatric unit.
   4. Report this behavior to the client abuse committee.

6. Which client should the psychiatric nurse working in a mental health clinic refer to the psychiatric social worker?
   1. The client who was raped and wants help to be able to get on with her life.
   2. The client who is scheduled for the first electroconvulsive therapy treatment.
   3. The client who reports having difficulty going to work every day.
   4. The client who is unable to buy the prescribed antipsychotic medications.

7. The psychiatric nurse has taken 15 minutes extra for the lunch break two times in the last week. Which action should the female clinical manager implement?
   1. Take no action and continue to watch the nurse's behavior.
   2. Document the behavior in writing and place in the nurse's file.
   3. Tell the nurse to check in and out with her when taking lunch.
   4. Talk to the nurse informally about taking 45 minutes for lunch.

8. The client diagnosed with Alzheimer's disease is on a special unit for clients with cognitive disorders. Which assessment data would warrant immediate intervention by the psychiatric nurse?
   1. The client does not know his or her name, date, or place.
   2. The client is unable to dress himself or herself without assistance.
   3. The client is difficult to arouse from sleep.
   4. The client needs assistance when eating a meal.

9. The mother of a client recently diagnosed with schizophrenia asks the nurse, "I was afraid of my son. Will he be all right?" Which response by the psychiatric nurse supports the ethical principal of veracity?
   1. "I can see your fear; you are concerned your son will not be all right."
   2. "If your son takes medication, the symptoms can be controlled."
   3. "Why were you afraid of your son? Did you think he would hurt you?"
   4. "Schizophrenia is a mental illness and your son will not be all right."

10. The nurse is caring for clients in an outpatient psychiatric clinic. Which client would the nurse discuss with the health-care provider?
    1. The client diagnosed with bipolar disorder who is receiving carbamazepine (Tegretol), an anticonvulsant.
    2. The client diagnosed with schizophrenia who reports taking the antacid Maalox daily for heartburn.
    3. The client diagnosed with major depression who is receiving isoniazid (INH), an antituberculosis medication.
    4. The client diagnosed with anorexia nervosa who is receiving amitriptyline (Elavil), a tricyclic antidepressant.

11. The client in the psychiatric unit tells the nurse, "Someone just put a bomb under the couch in the lobby." Which action should the nurse implement first?
    1. Look under the couch for a bomb.
    2. Implement the bomb scare protocol.
    3. Have the staff evacuate the unit.
    4. Tell the client there is no bomb.

12. The new nurse on the psychiatric unit tells the charge nurse, "I don't like how the shift report is given." Which statement is the charge nurse's best response?
    1. "Since you're new I think you should try it our way before making any comments."
    2. "We have been doing the shift report this way since I started working here more than 5 years ago."
    3. "Have you discussed your concerns about the shift report with the other nurses?"
    4. "I would be happy to listen to any ideas you have on how to give the shift report."

13. The client on the psychiatric unit tells the nurse, "I am so bored. I hate just sitting on the unit doing nothing." Which intervention should the nurse implement?
    1. Explain that with time the client will be able to go to the activity area.
    2. Allow the client to ventilate feelings of being bored on the unit.
    3. Notify the psychiatric recreational therapist about the client's concerns.
    4. Tell the client that there is nothing that can be done about being bored.

14. The head nurse in a psychiatric unit in the county emergency department is assigning clients to the staff nurses. Which client should be assigned to the most experienced nurse?
    1. The client who is crying and upset because she was raped.
    2. The client diagnosed with bipolar disorder who is agitated.
    3. The client who was found wandering the streets in a daze.
    4. The client diagnosed with schizophrenia who is hallucinating.

15. The client diagnosed with anorexia is refusing to eat and is less than 20% of normal body weight for her height and structure. The client has not eaten anything since admission 2 days ago. Which action should the nurse implement?
    1. Notify the psychiatrist to request a court order to feed the client.
    2. Take no action because the client has the right to refuse treatment.
    3. Discharge the client because she is not complying with the treatment.
    4. Physically restrain the client and insert a nasogastric tube for feeding.

16. The client on a psychiatric involuntary admission is threatening to run away from the unit. Which intervention should the nurse implement first?
    1. Notify the police department of the client's threats.
    2. Place the unit on high alert for unauthorized departure.
    3. Talk to the client about the threat of running away.
    4. Have the client sign out against medical advice (AMA).

17. The nurse answers the client's phone in the lobby area and the person asks, "May I speak to Mr. Jones?" Which action should the nurse implement?
    1. Ask the caller who is asking for Mr. Jones.
    2. Tell the caller Mr. Jones cannot have phone calls.
    3. Request the caller to give the access code for information.
    4. Find Mr. Jones and tell him he has a phone call.

18. The client seeing the psychiatric nurse in the mental health clinic tells the nurse, "If I tell you something very important, will you promise not to tell anyone?" Which statement is the nurse's best response?
    1. "I promise I will not tell anyone if you don't want me to."
    2. "If it affects your care I will have to tell someone who can help."
    3. "If you don't want me to tell anyone, then please don't tell me."
    4. "Why do you not want me to tell anyone if it is so important?"

19. Which situation would warrant immediate intervention by the charge nurse on the psychiatric unit after receiving the A.M. shift report?
    1. The client diagnosed with paranoid schizophrenia who is delusional.
    2. The P.M. shift LPN called in to say he or she would not be able to work today.
    3. The male MHW reports losing his unit key and identification card.
    4. The unit secretary has HCP's orders that need to be co-signed.

20. The client enters a mental health clinic with a gun and is threatening to kill the nurse who told his wife to leave him. Which action should the nurse implement first?
    1. Instruct a staff member to call the local police department.
    2. Evacuate the clients and staff to a safe and secure place.
    3. Encourage the client to talk about his feelings of anger.
    4. Calmly and firmly ask the man to put the gun down on the floor.

1. 1. The nurse should determine the lithium level, but it is not the first intervention the nurse should implement.
   2. The nurse should assess the behavior that prompted the admission, but this is not the first intervention.
   3. **The nurse should first assess the client's physiologic needs because the client in the manic state may not have slept, bathed, or had anything to eat for days. The client's physiologic needs are priority.**
   4. Lithium takes 2 to 3 weeks to become therapeutic; therefore, a stat dose of lithium orally will not help the client's manic state. This is not the nurse's first intervention.

2. 1. A democratic manager is people oriented and emphasizes efficient group functioning. The environment is open and communication flows both ways, which includes having meetings to discuss concerns.
   2. This statement is that of an autocratic manager who uses an authoritarian approach to direct the activities of others.
   3. **This statement is that of a laissez-faire manager who maintains a permissive climate with little direction or control. Instructing the staff to handle the situation on their own does not support the staff.**
   4. This statement is taking control of the situation; therefore, this is not a statement indicating a laissez faire manager.

3. 1. Unless the client is anorexic and there is a court order, the nurse cannot force-feed a client.
   2. **This is client abuse, and the charge nurse must investigate the allegation immediately with the nurse. If the allegations are true, they should be documented in writing and reported to the client abuse committee.**
   3. The charge nurse should not ask the client about the situation first. The nurse and MHW should be involved in the investigation of the allegation. Then, if needed, the client can be asked about the situation.
   4. The charge nurse should investigate the allegations first and then, if needed, have the MHW write down the situation.

4. 1, 2, and 5 are correct.
   1. **The nurse should assess the client for any injury, side effects of medication, and general well-being every 2 to 4 hours.**
   2. **As soon as possible, the nurse must inform the client of what behavior will allow the client to be released from the seclusion room.**
   3. According to the Joint Commission Restraint and Seclusion Standards for Behavioral Health, the client's family is notified promptly of the initiation of restraint or seclusion.
   4. The nurse's goal is to release the client as soon as possible from the seclusion room. When the client has calmed down and is able to verbalize feelings and concerns in a rational manner, the client should be released. The seclusion order must be renewed every 24 hours, but the client should not be kept for 24 hours unless absolutely necessary.
   5. **Clients must be checked at least every 10 to 15 minutes in person and may be continuously monitored on video cameras.**

5. 1. **The nurse should first separate the MHW from the client; therefore, asking the MHW to go to the nurse's station would be the first intervention.**
   2. The nurse should not correct the MHW in front of the client and should not use the word "arguing"; therefore, this would not be an appropriate action.
   3. The psychiatric nurse should handle this situation immediately. If this is a pattern of behavior of the MHW, then the clinical manager should be notified.
   4. This behavior may or may not need to be reported to the client abuse committee, but if the nurse overhears the MHW and client arguing, the nurse should stop the behavior.

6. 1. The psychiatric social worker can refer clients, but the nurse should assess the client to see what type of help she wants.
   2. The psychiatric social worker does not perform or participate in ECT treatment; therefore, this client should not be referred.
   3. The nurse needs to assess the client to determine why the client is having difficulty going to work. For example, is it sedation secondary to medications?
   4. **The psychiatric social worker can assist with financial arrangements, referrals, and nonphysiologic concerns.**

7. 1. Two times in one week is becoming a pattern of behavior. The clinical manager should talk informally to the nurse to find out what is going on.

2. This is only the second time the nurse has taken 45 minutes for lunch and does not warrant formal counseling. The clinical manager should assess the situation before formally documenting the behavior.

3. This is very punitive behavior for the psychiatric nurse. The clinical manager should talk to the nurse before taking this type of action.

4. **The clinical manager should talk to the nurse informally and find out what is going on. This behavior cannot continue, but it is not behavior that requires anything more than informally finding out why the nurse has been late.**

8. 1. The client diagnosed with Alzheimer's disease would be expected to be confused; therefore, this would not warrant immediate intervention.

2. The client diagnosed with Alzheimer's disease has difficulty completing simple routine activities of daily living. This would not warrant immediate intervention.

3. **The client diagnosed with Alzheimer's disease should not be difficult to arouse from sleep. This is not a typical symptom of this disease and would warrant immediate intervention from the nurse.**

4. The client diagnosed with Alzheimer's disease has difficulty completing simple routine activities of daily living. This would not warrant immediate intervention.

9. 1. This is a therapeutic response that helps the client to ventilate feelings, but this statement does not support the ethical principle of veracity.

2. **Veracity is the ethical principle "to tell the truth." The truth is that schizophrenia is a thought disorder caused by a chemical imbalance of the brain. Antipsychotic medication can control the client's hallucinations and delusions.**

3. This is interviewing the client, and this statement does not support the ethical principle of veracity.

4. Schizophrenia is a mental illness, but if the client takes the antipsychotic medication, the client may be able to work, get married, and live a productive life. This is a false statement.

10. 1. Tegretol is a medication that is often prescribed for clients diagnosed with bipolar disorder even though it is classified as an anticonvulsant. Many times, a medication

with a different classification is prescribed for another disease process.

2. **Antacids neutralize gastric acid and may reduce the effects of antipsychotic medications and lead to medication failure. The client diagnosed with schizophrenia would be on an antipsychotic medication; therefore, the nurse should discuss this client with the psychiatric HCP.**

3. The client receiving antitubercular medications must receive them to prevent resistant strains of tuberculosis and protect the community. The nurse would not need to discuss this client with the HCP.

4. Elavil has shown efficacy in promoting weight gain in clients with anorexia nervosa; therefore, the nurse would not discuss this medication with the HCP.

11. 1. **The nurse must know the bomb scare policy of the facility, and in many cases the nurse looks for the bomb but does not touch it if it is found. In some instances, the nurse should not attempt to look for a bomb, but because the client is on a psychiatric unit, the nurse should look for a suspicious-looking object before notifying the bomb squad and evacuating the clients.**

2. The nurse would implement the bomb scare protocol if there was a bomb or suspicious-looking bag, but the nurse should first investigate the comment because the client is on a psychiatric unit.

3. The nurse would evacuate the clients if a bomb or suspicious-looking bag was under the couch. The nurse should have the clients leave the lobby area, but not the unit.

4. Just because the client is in a psychiatric unit does not mean that someone did or did not put a bomb under the couch. The nurse should look under the couch and take appropriate action.

12. 1. The response is closed and does not allow the new nurse to voice her opinion and be part of the team.

2. The charge nurse should be open to change. Just because something has been done the same way for years does not mean it can't be done another way.

3. The charge nurse should not make the new nurse talk to the other nurses just because she doesn't like the way shift report is done.

4. The best response is to allow the new nurse to share any new ideas with the charge nurse. The charge nurse could then talk to the other staff members and take the change to the clinical manager to determine whether the change should be instituted.

13. 1. The client may eventually be able to go to the activity area, but while the client is confined to the unit, the nurse should refer the client to a recreational therapist to be provided with activities to alleviate boredom.
    2. Allowing the client to ventilate feelings will not help alleviate the client's boredom on the unit.
    3. **According to the NSCBN RN-NCLEX test blueprint, the nurse must be knowledgeable of the multidisciplinary team. The recreational therapist helps the client to balance work and play in his or her life and provides activities that promote constructive use of leisure or unstructured time.**
    4. The nurse should acknowledge the client's concern and contact the recreational therapist.

14. 1. A client who was raped would be expected to be upset and crying. This client would not require the most experienced nurse.
    2. The client who is diagnosed with bipolar disorder would be agitated in the manic state. This client would not require the most experience nurse.
    3. **The client who was found wandering in a daze has no diagnosis and requires an in-depth assessment. This client should be assigned to the most experienced nurse.**
    4. The client diagnosed with schizophrenia would have hallucinations if not taking antipsychotic medication. The client would not require the most experienced nurse.

15. 1. **When a person is admitted to a psychiatric unit, the client does not lose any rights. The client has a right to refuse treatment, but if the client is a danger to herself, then the psychiatric team must go to court and obtain an order to force-feed the client. This could be with nasogastric tube feedings or total parenteral nutrition.**
    2. The client has a right to refuse treatment, but if the client is a danger to herself, then the psychiatric team must intervene. If the client does not eat, the client will die.

3. If the client is discharged and dies, the psychiatric team will be responsible. If a person is mentally ill, the psychiatric team must protect the client.
    4. This is against the client's rights. The nurse cannot restrain a client without a court order.

16. 1. The nurse would notify the police department if the client ran away from the unit.
    2. **The nurse's first intervention is to place the unit on high alert, which includes putting signs on the exit doors warning all people coming in and out that there is a client threatening to leave the unit.**
    3. The nurse should talk to the client, but the first intervention is to prevent the client from making good on the threat of running away.
    4. The client who is on an involuntary admission loses the right to sign out of the psychiatric unit against medical advice (AMA).

17. 1. The nurse does not have a right to ask the caller for his or her name. Mr. Jones has a right to telephone calls.
    2. Mr. Jones retains all his civil rights when admitted to a psychiatric unit unless phone restriction is part of the individualized care plan.
    3. The access code for client information is requested when the caller is asking questions about the client. It is not used when the caller wants to talk directly to the client.
    4. **The nurse should find Mr. Jones and tell him he has a phone call. The client cannot have rights restricted unless it is a part of the client's individualized care plan. For example, the client may not be able to use the phone if he or she is calling 911 and making false reports.**

18. 1. The psychiatric nurse should not make promises he or she cannot keep. If the information must be shared with the health-care team, then the nurse will have to break a promise to the client. This will destroy the nurse-client relationship.
    2. **This is the nurse's best response. The nurse is being honest with the client but will keep the information confidential if it does not affect the client's care.**

3. The client may need to share information that is pertinent to the client's care and should not tell the client he or she cannot talk to the nurse.
4. Asking the client why may put the client on the defensive and he or she would not share the information.

19. 1. The client diagnosed with schizophrenia would be expected to be delusional; therefore, this situation would not warrant immediate intervention.
2. The charge nurse has the entire shift to arrange for another nurse to cover the LPN; therefore, this situation does not warrant immediate intervention.
3. **The loss of a unit key is priority because the nurse must determine when the MHW last had the key and determine whether it may be lost on the psychiatric unit. If a client finds the key, then the unit is no longer secure.**
4. The signing of HCP's orders is important, but it does not warrant immediate intervention.

20. 1. The local police department needs to be called, but the nurse must first talk to the man and attempt to diffuse the situation. This action tries to ensure safety for the man, the other clients, and the staff.
2. Ensuring safety of the other clients and staff is important, but the nurse should first attempt to make contact with the man.
3. The nurse should not encourage the client to talk about his feelings until the gun is removed. The anger may cause the client to shoot an innocent person accidentally or on purpose.
4. **The nurse should first try to talk to the client and diffuse the situation. This action is attempting to ensure the safety of the man, the other clients, and the staff.**

Women's Health Setting

11

"Science may have found a cure for most evils, but it has found no remedy for the worst of them all—the apathy of human beings."

—Helen Keller

ABBREVIATION LIST

C-section	Cesarean Section	**IVP**	Intravenous Push
CBC	Complete Blood Cell Count	**LPN**	Licensed Practical Nurse
CPS	Child Protective Services	**OB**	Obstetric
HCP	Health-Care Provider	**PPD**	Purified Protein Derivative
H&H	Hemoglobin and Hematocrit	**PMS**	Premenstrual Syndrome
		RN	Registered Nurse
HIV	Human Immunodeficiency Virus	**SIDS**	Sudden Infant Death Syndrome
ID	Identification	**UAP**	Unlicensed Assistive Personnel
IV	Intravenous		

PRACTICE QUESTIONS

Setting Priorities When Caring for Clients

1. Which client should the postpartum nurse assess first after receiving the A.M. shift report?
   1. The client who is complaining of perineal pain when urinating.
   2. The client who saturated multiple peri-pads during the night.
   3. The client who is refusing to have the newborn in the room.
   4. The client who is crying because the baby will not nurse.

2. Which newborn infant would warrant immediate intervention by the nursery nurse?
   1. The 1-hour-old newborn who has abundant lanugo.
   2. The 6-hour-old newborn whose respirations are 52.
   3. The 12-hour-old newborn who is turning red and crying.
   4. The 24-hour-old newborn who has not passed meconium.

3. The client in labor is showing late decelerations on the fetal monitor. Which intervention should the nurse implement first?
   1. Notify the health-care provider (HCP) immediately.
   2. Instruct the client to take slow, deep breaths.
   3. Place the client in the left lateral position.
   4. Prepare for an immediate delivery of the fetus.

4. The nurse walks into the client's room to check on the mother and her newborn. The client states another nurse just took her baby back to the nursery. Which intervention should the nurse implement first?
   1. Initiate an emergency Code Pink, indicating an infant abduction.
   2. Request the mother to describe the nurse who took the baby.
   3. Determine whether or not the infant was returned to the nursery.
   4. Ask the mother whether the nurse asked for the code word.

5. The nurse in the labor and delivery department is caring for a client whose abdomen remains hard and rigid between contractions and the fetal heart rate is 100. Which client problem is priority?
   1. Alteration in comfort.
   2. Ineffective breathing pattern.
   3. Risk for fetal demise.
   4. Fluid and electrolyte imbalance.

6. The nurse working in a women's health clinic is returning telephone calls. Which client should the nurse contact first?
   1. The 16-year-old client who is complaining of severe lower abdominal cramping.
   2. The 27-year-old primigravida client who is complaining of blurred vision.
   3. The 48-year-old perimenopausal client who is expelling dark red blood clots.
   4. The 68-year-old client who thinks her uterus is falling out of her vagina.

7. The charge nurse has received laboratory results for clients on the postpartum unit. Which client would warrant intervention by the nurse?
   1. The client whose white blood cell count is 18,000 mm^3.
   2. The client whose serum creatinine level is 0.8 mg/dL.
   3. The client whose platelet count is 410,000 mm^3.
   4. The client whose serum glucose level is 280 mg/dL.

8. The nurse on the postpartum unit is administering AM medications. Which medication should the nurse administer first?
   1. The sliding scale insulin to the client diagnosed with type 1 diabetes.
   2. The stool softener to the client complaining of severe constipation.
   3. The non-narcotic analgesic to the client complaining of headache, rated as "3."
   4. The rectal suppository for the client complaining of hemorrhoidal pain.

9. The labor and delivery nurse is performing a vaginal examination and assesses a prolapsed cord. Which intervention should the nurse implement first?
   1. Place the client in the Trendelenberg position.
   2. Ask the father to leave the delivery room.
   3. Request the client not to push during contractions.
   4. Prepare the client for an emergency C-section.

10. Which newborn infant would the nursery nurse assess first?
    1. The 3-hour-old newborn who weighs 6 pounds and 2 ounces.
    2. The 4-hour-old newborn delivered at 42 weeks' gestation.
    3. The 6-hour-old newborn who is 22 inches long.
    4. The 8-hour-old newborn who was born at 40 weeks' gestation.

Delegating and Assigning Nursing Tasks

11. The female unlicensed assistive personnel (UAP) tells the nurse she has helped the 1-day postpartum client change her peri-pad three times in the last 4 hours. Which action should the nurse implement?
    1. Ask the UAP why the nurse was not notified earlier.
    2. Go to the room and check the client immediately.
    3. Instruct the UAP to massage the client's uterus.
    4. Document the finding in the client's chart.

12. The UAP is assisting the nurse in the newborn nursery. Which action by the UAP would warrant intervention?
    1. The UAP swaddles the infant securely in a blanket.
    2. The UAP uses gloves when changing the infant.
    3. The UAP is bathing the newborn with a bar of soap.
    4. The UAP wipes down the crib with a disinfectant.

13. The charge nurse is making assignment in the labor and delivery department. Which client should be assigned to the most experienced nurse?
    1. The 26-week gestational client who is having Braxton Hicks contractions.
    2. The 32-week gestational client who is having triplets and is on bed rest.
    3. The 38-week gestational client whose contractions are 3 minutes apart.
    4. The 39-week gestational client who has late decelerations on the fetal monitor.

14. Which task should the nurse on the postpartum unit delegate to the UAP?
    1. Instruct the UAP to prepare a sitz bath for the client.
    2. Ask the UAP to call the laboratory for a stat complete blood cell (CBC) count.
    3. Tell the UAP to show the mother how to breast-feed.
    4. Have the UAP check the client's fundus.

15. A nurse from the medical-surgical unit is assigned to the postpartum unit. Which client should the charge nurse assign to the medical-surgical nurse?
    1. The client who has developed mastitis and is trying to breast-feed.
    2. The client who had a vaginal hysterectomy and oophorectomy.
    3. The client who is having difficulty bonding with her infant.
    4. The unmarried client who is giving her child up for adoption.

16. The UAP responds to a code in the newborn nursery. Which task should the house supervisor delegate to the UAP?
    1. Tell the UAP to sit with the family in the waiting room.
    2. Give medication to the nurse from the crash cart.
    3. Assist the nurse anesthetist with intubation.
    4. Instruct the UAP to obtain supplies for the code.

17. Which action by the nursery nurse would warrant immediate intervention by the charge nurse?
    1. The nurse allows an experienced volunteer to rock an infant.
    2. The nurse puts a gloved finger into the newborn's mouth.
    3. The nurse performs the Ortoloni maneuver on the newborn.
    4. The nurse requests the LPN to bathe the newborn infant.

18. The RN and UAP are caring for clients on a postpartum unit. Which task would be most appropriate for the RN to assign to the UAP?
    1. Perform an in-and-out catheterization.
    2. Complete the client's discharge instructions.
    3. Escort the client to the car and check for a car seat.
    4. Spray anesthetic foam on the client's episiotomy.

19. The charge nurse is making assignments on the postpartum unit. Which client should be assigned to the LPN?
    1. The client who has delivered her sixth baby and has just returned to her room.
    2. The client who had a C-section yesterday and is running a low-grade fever.
    3. The client who had a vaginal delivery this morning and has foul-smelling lochia.
    4. The client who is 1-day post vaginal delivery who is ambulating in the hall.

20. The nurse and UAP are caring for babies in the newborn nursery. Which action by the UAP would warrant immediate intervention?
    1. The UAP does not check the mother's identification (ID) band with the infant's ID band.
    2. The UAP brings the mother a full package of newborn diapers.
    3. The UAP applies baby lotion to the newborn while the mother is watching.
    4. The UAP tells the father to support the newborn's head.

Managing Clients and Nursing Staff

21. The client being seen in the obstetric (OB) clinic tells the nurse, "I don't think it is right that the judge is making me get a contraceptive implant just because they don't think I am a good mother." Which ethical principle does the requirement violate?
    1. Autonomy.
    2. Justice.
    3. Fidelity.
    4. Beneficence.

22. The client in labor is diagnosed with pregnancy-induced hypertension and has pre-eclampsia. Which interventions should the nurse implement? Select all that apply.
    1. Monitor the intravenous (IV) magnesium sulfate.
    2. Check the client's telemetry monitor.
    3. Assess the client's deep tendon reflexes.
    4. Administer furosemide (Lasix) intravenous push (IVP).
    5. Notify the nursery when delivery is imminent or has occurred.

23. The father of a newborn infant tells the nurse excitedly, "Someone just took our baby and they didn't know the code word." Which action should the nurse implement first?
    1. Tell the father to remain calm and go back to his wife.
    2. Assign staff members to block all exits from the unit.
    3. Page a Code Pink, indicating an infant abduction.
    4. Question the father about what exactly happened in the room.

24. The client who delivered twins 3 days ago calls the women's health clinic and tells the nurse, "I am having hip pain that makes it difficult for me to walk." Which statement is the nurse's best response?
    1. "I am going to make you an appointment to see the HCP today."
    2. "This often occurs a few days after delivery and will go away with time."
    3. "Are you performing the Kegel exercises 10 to 20 times a day?"
    4. "The pain may decrease if you empty your bladder every 2 hours."

25. The 36-week gestational client has just delivered a stillborn infant. Which intervention should the nurse implement?
    1. Call the sudden infant death syndrome support group.
    2. Refer the client to the maternal child case manager.
    3. Notify the hospital chaplain of the fetal demise.
    4. Contact Child Protective Services.

26. The client who is 20 weeks' gestation comes to the women's health clinic, and the nurse notices bruises on her abdomen and back. Which response is most appropriate for the nurse?
    1. "Please tell me who is abusing you."
    2. "This could cause you to lose your baby."
    3. "How did you get these bruises?"
    4. "Do you feel safe in your home?"

27. The boyfriend comes to the postpartum unit and demands his girlfriend's room number. The nurse can smell alcohol on the man's breath, and he is acting erratically. Which action should the nurse implement?
    1. Explain to the client her boyfriend is causing problems.
    2. Give the boyfriend the client's room number.
    3. Contact hospital security to come to the unit.
    4. Tell the boyfriend that he can't be here if he is drunk.

28. The nurse is caring for a postpartum client who is a Jehovah's Witness and needs a RhoGAM injection. Which question should the nurse ask the client?
    1. "RhoGAM is a blood product. Do you want the injection?"
    2. "Do you know what type blood your husband has?
    3. "Did you know that you have Rh-negative blood?"
    4. "Do you know whether your insurance will pay for the shot?"

29. The nurse is administering medications to clients on a postpartum floor. Which medication should the nurse question administering?
    1. The rubella vaccine to the postpartum client who has a negative titer.
    2. The yearly flu vaccine to a client who reports an allergy to eggs.
    3. The PPD to a client who suspects she was exposed to tuberculosis.
    4. The hepatitis B vaccine to a client who is breast-feeding.

30. Which client would the newborn nursery nurse assess first after receiving shift report?
    1. The newborn who has chignon.
    2. The newborn with caput succedaneum.
    3. The newborn who has a cephalhematoma.
    4. The newborn who has a port-wine stain.

Setting Priorities When Caring for Clients

1. 1. This pain may be related to an episiotomy or perineal tear, but this client is not priority over a client who may be hemorrhaging.
   2. Saturating multiple peri-pads indicates heavy bleeding, which may indicate hemorrhaging. The nurse should assess this client first.
   3. The nurse needs to assess this client for possible maternal/infant bonding problems, but this is a psychosocial issue that should be addressed after a physiologic issue, such as possible hemorrhaging.
   4. This client is going to require some time to be taught, but this is not priority over a client who is hemorrhaging.

   MAKING NURSING DECISIONS: The test taker should apply some systematic approach when answering a priority question. Maslow's Hierarchy of Needs should be used when determining which client to assess first. The test taker should start at the bottom of the pyramid, and physiologic needs are priority.

2. 1. The newborn with lanugo is normal and would not warrant immediate intervention by the nurse.
   2. The normal respiratory rate for a newborn is 30 to 60; therefore, this would not warrant immediate intervention.
   3. The newborn who is turning red when crying is not in distress; therefore, this would not warrant immediate intervention.
   4. The newborn who has not passed meconium 24 hours after birth must be evaluated for intestinal obstruction or a congenital abnormality. This could be caused by an imperforate anus, Hirschsprung's disease, cystic fibrosis, or several other possibilities. This newborn warrants immediate intervention.

   MAKING NURSING DECISIONS: When deciding which client to assess first, the test taker should determine whether the signs/symptoms the client is exhibiting are normal or expected for the client situation. After eliminating the expected options, the test taker should determine which situation is more life threatening.

3. 1. The nurse should first intervene to increase blood supply to the fetus; therefore, notifying the HCP is not the nurse's first intervention.
   2. Slow, deep breaths may help decrease the mother's anxiety, but the nurse's first intervention is to increase blood supply to the fetus.
   3. The left lateral position will improve placental blood flow and oxygen supply to the fetus. This should be the nurse's first intervention.
   4. The nurse should prepare for an emergency C-section, but this is not the nurse's first intervention.

   MAKING NURSING DECISIONS: When the test taker is deciding when to notify an HCP, the test taker should look at the other three options and determine whether one of the options should be implemented prior to notifying the HCP. Another option may, for example, provide information the HCP will need in order to make a decision.

4. 1. Once the nurse definitely determines the infant is not in the nursery, then a Code Pink should be initiated. This notifies all hospital personnel of a possible infant abduction.
   2. This will be done if the infant was not returned to the nursery, but this is not the first intervention.
   3. The nurse should first determine whether another staff member returned the infant to the nursery. The nurse should not call a false alarm.
   4. There are many safety precautions to prevent infant abductions, and most facilities have a code word that is changed daily. The mother must ask anyone who wants to take the infant out of the mother's room for the code word. This is not the nurse's first intervention.

5. 1. Pain for the mother is a priority, but it is not priority over potential death of the fetus.
   2. The client is not having trouble breathing; therefore, this would not be a priority problem. Altered gas exchange would be an appropriate problem for the fetus.

3. The client is exhibiting signs of abruptio placentae, and a decreased heart rate indicates a compromised fetus. This problem will lead quickly to death of the fetus. Therefore, it is the priority problem.

4. All pregnant women experience an increase in fluid volume status and some resulting electrolyte imbalance; therefore, this is not a priority problem.

6. 1. The client with severe lower abdominal cramping should be called to determine whether she is currently menstruating, but this is not priority over a pregnant client with symptoms of pre-eclampsia.

2. Blurred vision is a symptom of pre-eclampsia, and this is the client's first pregnancy. This client should be contacted first and told to come into the clinic for further evaluation.

3. The expulsion of dark red blood clots indicates the client is going through menopause. This is not a life-threatening situation because dark red blood does not indicate frank bleeding.

4. This is uncomfortable for the client and indicates the need for a hysterectomy or instructions in the insertion and use of a pessary device to hold the uterus in place, but it is not life threatening.

MAKING NURSING DECISIONS: When deciding which client to assess first, the test taker should determine whether the signs/symptoms the client is exhibiting are normal or expected for the client situation. After eliminating the expected options, the test taker should determine which situation is more life threatening.

7. 1. The white blood cell count rises normally during labor and post partum—up to 25,000; therefore, this does not warrant intervention.

2. The serum creatinine level is within normal limits; therefore, this client does not warrant immediate intervention.

3. Platelets show marked increase 3 to 5 days after birth, but the client who is 1 to 2 days post partum would have a slightly increased platelet count. Normal platelet count is 150,000 to 450,000, so this client's count is within normal limits.

4. This glucose level is elevated, and the nurse should investigate further as to why the glucose level is abnormal. The normal glucose level is 70 to 120 mg/dL.

8. 1. The client with type 1 diabetes must receive insulin prior to eating; therefore, this must be administered first.

2. The stool softener will take several days to soften the stool; therefore, this medication does not need to be administered first.

3. The client with a headache is not priority over a type 1 diabetic patient who needs sliding scale coverage. This client should receive medication after the insulin-dependent diabetic receives insulin.

4. The rectal suppository is administered to shrink the hemorrhoids and has a local anesthetic effect, but it would not be priority over the sliding scale insulin.

9. 1. A prolapsed cord is an emergency situation because the prolapsed cord could compromise the fetus's blood supply. Placing the client in the Trendelenberg position will cause the fetus to reverse back into the uterus, which will take the pressure off the umbilical cord. The safety of fetus is priority.

2. In emergency situations, the nurse may need to request visitors to leave the delivery room, depending on how visitors are acting during the crisis, but this is not the first intervention.

3. This is an appropriate intervention, but the nurse's priority is getting pressure off the umbilical cord.

4. The fetus is in distress and the nurse must prepare for an emergency C-section, but it is not the nurse's first intervention.

10. 1. The newborn who weighs 6 pounds and 2 ounces is within normal weight for a newborn; therefore, the nurse would not need to assess this baby first.

2. The newborn delivered at 42 weeks is postmature and is at risk for hypoglycemia and hypothermia because the placenta begins to deteriorate after 40 weeks and subcutaneous fat is utilized to support the infant's life. The nurse should assess this baby first just because of the 42-week gestation.

3. The newborn who is 22 inches long is longer than most infants, but this infant would not need to be assessed first.

4. The newborn delivered at 40 weeks gestation is within normal gestation time; therefore, the nurse would not need to assess this baby first.

MAKING NURSING DECISIONS: When deciding which client to assess first, the test taker should determine whether the signs/symptoms the client is exhibiting are

normal for the client situation. After eliminating the expected options, the test taker should determine which situation is more life threatening.

Delegating and Assigning Nursing Tasks

11. 1. The nurse should first assess the client to determine whether the UAP was negligent in reporting before talking to the UAP.
    2. This client may or may not be experiencing excessive bleeding, but the nurse's first intervention is to assess the client.
    3. Excessive bleeding could indicate the uterus is boggy, which would require the nurse to massage the uterus. This assessment and intervention cannot be delegated to a UAP.
    4. The nurse should not document any information before verifying the client situation.

    MAKING NURSING DECISIONS: Any time the nurse receives information from another staff member about a client who may be experiencing a complication, the nurse must assess the client. The nurse should not make decisions about client's needs based on another staff member's information.

12. 1. The infant should be securely swaddled in a blanket to maintain body heat.
    2. The UAP should wear nonsterile gloves when being exposed to blood or body fluids.
    3. When a bathing a newborn, soap is not necessary. Soap can be very drying to the skin; therefore, this action warrants intervention by the nurse.
    4. The UAP should wipe the crib with disinfectant to decrease the potential for contamination.

13. 1. Braxton Hicks contractions are irregular contractions of the uterus throughout the pregnancy and are not true labor. This client would not need to be assigned to the most experienced nurse.
    2. The client having triplets on bed rest is not in imminent danger; therefore, this client would not need the most experienced nurse.
    3. This client is progressing normally and would not require the most experienced nurse.
    4. Late decelerations on the fetal monitor indicate fetal distress; this

is a life-threatening emergency, and an emergency C-section may be necessary. The charge nurse should assign the most experienced nurse to this client.

MAKING NURSING DECISIONS: The test taker must determine which client is the most unstable and assign this client to the most experienced nurse.

14. 1. The UAP can provide hygiene care to the client. A sitz bath requires the UAP to check the temperature of the water and does not require nursing judgment.
    2. The UAP's primary responsibility is direct client care. The unit secretary, not the UAP, should call the laboratory.
    3. The nurse cannot delegate teaching to the UAP.
    4. The nurse cannot delegate assessment; therefore, the UAP cannot check the client's fundus.

    MAKING NURSING DECISIONS: The nurse cannot delegate assessment, evaluation, teaching, administration of medications, or care of an unstable client to a UAP.

15. 1. A client with mastitis who is trying to breast-feed requires a nurse experienced in the postpartum unit who can teach the client about breast-feeding and assess for complications.
    2. This is a routine surgical procedure that would not require the nurse to have any specialized postpartum experience. This client would be most appropriate to assign the float nurse who has experience on the medical-surgical unit.
    3. A client who is having difficulty bonding would require a nurse with experience in the postpartum unit to care for the client as well as document pertinent information if bonding does not occur.
    4. There are many legal issues surrounding an adoption as well as caring for the mother who is giving up her child; this client should be assigned a nurse more experienced in postpartum care.

    MAKING NURSING DECISIONS: The test taker must determine which client requires the least amount of specialized knowledge and assign the float nurse to that client. Remember, legal issues, teaching, and psychosocial concepts require the more experienced nurse.

16. 1. An experienced nurse, a chaplain, or social worker should be assigned to sit with the family during this crisis.

2. Even though the UAP is not administering the medication, the UAP should not be handing the nurse medication in a crisis situation.
3. The UAP cannot assist with intubation; this must be assigned to a nurse or respiratory therapist.
4. **The UAP can stand by and be ready to obtain any supplies needed for the code. This would be a most appropriate task to delegate in an emergency situation.**

17. 1. Volunteers are often asked to rock irritable infants so that the nurse can have more time to perform higher-level nursing care to the infants. This action would not warrant immediate intervention by the charge nurse.
2. The nurse is using palpation to determine whether the newborn has a cleft palate. This assessment is within the scope of the newborn nursery nurse.
3. **The Ortoloni maneuver is performed to assess developmental hip dysplasia. A pediatrician or a nurse practitioner only should perform this maneuver because it can cause further damage if it is done incorrectly.**
4. The LPN can bathe a newborn infant; therefore, this would not warrant immediate intervention by the charge nurse.

18. 1. This client is unable to urinate, which may or may not be a complication of the delivery/anesthesia. Catheterization is a sterile procedure, and many facilities do not allow the UAP to perform sterile procedures. The nurse should not delegate this task.
2. This is teaching, and the nurse cannot delegate teaching to the UAP.
3. **The infant must be transported in a car safety seat. Many facilities will lend or give the client a car seat if one is not available. The UAP can determine whether there is a car seat and take the appropriate action if there is not one.**
4. Anesthetic foam is topical medication, and the nurse cannot delegate medication administration to the UAP.

MAKING NURSING DECISIONS: The nurse cannot delegate assessment, evaluation, teaching, medications, or an unstable client to a UAP.

19. 1. The more pregnancies the client has had, the more likely it will be that the uterus will not contract to prevent bleeding. The RN should be assigned to this client.

2. A client with a fever and a surgical incision may be experiencing a complication and should be assigned to an RN.
3. Foul-smelling lochia indicates the client has an infection; therefore, this client should not be assigned to the LPN.
4. **The client who is ambulating is stable and not exhibiting any complications; therefore, this client should be assigned to the LPN.**

MAKING NURSING DECISIONS: The test taker must determine which client is the most stable, which makes this an "except" question. Three clients are either unstable or have potentially life-threatening conditions.

20. 1. **The Joint Commission and safety standards mandate that all hospital personnel must check the parent's ID band with the infant's ID band before releasing the infant to the care of the mother or father.**
2. The UAP can bring diapers to the mother; therefore, this would not warrant immediate intervention.
3. The UAP can put lotion on the infant while the mother is watching because this is not teaching.
4. This may be teaching, but the UAP is making sure the newborn is safe; therefore, this action would not warrant immediate intervention.

Managing Clients and Nursing Staff

21. 1. **This requirement is violating the client's autonomy, which is a client's right to self-determination without outside control. This approach has been used as a condition of probation, to allow women accused of child abuse/neglect to get out of a jail term.**
2. Justice is the duty to treat all clients fairly, without regard to age, socioeconomic status, and other variables.
3. Fidelity is the duty to be faithful to commitments.
4. Beneficence is the duty to do good actively for the clients.

MAKING NURSING DECISIONS: The nurse must be cognizant of ethical principles that guide nursing and health-care practice. The judge is acting under legal guidelines that can supersede the client's rights.

22. 1, 3, and 5 are correct.
   1. Magnesium sulfate, a uterine relaxant, is the drug of choice to help prevent seizures. The medication relaxes smooth muscles and reduces vasoconstriction, thus promoting circulation to the vital organs of the mother and increasing placental circulation to the fetus.
   2. The mother is not placed on telemetry, but continuous electronic fetal monitoring is required to identify fetal heart rate patterns that suggest fetal compromise.
   3. The deep tendon reflexes are monitored to determine the effectiveness of the magnesium sulfate.
   4. After delivery, the mother will excrete large volumes of fluid, a sign of recovery from pre-eclampsia. However, the loop diuretic Lasix would not be given before delivery because it may lead to hypovolemia.
   5. The nursery should be notified of the delivery so it will be prepared for the neonate. Because the client is in labor, the baby will be born within a reasonable time frame.

23. 1. The nurse should encourage the father to remain calm for his wife in this crisis situation, but this is not the first intervention.
   2. Assigning staff members is part of the Code Pink protocol, but it is not the nurse's first intervention.
   3. The nurse's first intervention is to call a Code Pink. Then, the nurse should institute all other nursing interventions. The infant's safety is priority.
   4. The nurse should question the father for exact details, but the nurse should first call the Code Pink so that the person who took the infant can be found.

   MAKING NURSING DECISIONS: The nurse is responsible for knowing and complying with hospital protocols as well as the local, state, and federal standards of care.

24. 1. This pain is normal and does not require seeing the HCP today.
   2. During the first few days after delivery, levels of the hormone relaxin gradually subside, and the ligaments and cartilage of the pelvis return to their pre-pregnancy position. These changes cause hip and joint pain that interfere with ambulation. The mother should understand that the pain is temporary and does not indicate a problem.

3. Kegel exercises tone up the client's peritoneal muscles after a pregnancy. These exercises would not help hip and joint pain.
   4. Emptying the bladder will not help the client's joint and hip pain.

25. 1. SIDS occurs to infants who are living, not to infants in utero.
   2. The case manager is responsible for coordinating care between disciplines for clients with chronic illnesses. This client has lost a baby and would not need a referral to a case manager.
   3. According to the NCSBN NCLEX-RN test blueprint, management of care includes appropriate use of referrals. The chaplain is responsible for intervening in a case where there is spiritual distress. A loss of a child is devastating.
   4. Child Protective Services (CPS) are notified only if the child is being abused. This baby died in utero; therefore, CPS would not be notified, except in states where the mother is a drug abuser or has chronic alcoholism.

26. 1. This statement is making the assumption the client is being abused—which is probably true—but the nurse should not put words in the client's mouth. Because this is a legal issue, the nurse cannot suggest in any manner, verbally or physically, to the client that abuse is occurring. If the client is being abused and decides to file charges, then the accused can use the defense that indeed he or she was not abusing the client and the client decided to consider his or her actions as abuse only after the nurse suggested it.
   2. This is a true statement, but it is judgmental and would not encourage a therapeutic relationship with the client.
   3. Research indicates that abusive situations escalate during pregnancy, particularly with the woman being hit in the abdominal area; therefore; this question is not necessary. These bruises indicate that abuse is occurring.
   4. The nurse's best intervention is to assess the safety of the client and infant and provide information to the client about a safe haven.

   MAKING NURSING DECISIONS: The nurse is responsible for knowing and complying with local, state, and federal standards of care.

27. 1. The nurse should not upset the client by telling her the boyfriend is creating problems.
    2. The nurse should not allow a person displaying this behavior to remain on the unit.
    3. **The nurse should first contact hospital security to intervene and escort the boyfriend off the unit.**
    4. Confronting a drunken individual could escalate the situation. The nurse should contact security to take care of this situation.

28. 1. **Jehovah's Witnesses do not believe in accepting blood products, but it is the individual's choice. The nurse is a client advocate and should make sure the client is aware that without the injection her next pregnancy could result in erythroblastosis fetalis. However, with the injection her religious belief may be compromised because RhoGAM is a blood product.**
    2. The father of the baby is Rh-positive or the baby would not be Rh-positive and the mother would not require the RhoGAM injection. The baby's blood type determines whether the mother needs the RhoGAM injection.
    3. When administering RhoGAM to the client, this question is not pertinent. RhoGAM is prescribed only for Rh-negative mothers who have Rh-positive babies or within 72 hours of a miscarriage.
    4. The client's insurance status is not pertinent information for the nurse caring for the client.

    MAKING NURSING DECISIONS: Any time there is a cultural or religious factor in the question, the test taker should be aware that this will affect the correct answer.

29. 1. The nurse would not question administering this medication because a negative titer means the client is not immune to rubella (German measles). This vaccine prevents rubella infection and possible severe congenital defects in a fetus in a subsequent pregnancy.
    2. **The flu vaccine is made using duck eggs; therefore, the nurse should question the administration of this vaccine to a client who is allergic to eggs.**
    3. A positive PPD test determines whether the client was exposed to tuberculosis.
    4. The nurse would not question administering the hepatitis B vaccine to a mother who is breast-feeding because 1-day-old infants receive the vaccine.

30. 1. A chignon is newborn scalp edema created by vacuum extraction and will resolve within a few days of delivery. This infant would not need to be assessed first.
    2. Caput succedaneum appears over the vertex of the newborn's head as a result of pressure against the mother's cervix during labor. The edematous area crosses suture lines, is soft, and varies in size. It resolves quickly and disappears within 12 hours to several days after birth. This newborn would not need to be seen first.
    3. **A cephalhematoma results when there is bleeding between the periosteum and the skull from pressure during birth. The firm swelling is not present at birth but develops within the first 24 to 48 hours. Any time a client is bleeding, it warrants intervention by the nurse.**
    4. A port-wine stain, nevus flammeus, is a permanent, flat, reddish purple mark that varies in size and location and does not blanch with pressure. This would not require immediate intervention from the nurse.

COMPREHENSIVE EXAMINATION

1. The nurse volunteering in a free clinic has been caring for a female client for several weeks. The client states, "My husband and I been trying to have a baby for 6 years. What can we do?" Which statement is the nurse's best response?
   1. "You should discuss your concerns with the doctor when he comes in."
   2. "Infertility treatments are very expensive and you would have to pay for it."
   3. "You are concerned because you have not been able to get pregnant."
   4. "Have you tried the rhythm method to try and conceive a child?"

2. Which client should the labor and delivery nurse assess first after receiving report?
   1. The client who is 10 cm dilated and 100% effaced.
   2. The client who is exhibiting early decelerations on the fetal monitor.
   3. The client who is vacillating about whether or not to have an epidural.
   4. The client who is upset because her obstetrician is on vacation.

3. The nurse is caring for clients in a women's health clinic. Which client warrants intervention by the nurse?
   1. The pregnant client who has a hematocrit and hemoglobin of 11/33.
   2. The pregnant client who has a fasting blood glucose level of 110 mg/dL.
   3. The pregnant client who has 3+ proteins in her urine.
   4. The pregnant client who has a white blood cell count of 11,500 mm^3.

4. The client is 1-day post partum, and the nurse notes the fundus is displaced laterally to the right. Which nursing intervention should be implemented first?
   1. Prepare to perform an in-and-out catheterization.
   2. Assess the bladder using the bladder scanner.
   3. Massage the client's fundus for 2 minutes.
   4. Assist the client to the bathroom to urinate.

5. While making rounds, the charge nurse notices the client's chart has been left on the bedside table. Which action should the charge nurse implement first?
   1. Ask the client's nurse who left the chart at the bedside.
   2. Leave the chart at the bedside until talking to the nurse.
   3. Tell the nurse this could be a violation of HIPAA.
   4. Take the client's chart back to the nurse's station.

6. The 27-year-old female client is being scheduled for a chest x-ray. Which question should the nurse ask the client?
   1. "Have you ever had a chest x-ray before?"
   2. "Is there any chance you may be pregnant?"
   3. "When was the date of your last period?"
   4. "Do you have any allergies to shellfish?"

7. The clinical manager is reviewing hospital occurrence reports and notes that the nurse on the postpartum unit has documented three medication errors in the last 2 months. Which action should the clinical manager implement first?
   1. Initiate the formal counseling procedure for multiple medication errors.
   2. Continue to monitor the nurse for any further medication errors.
   3. Discuss the errors with the nurse to determine whether there is a medication system problem.
   4. Arrange for the nurse to attend a medication administration review course.

8. The nursery nurse is assessing newborns. Which newborn would require immediate intervention by the nurse?
   1. The newborn who remains in the fetal position when lying supine.
   2. The newborn whose toes flare out when the lateral heel is stroked.
   3. The newborn whose head turns toward the cheek being stroked.
   4. The newborn who extends the arms when hearing a loud noise.

9. The client on the postpartum unit tells the nurse, "My husband thinks he is the father of my baby but he is not. What should I tell him?" Which response supports the ethical principal of nonmalfeasance?
   1. "You should tell him the truth before he becomes attached to the infant."
   2. "How do you think your husband will feel if he knows he is not the father?"
   3. "I know my husband would want to know if my child was his or not."
   4. "Do you know what the real father is planning on doing about the baby?"

10. The chief nursing officer of the hospital instructed the clinical manager of the postpartum unit to research a change in the system of delivery of care. Which statement best describes modular nursing?
    1. Nurses are designated the primary responsible persons for client care.
    2. A nurse and a UAP are assigned a group of postpartum clients.
    3. Nursing staff members are divided into groups responsible for client care.
    4. Nurses are assigned specific tasks rather than specific clients.

11. Which action by the postpartum clinical manager would be most effective in producing a smooth transition to the new medication delivery system?
    1. Counsel any nurses who cannot adapt to the change.
    2. Ask the staff to vote on accepting the new system.
    3. Have an open-door policy to discuss the change.
    4. Send written documentation of the change by hospital e-mail.

12. During an interview, the pregnant client at the women's health clinic hesitantly tells the nurse, "I think I should let someone know that I can't stop eating dirt. I crave it all the time." Which action should the nurse implement first?
    1. Explain that the behavior is normal.
    2. Ask whether the client is taking the prenatal vitamins.
    3. Check the client's hemoglobin and hematocrit.
    4. Determine whether there is a history of pica in the family.

13. The client who is 16 weeks pregnant calls and tells the office nurse, "My husband's insurance has changed and they say I can't use you anymore." Which statement is the nurse's best response?
    1. "If we continue to see you it will cost you a lot more money."
    2. "Because you are already pregnant your insurance company must pay."
    3. "You are concerned you don't want to change doctors at this time."
    4. "Can your husband get a supplemental policy to cover this pregnancy?"

14. The 16-year-old mother of a 1-day-old infant wants her son circumcised. Which intervention should the nurse implement?
    1. Request the client's mother sign the permit.
    2. Determine whether the insurance will pay for the procedure.
    3. Refer the client to the social worker to apply for Medicaid.
    4. Have the 16-year-old client sign for informed consent.

15. The clinical manager is presenting a lecture on collective bargaining. One of the nurse participants asks, "What happens if nurses decide to go on strike?" Which statement is the clinical nurse manager's best response?
    1. "The UAPs and managers will have to take care of the clients."
    2. "If nurses go on strike it is considered abandonment of the clients."
    3. "The clients will get better care once the nurses' demands are met."
    4. "The nurses must give a 10-day notice before a strike takes place."

16. Which client should the newborn nurse refer to the hospital ethics committee?
    1. The newborn who is anencephalic whose parents want everything done.
    2. The newborn whose 16-year-old mother wants to place the infant up for adoption.
    3. The newborn whose mother is a known cocaine user and is HIV positive.
    4. The newborn who needs a unit of blood and the parents are refusing consent.

17. The client has delivered a 37-week gestation infant whose cord was wrapped around the neck. The infant died in utero. Which interventions should the nurse implement? Select all that apply.
    1. Allow the mother to hold and cuddle the infant.
    2. Have the mother transferred to the medical unit.
    3. Encourage the father to talk about his child to the nurse.
    4. Recommend to the parents that the child be cremated.
    5. Discourage the client from giving the infant a name.

18. Which action would be most important for the clinical manager to take regarding a primary nurse who has received numerous compliments from the clients and their families about the excellent care she provides?
    1. Ask the nurse what she does that makes her care so special.
    2. Document the comments on the nurse's performance evaluation.
    3. Acknowledge the comments with a celebration on the station.
    4. Take no action because excellent care is expected by all nurses.

19. The client asks the nurse in the women's health clinic, "I am so miserable during my premenstrual syndrome I can't even go to work. Please help me." Which interventions should the nurse implement? Select all that apply.
    1. Increase the amount of colas and coffee daily.
    2. Avoid simple sugars such as cakes and candy.
    3. Drink at least two glasses of red wine nightly.
    4. Decrease the intake of foods high in salt.
    5. Adhere to a regular schedule for sleep.

20. The nurse is completing the admission assessment on a 12-weeks-pregnant client who is visiting the women's health clinic. The client tells the nurse, "I am a vegan and will not drink any milk or eat any meat." Which intervention should the nurse implement?
    1. Recommend the client eat grains, legumes, and nuts daily.
    2. Suggest that the client eat at least two eggs every day.
    3. Discuss not adhering to the vegan diet during pregnancy.
    4. Explain that a vegan diet does not require iron supplements.

1. 1. The HCP in a free clinic would not be able to refer this client to an infertility clinic because of cost. The nurse can discuss this with the client.
   2. If the couple has not been able to conceive in 6 years, then a referral to an infertility clinic would be appropriate, but the tests and treatment for infertility are very expensive. The client is being seen in a free clinic, which indicates a lack of funds. The nurse has a relationship with this client over the time period "several weeks." The nurse should answer the client's question.
   3. This is a therapeutic response, which does not answer the client's question "What can we do?"
   4. If the client has not conceived in 6 years, this is not a probable solution to the client's concern.

2. 1. The client who is 10 cm dilated and 100% effaced is ready to deliver the fetus; therefore, the nurse should assess this client first.
   2. Early decelerations are not associated with fetal compromise and require no added interventions; therefore, this client would not need to be assessed first.
   3. This client does not have an immediate need; therefore, the nurse should not assess this client first.
   4. This is causing distress to the mother, but there is nothing the nurse can do about this situation. The on-call obstetrician will have to deliver the fetus.

3. 1. The pregnant client has an increased circulating blood volume, which results in a slight decrease of the hemoglobin and hematocrit; therefore, this client would not warrant intervention.
   2. The normal fasting blood glucose level is 70 to 120 mg/dL; therefore, this client does not warrant intervention by the nurse.
   3. Protein in the urine indicates the client is at risk for pregnancy-induced hypertension; therefore, this client warrants intervention and further assessment by the nurse.
   4. The white blood cell count increases during pregnancy; the normal range is 5000 to 12,000 and rises during labor. This client does not warrant intervention.

4. 1. If the client is unable to urinate, then the nurse will have to perform an in-and-out catheterization to empty the bladder. However, the nurse should implement the least invasive intervention.
   2. The nurse could use a bladder scanner to determine whether the bladder was full, but the first intervention is to ask the client to urinate.
   3. Massaging the fundus will not put the fundus in a midline position until the bladder is empty.
   4. The number 1 reason for a displaced fundus is a full bladder. The nurse should always do the least invasive procedure, which is to ask the client to attempt to void. The emptying of the bladder should allow the fundus to return to the midline position.

5. 1. Anyone could have left the client's chart at the bedside, such as the HCP or the radiology technician. The charge nurse should first determine the facts before taking further action.
   2. The charge nurse should take the client's chart back to the nurse's station.
   3. This could be a violation of HIPAA because anyone entering the client's room could read the client's chart, but this is not the charge nurse's first intervention.
   4. The charge nurse should first take the client's chart back to the nurse's station and then determine why and who left it at the client's bedside.

6. 1. The nurse really does not need to know when the client had her last chest x-ray when scheduling this chest x-ray.
   2. The nurse should ask whether the client may be pregnant because if there is a chance of pregnancy, the client should not have an x-ray. Any time a female client is of childbearing age and is having any type of x-ray, this question should be asked.
   3. The date of the client's last period would not affect the client's having a chest x-ray.
   4. This question would be asked if the client was receiving some type of contrast or dye.

7. 1. The clinical manager should first talk to the nurse to determine what is causing the medication error.
   2. Three medication errors in a short period of time require the clinical manager to investigate the cause.

3. This should be the clinical manager's first intervention, to assess whether the system is responsible for the medication errors or whether it is a nursing error problem. For example, a system error problem would be that the medication is not available at the prescribed time.

4. This may be needed, but it is not the nurse's first intervention. If the clinical manager determines the nurse is at fault, then this could be a possible action.

8. 1. When the infant is placed in the supine position, the infant should extend the arm and leg on the side to which the head is turned and then flex the extremities on the other. This is known as the tonic-neck reflex or fencing reflex, which is normal for the newborn. The newborn remaining in a fetal position when supine warrants further intervention to assess for neurological problems.

2. The Babinski reflex is elicited by stroking the lateral sole of the foot from the heel forward. Normal reflex is that the toes flare outward and the big toe dorsiflexes. This is a normal response for an infant but is abnormal in an adult, indicating neurological deficit in the adult. Therefore, this does not warrant immediate intervention.

3. This is the rooting reflex, which is normal for a newborn. This would not warrant immediate intervention.

4. The Moro reflex or the startle reflex is a sharp extension and abduction of arm with thumbs and forefingers in a C-position followed by flexion and adduction to embrace position. This response occurs with loud noise or when the newborn is startled. This would not warrant immediate intervention.

9. 1. This is the ethical principle of veracity, which is truth telling.

2. Nonmaleficence is the duty to do no harm. Many ethicists think that the principle of nonmaleficence has priority over other ethical principles except for autonomy. Nonmaleficence allows the nurse to answer a question or make a decision that does not create further complications for the client.

3. This is paternalism, which is giving advice and telling the client what is best for her.

4. This is an assessment question that could guide the nurse in helping the client make a decision, but it does not demonstrate the ethical principle of nonmaleficence.

10. 1. This statement describes primary care, which is a type of nursing care delivery.

2. Modular nursing is frequently called care pairs, in which nurses are paired with other less well-trained caregivers to provide nursing care to group clients.

3. This statement describes team nursing, which is a type of nursing care delivery.

4. This statement describes functional nursing, in which there is a charge nurse, a medication nurse, and a treatment nurse.

11. 1. Threatening and attempting to manipulate the staff will create distrust and anger, which will not facilitate a smooth transition for the medication delivery system.

2. This action is not fair because the new system is being implemented whether the staff members vote for it or not. There are situations, resulting from financial or other constraints, that require the clinical manager to implement a change without the input of the staff.

3. To be an effective change agent, the manager needs to develop a sense of trust, establish common goals, and facilitate effective communication.

4. Sending the documentation by hospital e-mail is pertinent to ensure all staff members receive the information, but it is not effective in producing a smooth transition and reduction of resistance to the change.

12. 1. This behavior may be normal for some individuals and may not be detrimental to the infant or mother, but the nurse must investigate the situation first before making this statement.

2. Clay and dirt in the gut may decrease the absorption of nutrients such as iron. Therefore, asking this question is appropriate, but the first intervention should be to determine whether there are complications related to pica.

3. Pica, ingesting substances not normally considered food, may decrease the intake of food and therefore essential nutrients. Iron deficiency was once thought to be a cause of pica but is now considered a result. The nurse must first assess to determine whether the behavior is detrimental to the mother or infant before further action is taken.

4. Pica may be related to cultural beliefs about materials that will ensure a healthy mother and infant. This should not be the nurse's first intervention. The safety of

mother and fetus is priority. If the H&H is within normal limits, the nurse should support the cultural belief.

13. 1. Insurance companies contract with certain providers to provide care to the client at a reduced rate. Using this doctor, who is not a preferred provider of care, will result in a greater out-of-pocket expense for the client.
2. This is not a true statement, and the nurse should not give the client false information, especially about money.
3. This therapeutic response is to encourage the client to ventilate feelings. This client needs factual information.
4. Most insurance companies will not cover a preexisting condition for 1 year after the policy is initiated; therefore, this pregnancy may not be covered.

14. 1. The 16-year-old client must sign for her child's care. The grandmother does not have the authority to sign informed consent for the procedure.
2. The cost of the procedure should not be a factor for the nurse when discussing a medical procedure with the client.
3. The client is not requesting assistance to pay the medical bills; therefore, this intervention is not appropriate.
4. A 16-year-old mother has the right to make decisions for her child; therefore, the mother must sign the informed consent for the procedure.

15. 1. The UAPs may or may not cross the picket line, and the managers will not be able to provide care to all the clients. This is not the best response.
2. Abandonment is leaving the shift without notifying the supervisor after accepting the assignment. Going on strike with a 10-day notice is not abandonment.
3. This may or may not be a true statement; therefore, it is not the best response.
4. Federal law requires that there must be a 10-day notice before going on a strike. This gives the hospital a chance to prepare for the strike and make changes to ensure client safety.

16. 1. Anencephaly is a congenital abnormality that entails an absence of all or a major part of the brain. The infant has no chance of life outside of a health-care institution. The health-care team refers situations to the ethics committee to help resolve dilemmas when caring for clients.

2. This is not an ethical dilemma because the 16-year-old client has a right to place her infant up for adoption. This would not need to be referred to an ethics committee.
3. If the nurse wants to take the child away from the mother, then this must be reported to Child Protective Services. Therefore, this is not an ethical dilemma. The nurse has a law that directs the decision. This would not need to be referred to an ethics committee.
4. This is a legal issue, not an ethical issue. The health-care team can request the hospital attorney to take these parents to court and request a court order to administer blood. The parents do not have the right to refuse life-sustaining treatment for their child.

17. 1, 2, and 3 are correct.
1. The mother should be encouraged to hold and cuddle the infant to help with the grieving process.
2. The mother should not be required to stay on a unit where she can hear crying infants and happy families. This is a very cruel action to take. The nurse should transfer the client to another unit.
3. The nurse should remember the father has lost the baby, too. Acknowledging and encouraging the father to talk about his loss will help with his grieving process.
4. The nurse should not impose his or her beliefs about funerals on the client. This is a boundary crossing violation.
5. Grief support groups recommend giving the infant a name because it acknowledges the infant's existence.

18. 1. The clinical manager could ask the primary nurse why she provides such excellent care, but it is not the most important action. Excellence in care should be documented in writing in nurse's personnel file to support merit raises, transfers, and promotions.
2. The clinical manager should recognize the comments of clients/families during the performance evaluation. Excellence in care should be documented in writing in nurse's personnel file to support merit raises, transfers, and promotions. Many health-care facilities have employee recognition programs.
3. This is a possible action, but this could single out the nurse and cause dissension among the other staff. Parties on the unit

should celebrate the unit's accomplishments, not a single individual.
4. Excellent care is the expectation of all clinical managers, but when the multiple clients/families recognize the nurse's care, then there should be documentation in the nurse's personnel file.

19. 2, 4, and 5 are correct.
1. The client should decrease the amount of caffeine, which includes coffee, teas, cola, and chocolate, because caffeine increases irritability, insomnia, anxiety, and nervousness.
2. **Avoiding simple sugars will prevent rebound hypoglycemia, which will exacerbate the signs/symptoms of PMS.**
3. Alcohol is a central nervous system depressant and aggravates the depression associated with PMS. This is not an appropriate intervention.
4. **Decreasing the intake of salt will decrease fluid retention, thereby decreasing edema.**
5. **Insomnia is a symptom of PMS, and a regular schedule for sleep will help decrease the severity of the PMS.**

20. 1. Vegans are individuals who avoid animal proteins, which are complete proteins that contain all the essential amino acids the body cannot synthesize from other sources. Vegetable proteins lack one or more of the essential amino acids, so the vegan must combine different plant proteins, grains, legumes, and nuts, to allow for intake of all essential amino acids. Vegans avoid all animal products and have difficulty meeting adequate nutritional protein needs.
2. Vegans avoid animal products, and if she does not drink milk she will not eat eggs.
3. The nurse should assist the client in adhering to cultural, spiritual, or personal beliefs, not try to talk the client into changing her beliefs unless it is a danger to the fetus or the mother.
4. A vegan diet requires extra iron supplements; iron in the vegetarian diet is poorly absorbed because of the lack of heme iron that comes from meat.

End of Life Issues

12

"People are like stained-glass windows. They sparkle and shine when the sun is out, but when the darkness sets in, their true beauty is revealed only if there is light from within."

—Elisabeth Kübler-Ross

ABBREVIATION LIST

ac	before a meal	**MAR**	Medication Administration Record
ADLs	Activities of Daily Living	**P**	Pulse
BP	Blood Pressure	**PEG**	Percutaneous Endoscopic Gastrostomy
CBC	Complete Blood Cell Count		
CPR	Cardiopulmonary Resuscitation	**PO**	Per Os (by Mouth)
DNR	Do Not Resuscitate	**PRN**	As Needed
EBP	Evidence-Based Practice	**PT**	Prothrombin Time
HH	Home Health	**R**	Respiration
HCP	Health-Care Provider	**RN**	Registered Nurse
INR	International Normalized Ratio	**R/O**	Rule Out
IV	Intravenous	**TID**	Three Times Daily
IVP	Intravenous Push	**UAP**	Unlicensed Assistive Personnel
IVPB	Intravenous Piggy Back	**WBC**	White Blood Cell
LPN	Licensed Practical Nurse		

PRACTICE QUESTIONS

Setting Priorities When Caring for Clients

1. The home health (HH) hospice nurse is making rounds. Which client should the nurse assess first?
   1. The client with end-stage heart failure who has increasing difficulty breathing.
   2. The client whose family has planned to surprise her with an early birthday party.
   3. The client who is complaining of being tired and irritable all the time.
   4. The client with chronic lung disease who has not eaten for 3 days.

2. A client diagnosed with cancer and receiving chemotherapy is brought to the emergency department after vomiting bright red blood. Which intervention should the nurse implement first?
   1. Check to see which antineoplastic medications the client has received.
   2. Start an IV of normal saline with an 18-gauge intravenous catheter.
   3. Investigate to see whether the client has a do not resuscitate (DNR) order written.
   4. Call the oncologist to determine what lab work to order.

3. The nurse is called to the room of a male client diagnosed with lung cancer by the client's wife because the client is not breathing. The client has discussed being a DNR but has not made a decision. Which interventions should the nurse implement first?
   1. Ask the spouse whether she wants the client to be resuscitated.
   2. Tell the spouse to leave the room and then perform a slow code.
   3. Assess the client's breathing and call a code from the room.
   4. Notify the oncologist the client has arrested.

4. The nurse is preparing to perform a dressing change on a female client who has end-stage renal disease and notes the client's husband silently holding the client's hand and praying. Which action should the nurse implement first?
   1. Continue to prepare for the dressing change in the room.
   2. Call the chaplain to help the client and spouse pray.
   3. Quietly leave the room and come back for the dressing change.
   4. Ask the husband whether he would like the nurse to join in the prayer.

5. The nurse is administering medications on a medical unit. Which medication should the nurse question administering?
   1. Warfarin (Coumadin), an anticoagulant, to a client with a prothrombin time (PT) of 14 and an international normalized ratio (INR) of 1.6 mg/dL.
   2. Digoxin (Lanoxin), a cardiac glycoside, to a client with a potassium level of 2.7 mEq/L.
   3. Levothyroxine (Synthroid), a thyroid hormone, to a client with bradycardia who complaints of being cold.
   4. Theophylline (Theodur), a methylxanthine, to a client who does not have wheezes or crackles in the lungs.

6. The hospice nurse is writing a care plan for a client diagnosed with type 2 diabetes mellitus who has peripheral neuropathy. Which client problem has priority for the client?
   1. Altered glucose metabolism.
   2. Anticipatory grieving.
   3. Alteration in comfort.
   4. Spiritual distress.

7. The female client who is dying asks to see her son, but the son refuses to come to the hospital. Which action should the nurse implement first?
   1. Call the son and tell him he must come to see his mother before it is too late.
   2. Ask the social worker to call the son and see whether the son will come to the hospital.
   3. Check with the family to see whether they can discuss the issue with the son.
   4. Do nothing because to intervene in a private matter would be boundary crossing.

8. The nurse is caring for clients on an oncology unit. Which client should the nurse assess first?
   1. The client diagnosed with leukemia who is afebrile and has a white blood cell (WBC) count of 100,000 mm³.
   2. The client who has undergone four rounds of chemotherapy and is nauseated.
   3. The client diagnosed with lung cancer who has absent breath sounds in the lower lobes.
   4. The client diagnosed with rule out (R/O) breast cancer who had a negative biopsy this A.M.

9. The nurse caring for clients on an oncology unit is administering medications. Which medication should the nurse administer first?
   1. The antinausea medication to the male client who thinks he may get sick.
   2. The pain medication to the female client who has pain she rates a "2."
   3. The loop diuretic to the female client who had an output greater than the intake.
   4. The nitroglycerin paste to the male client who is diagnosed with angina pectoris.

10. The staff nurse is caring for a client who was diagnosed with pancreatic cancer during an exploratory laparotomy. Which client problem is priority for postoperative day 1?
    1. Ineffective coping.
    2. Fluid and electrolyte imbalance.
    3. Risk for infection.
    4. Potential for suicidal thoughts.

Delegating and Assigning Nursing Tasks

11. The hospice nurse is working with a volunteer. Which task could the nurse delegate to the volunteer?
    1. Sit with the client while he or she reminisces about life experiences.
    2. Give the client a sponge bath and rub lotion on the bony prominences.
    3. Provide spiritual support for the client and family members.
    4. Check the home to see that all necessary medical equipment is available.

12. The nurse delegates postmortem care to the unlicensed assistive personnel (UAP). The UAP tells the nurse that the UAP has never performed postmortem care. Which is the best response by the nurse to the UAP?
    1. "It can be uncomfortable. I will go with you and show you what to do."
    2. "The client is already dead. You cannot hurt him now."
    3. "There is nothing to it; it is just a bed bath and change of clothes."
    4. "Don't worry. You can skip it this time but you need to learn what to do."

13. The UAP tells the nurse that the client is complaining of chest pain. Which task should the nurse delegate to the UAP?
    1. Call the health-care provider (HCP) and report the client's chest pain.
    2. Give a client some acetaminophen (Tylenol) while the nurse checks the client.
    3. Get the client's medical records and bring them to the client's room.
    4. Notify the client's family of the onset of chest pain.

14. The registered nurse (RN) and licensed practical nurse (LPN) are caring for a group of clients. Which nursing task should not be assigned to the LPN?
    1. Feed the client who has an IV in both forearms.
    2. Assess the client diagnosed with stage IV heart failure.
    3. Discharge the client who had a negative breast biopsy.
    4. Administer the intravenous piggy back (IVPB) antibiotic ceftriaxone (Rocephin).

15. The hospice nurse is discussing the clients' care with the UAP. Which statement contains the best information about caring for dying clients?
    1. "Perform as much care for the clients as possible to conserve their strength."
    2. "Do not get too attached to the clients because it will hurt when they die."
    3. "Be careful not to promise to withhold health-care information from the team."
    4. "Clients may want to talk about their life, but you should discourage them."

16. The client on telemetry has the following strip on the monitor. Which action should the telemetry nurse delegate to the UAP?

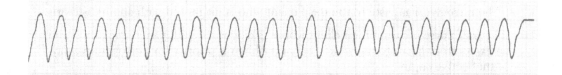

    1. Have the UAP call the operator and announce the code.
    2. Tell the UAP to answer the other call lights on the unit.
    3. Send the UAP to the room to start rescue breaths.
    4. Ask the family to step out of the room during the code.

17. The charge nurse observes the UAP crying after the death of a client. Which is the charge nurse's best response to the UAP?
    1. "If you cry every time a client dies, you won't last long on the unit."
    2. "It can be difficult when a client dies. Would you like to take a break?"
    3. "You need to stop crying and go on about your responsibilities."
    4. "Did you not realize that clients die in a health-care facility?"

18. The hospice nurse overseeing the care of a client in a long-term care facility is confronted by the nursing staff who want to send the client to the hospital for treatment. Which action should the nurse implement first?
    1. Check with the client to see whether the client wants to go to a hospital.
    2. Explain that the client can be kept comfortable at the long-term care facility.
    3. Discuss the hospice concept of comfort measures only with the staff.
    4. Call a client care conference immediately to discuss the conflict.

19. The nurse administered pain medication 30 minutes ago to a client diagnosed with terminal cancer. Thirty minutes after the medication, the client tells the nurse "I don't think you gave me anything. My pain is even worse than before." Which intervention should the nurse implement? Select all that apply.
    1. Attempt to determine whether the client is experiencing spiritual distress.
    2. Ask the client to rate the current pain on the numeric pain scale.
    3. Reposition the client to relieve pressure on the pain site.
    4. Call the HCP to request an increase in pain medication.
    5. Explain to the client he or she should relax and let the medication take effect.

20. Which nurse should be assigned to a dying client who is having frequent symptoms of distress?
    1. The UAP who can be spared to sit with the client.
    2. The LPN who has grown attached to the family.
    3. The RN who has experience as a hospice nurse.
    4. The RN who graduated 2 months ago.

Managing Clients and Nursing Staff

21. The wife of a client diagnosed as terminal is concerned that the client is not eating or drinking. Which is the nurse's best response?
    1. "I will start an IV if your husband continues to refuse to eat or drink."
    2. "You should discuss placing a PEG feeding tube in your husband with the HCP."
    3. "This is normal at the end of life; the dehydration produces a type of euphoria."
    4. "You are right to be concerned. Would you like to talk about your worry?"

22. The client has just been told that the medical condition cannot be treated success-fully and the client has a life expectancy of about 6 months. Which referral would the nurse make at this time?
    1. To a home health nurse.
    2. To the client's pastor.
    3. To a hospice agency.
    4. To the social worker.

23. The hospice client asks the nurse, "What should I do about my house? My son and daughter are fighting over it." Which statement is the nurse's best response?
    1. "I think you should tell your children that you will leave the house to a charity."
    2. "I would sell the house and go on an extended vacation and spend the money."
    3. "What would you want to happen to your house? It is your decision."
    4. "Wait and let your children fight over the house after you are gone."

24. During the morning assessment, the client diagnosed with cancer complains of nausea most of the time. Based on the client's MAR, which intervention should the day nurse implement first?

Client's Name: Mr. B	Admit Number: 543216		Allergies: NKDA	
Date: Today	Height: 69 inches Weight: 74.2 kg 163 pounds		Diagnosis: Cancer of the Pancreas	
Medication	0701–1500	1501–2300	2301–0700	
Morphine sulfate 2 mg IVP q 2 hours prn				
Promethazine (Phenergan) 12.5 mg IVP q 4 hours prn				
Prochlorperazine (Compazine) 5 mg PO TID prn				
Hydrocodone (Vicodin) 5 mg PO q 4–6 hours prn				
Nurse's Name/Initials	Day Nurse RN/ DN			

   1. Administer the prescribed antiemetic promethazine (Phenergan) prn.
   2. Administer the prescribed antiemetic prochlorperazine (Compazine) ac.
   3. Discuss changing the order for Compazine to routine with the HCP.
   4. Assess the client to see whether pain is the cause of the nausea.

25. The unit manager is evaluating the staff nurse. Which data should be included in the nurse's yearly evaluation?
    1. The fact that the nurse clocked in late to work twice in the last year.
    2. The complaint that the nurse did not answer a call light during a code.
    3. The number of times the nurse switched shifts with another nurse.
    4. The appropriateness of the nurse's written documentation in the charts.

26. The hospice nurse is providing follow-up care with the family member of a deceased client. Which intervention is priority?
    1. Attend the client's funeral service or visitation.
    2. Check on the family 1 to 2 months after the death.
    3. Make sure the arrangements are what the client wanted.
    4. Help the family member dispose of belongings as soon as possible.

27. The nurse is attempting to start an intravenous (IV) line in an elderly client who is dehydrated. After two unsuccessful attempts, which action should the nurse implement?
    1. Keep trying to get a patent IV access.
    2. Ask the HCP to order oral fluid replacement.
    3. Ask a second nurse to attempt to start the IV.
    4. Place cold packs on the client's arms for comfort.

28. The neurologist has explained to the family of a 22-year-old client placed on a ventilator after a motor vehicle accident that the client does not have any brain function. Which referral is appropriate at this time?
    1. A local funeral director.
    2. A hospice agency.
    3. A home health nurse.
    4. A tissue and organ bank.

29. The male client who is dying asks the nurse to explain what will happen to his body when death occurs. Which is the nurse's best response?
    1. "Death is a unique experience, but I can explain to you about how the body stops functioning."
    2. "You will begin to have trouble breathing and then you will not be able to swallow your saliva."
    3. "This must be troubling you. Would you like to discuss how you feel about the dying process?"
    4. "That is a gruesome topic. You need to concentrate on getting well and not on what happens when you die."

30. The family member of a deceased client tells the nurse, "I am new here and don't know any funeral home. Which one should I choose?" Which is the nurse's best response?
    1. "I think you should check with the chaplain for the best funeral home."
    2. "I can get you some numbers of funeral homes in the area so you can choose."
    3. "Funeral homes charge a lot of money. I would have the body cremated."
    4. "The charge nurse will tell you the funeral homes that give us good service."

Setting Priorities When Caring for Clients

1. 1. This client may need oxygen or an intervention to keep the client comfortable. This client should be seen first.
   2. This client does not have priority over difficulty breathing.
   3. This client does not have priority over difficulty breathing.
   4. This client does not have priority over difficulty breathing.

   MAKING NURSING DECISIONS: The test taker should apply some systematic approach when answering priority questions. Maslow's Hierarchy of Needs should be used when determining which client to assess first. The test taker should start at the bottom of the pyramid, where physiologic needs are priority.

2. 1. The medications are not important at this time. The client is bleeding.
   2. **The client is at risk for shock. The nurse should take steps to prevent vascular collapse. Starting the IV is the priority.**
   3. This is not important in the emergency department.
   4. Prevention of circulatory collapse is the priority. The nurses could anticipate an order for a complete blood count (CBC) and a type and crossmatch.

   MAKING NURSING DECISIONS: The test taker must be aware of the setting, which dictates the appropriate intervention. The adjectives will cue the test taker to the setting, in this case, the emergency department. The test taker must also remember the nurse's scope of practice. Starting an IV with normal saline is within a nurse's scope of practice.

3. 1. It is too late to ask this question. This decision must be made prior to an arrest situation.
   2. The nurse should not hesitate to call a code, and a full code must be performed, not a slow code.
   3. **These are the first steps of a code.**
   4. This should be done by someone at the desk, not by the nurse responding to the emergency.

   MAKING NURSING DECISIONS: The nurse must react immediately in an emergency

situation and should not hesitate. The nurse should immediately begin cardiopulmonary resuscitation (CPR) and follow the hospital's protocol.

4. 1. This is a private moment between the client and the spouse; the nurse should not impose on the situation.
   2. The client and spouse did not ask for help; the nurse should not assume that help is needed.
   3. **This is a private moment and should be respected by the nurse. The nurse should allow the client and spouse quiet time together.**
   4. This is a private moment between the client and the spouse; the nurse should not impose on the situation.

   MAKING NURSING DECISIONS: The nurse must be aware of spiritual needs and help to support the client's needs whenever possible.

5. 1. The INR is not at a therapeutic level yet; the nurse should administer this medication.
   2. **This potassium level is very low. Hypokalemia potentiates dysrhythmias in clients receiving digoxin. This nurse should discuss potassium replacement with the HCP before administering this medication.**
   3. Bradycardia and complaints of being cold are symptoms of hypothyroidism. Synthroid is administered to clients who do not produce enough thyroid hormone. The nurse should administer this medication.
   4. This information supports that the Theo-dur is working effectively. The nurse should administer this medication.

   MAKING NURSING DECISIONS: The test taker must know normal laboratory data. See Appendix A for normal laboratory data.

6. 1. The client may be diagnosed with diabetes, but at the end of life this is not the priority nursing diagnosis. In fact, as a comfort measure, many clients are allowed to eat whatever they wish occasionally without regard to the carbohydrates.
   2. This is a psychosocial diagnosis and not a priority over the physiologic problems.

3. The client has peripheral neuropathy, which produces shooting pain in the extremities. The priority at the end of life is to keep the client comfortable.
4. This is a psychosocial diagnosis and not a priority over the physiologic problems.

MAKING NURSING DECISIONS: The test taker must be aware of the setting, which dictates the appropriate intervention. The "hospice nurse" tells the test taker that this client has a prognosis of less than 6 months to live. Comfort measures are very important at the end of life.

7. 1. The son has a right to refuse to come to the hospital regardless of what the nurse thinks the son should do. The nurse is unaware of the family dynamics that led to this dilemma.
2. This is only placing another health-care professional in the picture and would not be the best option.
3. Other family members are more likely to understand the family dynamics and would be the best ones to intervene in the situation.
4. The nurse should attempt to assist in reconciliation between the client and her son if possible.

8. 1. This is an expected lab value for a client diagnosed with leukemia. The client's bone marrow is overproducing immature white blood cells and clogging the bloodstream.
2. This client is complaining of nausea, which is an uncomfortable experience. The nurse should attempt to intervene and treat the nausea. This client should be seen first.
3. Absent breath sounds are expected in a client diagnosed with lung cancer.
4. A negative biopsy is a good result. This client does not need to be seen first.

MAKING NURSING DECISIONS: When deciding which client to assess first, the test taker should determine whether the signs/symptoms the client is exhibiting are normal or expected for the client situation. After eliminating the expected options, the test taker should determine which situation is unexpected or causing the client distress.

9. 1. Anticipatory nausea is a very real problem for clients diagnosed with cancer and undergoing treatment. If this problem is not rectified quickly and progresses to vomiting, the client may not get relief. This medication should be administered first.

2. This is considered mild pain and can be treated after the anticipatory nausea.
3. This is expected and indicates the medication is working. This medication does not have priority.
4. This is a routine medication and can be administered after the nausea and pain medications. Sublingual nitroglycerin is administered for acute chest pain, angina.

10. 1. Ineffective coping is a psychological problem that would not have priority on the first day after major abdominal surgery.
2. After major trauma, the body undergoes a fluid shift. The possibility of fluid and electrolyte imbalance is the top priority problem for 1 day after major abdominal surgery.
3. This could be a priority, but a potential or risk is not priority over an actual problem.
4. A potential psychological problem would not have priority on the first day after major abdominal surgery.

MAKING NURSING DECISIONS: When the test taker is deciding which client problem is priority, physiologic problems usually are priority, and an actual problem is priority over a potential problem.

Delegating and Assigning Nursing Tasks

11. 1. Encouraging the client to review his or her life experiences assists the client to come to a closure of his or her life. This is an important intervention that the volunteer can perform.
2. This is the job of the UAP, not a volunteer.
3. This is the job of the chaplain, not the volunteer.
4. This is the job of the nurse or occupational therapist, not the volunteer.

MAKING NURSING DECISIONS: When the test taker is deciding which option is the most appropriate task to delegate/assign, the test taker should choose the task that allows each staff member to function within his or her full scope of practice. Do not assign a task to a staff member that falls outside the staff member or volunteer's expertise.

12. 1. The nurse should provide instruction and support to the UAP. This is the best response.
2. This is a callous statement and does not help the UAP learn to provide postmortem care.

3. This is not hearing the UAP's concern.
4. The nurse should assist the UAP to learn to perform the duties of a UAP, not circumvent the workload.

13. 1. If the HCP is called, the nurse should perform this task, not the UAP. A UAP cannot take a telephone order; only a licensed nurse can take telephone orders.
   2. The UAP cannot administer a medication, not even Tylenol.
   3. **The nurse should immediately go to the client's room and assess the client. Sometimes the nurse may need the client's chart and medical administration record (MAR) to assist in the assessment of findings. The UAP can bring these documents to the room.**
   4. The UAP should not be asked to relay such information. This is the nurse's or HCP's responsibility.

   MAKING NURSING DECISIONS: When the test taker is deciding which option is the most appropriate task to delegate/assign, the test taker should choose the task that allows each staff member to function within his or her full scope of practice. Do not assign a task to a staff member that requires a higher level of expertise than that staff member has. Conversely, do not assign a task to a staff member when that task could be performed by a staff member with a lower level of expertise.

14. 1. The LPN can feed a client who is stable but unable to feed himself or herself because of medical equipment. This is an appropriate task to assign.
   2. **The nurse cannot assign assessment. This is the inappropriate task to assign to the LPN.**
   3. The LPN can discharge a client who had a minor procedure and who does not require extensive teaching.
   4. The LPN can administer a routine IVPB medication.

   MAKING NURSING DECISIONS: When the test taker is deciding which option is the most appropriate task to delegate/assign, the test taker should choose the task that allows each staff member to function within his or her full scope of practice. Do not assign a task to a staff member that requires a higher level of expertise or could be delegated/assigned to a staff member with a lower level of expertise.

15. 1. The UAP should encourage the client to remain independent as long as possible. If the client is unable to perform activities of daily living (ADLs), then the UAP should perform the tasks.
   2. This may be true, but the UAP cannot and should not distance himself or herself from the clients. The UAP should maintain a professional relationship with the clients.
   3. **This is an important statement for the UAP to understand. If information revealed to the UAP is necessary to provide appropriate care to the client, then the information must be shared on a need-to-know basis with the health-care team.**
   4. Clients should be encouraged to discuss their life because life review may help clients accept their death.

16. 1. The nurse in the client's room notifies the hospital operator of a code situation.
   2. **Answering the call lights of the other clients on the unit can be delegated to the UAP.**
   3. In a hospital, the respiratory therapist assumes the responsibility for ventilations.
   4. The nursing supervisor is responsible for requesting the family to leave the room. The UAP does not have the authority to make this request.

   MAKING NURSING DECISIONS: When the test taker is deciding which option is the most appropriate task to delegate/assign, the test taker should choose the task that allows each member of the staff to function within his or her full scope of practice. Do not assign a task to a staff member that requires a higher level of expertise or which a staff member with a lower level of expertise could perform.

17. 1. Crying at a death is a universal human response. Although the statement may be true, the nurse should recognize the UAP's need for a short time to compose himself or herself.
   2. **Hospital personnel are not immune to human emotions. The UAP needs a short time to compose himself or herself. The nurse should offer the UAP compassion. If this occurred with every death, the UAP could be counseled to transfer to a different area of the hospital.**
   3. This is not accepting the UAP's feelings.
   4. This is not accepting the UAP's feelings.

18. 1. Clients receiving hospice can decide to discontinue the service and resume standard health-care practices and treatments whenever they wish. The nurse should assess the client's wishes before continuing.
    2. This is true, but if the client wants to be treated, it is the client's decision. If the client does not want treatment, then the nurse should discuss the client's wishes with the long-term care facility staff.
    3. If the client does not want treatment, then the nurse should discuss the client's wishes with the long-term care facility staff.
    4. If the staff continues to try to get the client to accept futile treatment, a client conference should be called. This is not the first action for the hospice nurse because a client conference is a scheduled event and would not take place immediately.

    MAKING NURSING DECISIONS: **This question requires the test taker to have a basic knowledge of hospice and hospice goals. The nurse must also be aware of basic referrals.**

19. 1, 3, and 4 are correct.
    1. Spiritual distress can greatly affect the perception of pain. If the client is not receiving relief from pain medication, the nurse should explore other variables that could affect the perception of pain.
    2. Clients experiencing chronic pain may or may not be able to rate their pain on a pain scale. The client has provided all the information about the pain that is currently needed. The pain is greater than it was before the medication.
    3. This is an alternative to medication that may provide some minimal relief while other interventions are being attempted.
    4. The nurse should notify the HCP that the current pain regimen is not effective.
    5. This is a condescending statement and would tend to agitate the client more than help.

20. 1. The charge nurse should not assign a UAP to care for a client in spiritual distress. This is outside of the UAP's ability to function.
    2. The charge nurse should not delegate or assign care based on a personal relationship of the nurse with the family. The nurse most qualified to care for the client's needs should be assigned to the client.
    3. A hospice nurse has experience in managing symptoms associated with

the dying process. This is the best nurse to care for this client.
    4. A new graduate would not have the experience or knowledge to manage the symptoms as effectively as an experienced hospice nurse.

    MAKING NURSING DECISIONS: **When the test taker is deciding which option is the most appropriate task to delegate/assign, the test taker should choose the task that allows each member of the staff to function within his or her full scope of their abilities.**

Managing Clients and Nursing Staff

21. 1. The body naturally begins to slow down, and clients may not wish to take in liquids or nourishment. This can produce a natural euphoria and make the dying process easier on the client. IV fluids would interfere with this process and would increase secretions the client cannot handle, thus making the client more uncomfortable.
    2. A PEG feeding tube would increase the intake of the client and would increase secretions the client cannot handle. This can require suctioning the client and further augmenting the client's discomfort.
    3. Refusal to take in food and liquids produces a natural euphoria and makes the dying process easier on the client. This is an appropriate teaching statement.
    4. This is a therapeutic response, but factual information is needed by the wife to accept the process.

22. 1. The home health nurse may be a possibility if a hospice organization is not available, but hospice is the best referral.
    2. The nurse would not refer the client to his or her own pastor. The nurse could place a call to notify the pastor at the client's request, but this would not be considered a referral.
    3. One of the guidelines for admission to a hospice agency is a terminal process with a life expectancy of 6 months or less. These organizations work to assist the client and family to live life to its fullest while providing for comfort measures and a peaceful, dignified death.
    4. The hospital social worker is not an appropriate referral at this time.

MAKING NURSING DECISIONS: The nurse must be knowledgeable about appropriate referrals and implement the referral to the most appropriate person/agency.

23. 1. This is advising and crossing professional boundaries. The nurse should not try to influence the client in these types of concerns.
    2. This is advising and crossing professional boundaries. The nurse should not try to influence the client in these types of concerns.
    3. This response allows the client to make his or her own decision. It validates that the nurse heard the concern but does not advise the client.
    4. This is advising and crossing professional boundaries. The nurse should not try to influence the client in these types of concerns.

MAKING NURSING DECISIONS: The nurse must always remember that nurses have positions of authority in a health-care environment. Nurses must maintain professional boundaries at all times and refuse to cross professional boundaries.

24. 1. The nurse could administer the Phenergan as a one-time medication administration or whenever the client asks for it, but this is not a proactive intervention.
    2. Administering the prn Compazine prophylactically before meals is a proactive stance and assists the client in maintaining his or her nutrition. This is the best action. If the client responds well to the regimen, the nurse should discuss changing the order to become a routine medication.
    3. If the client responds well to the prn Compazine, the nurse should discuss changing the order to become a routine medication instead of just prn.
    4. The client did not complain of pain. Nausea can be caused by pain, but it can also be caused by any number of other reasons. The nurse should be concerned with controlling the symptom.

25. 1. Clocking in late twice in a year's time is not a pattern of behavior.
    2. The nurse involved in a code would not be able to leave the code to answer a call light.
    3. The nurse has covered himself or herself or may be changing to cover someone else. This action is assuming responsibility for the client care on the unit and does

not require a mention in the evaluation unless the nurse is changing at the request of management.
    4. The nurse's care is being evaluated including the nurse's documentation. The completeness of documentation should be included in the evaluation.

26. 1. This is a nice gesture, but the priority is to provide support when the family and friends have returned to their own lives.
    2. The family and friends will have returned to their own lives 1 to 2 months after a family member has died. This is when the next of kin needs support from the hospice nurse. Hospice will follow up with the significant other for up to 13 months.
    3. This is the family's responsibility, not that of the hospice nurse.
    4. This is not the nurse's responsibility and should be discouraged for a short period of time. In the immediate grieving period, the significant other may get rid of possessions that later he or she may wish had been kept.

27. 1. The nurse should not continue to attempt IV access if there is another nurse available who may be able to insert the IV line successfully.
    2. The client needs IV replacement at this time.
    3. After two attempts, the nurse should arrange for a second nurse to attempt the placement.
    4. Cold packs would cause the circulatory system to contract and make it more difficult to start an IV line. Hot packs dilate the blood vessels.

28. 1. The family should designate a funeral home of their choice. The nurse does not make this referral.
    2. Hospice is for clients who are dying, but this client is considered brain dead.
    3. A home health nurse cannot help this client or family.
    4. A 22-year-old client who experienced a traumatic brain death may be a good candidate for organ donation. Most tissue and organ banks prefer to be the ones to approach the family. This is the best referral.

MAKING NURSING DECISIONS: The nurse is responsible for being knowledgeable of referrals in common situations.

29. 1. This is the nurse's best response.
    2. This may or may not happen to the client. The nurse should be truthful in answering a client's question but should avoid disclosing too much information.
    3. The client is asking for information. The nurse should answer the client's question.
    4. This is ignoring the client's concerns and is condescending.

    MAKING NURSING DECISIONS: The nurse should use the ethical principle of veracity and attempt to be honest with the client, but it is not necessary to disclose all the nurse knows. The test taker should not choose a therapeutic response when the client is asking for information.

30. 1. No hospital personnel should attempt to choose a funeral home for the client. The chaplain may provide a list of facilities in the community from which the family can choose.
    2. **This is the best response. The nurse should not try to influence the family because this can cause trouble for the nurse later if the family is not satisfied with the funeral home, arrangement, or cost.**
    3. This is advising, and the nurse should not cross this boundary.
    4. No hospital personnel should attempt to choose a funeral home for the client's family.

COMPREHENSIVE EXAMINATION

1. The client on the medical unit died unexpectedly, and the nurse must notify the significant other. Which statement made by the nurse is the best over the telephone?
   1. "I am sorry to tell you, but your loved one has died."
   2. "Could you come to the hospital? The client is not doing well."
   3. "The HCP has asked me to tell you of your family member's death."
   4. "Do you know whether the client wished to be an organ donor?"

2. The nurse has been pulled from a medical unit to work on an oncology unit for the shift. Which client should the charge nurse assign to the medical unit nurse?
   1. The client diagnosed with a spontaneous pneumothorax who has a chest tube.
   2. The client receiving a continuous infusion of an antineoplastic agent.
   3. The client newly diagnosed with cancer who is deciding on treatment options.
   4. The client who has been on the unit for weeks and is difficult to care for.

3. The charge nurse in an intensive care unit assigns three clients to the staff nurse. Which action should the staff nurse implement first?
   1. Refuse to take the assignment and leave the hospital immediately.
   2. Tell the supervisor that he or she is concerned about the unsafe assignment.
   3. Document his or her concerns in writing and give it to the supervisor.
   4. Take the assignment for the shift but turn in his or her resignation.

4. The female family member of the client experiencing a cardiac arrest refuses to leave the client's room. Which intervention should the administrative supervisor implement?
   1. Stay with the family member and explain what the team is doing.
   2. Call hospital security to escort the family member out of the room.
   3. Ask the HCP whether the family member can stay.
   4. Ignore the family member unless she becomes hysterical.

5. At 2230, the nurse is preparing to administer pain medication to a male client who rates his pain as a "4" on the numeric pain scale. Which medication should the nurse administer?

Client: Mr. C	Admit Number: 432165		Allergies: Ibuprofen
Date: Today	Height: 65 inches Weight: 64.2 kg 141.2 pounds		Diagnosis: Unresectable brain tumor Please take out double spacing and keep MAR on one page
Medication	**0701-1500**	**1501-2300**	**2301-0700**
Morphine sulfate 2 mg IVP q 2 hours PRN	0930 DN		
Promethazine (Phenergan) 12.5 mg IVP q 4 hours PRN		1845 EN	
Prochlorperazine (Compazine) 5 mg PO TID PRN			
Hydrocodone (Vicodin) 5 mg PO q 4-6 hours PRN		1730 EN	
Ibuprofen (Motrin) 600 mg PO q 3-4 hours PRN			
Nurse's Name/ Initials	**Day Nurse RN/ DN**	**Evening Nurse RN/EN**	**Night Nurse RN/NN**

1. Administer morphine 2 mg IVP.
2. Administer promethazine 12.5 mg IVP.
3. Administer hydrocodone 5 mg PO.
4. Administer ibuprofen 600 mg PO.

6. The labor and delivery nurse has assisted in the delivery of a 37-week fetal demise. Which intervention should the nurse implement?
1. Remove the baby from the delivery area quickly.
2. Tell the father to arrange to take the infant home.
3. Wrap the infant in a towel and place it aside.
4. Obtain a lock of the infant's hair for the parents.

7. The infection control nurse notices a rise in nosocomial infection rates on the surgical unit. Which action should the infection control nurse implement first?
1. Hold an in-service for the staff on the proper method of handwashing.
2. Tell the unit manager to decide on a corrective measure.
3. Arrange to observe the staff at work for several shifts.
4. Form a hospital-wide quality improvement project.

8. The male client presents to the emergency department with a complaint of chest pain but does not have the ability to pay for the services. Which should the emergency department nurse implement first?
   1. Place the client on a telemetry monitor and assess the client.
   2. Call an ambulance to transfer the client to a charity hospital.
   3. Have the client sign a form agreeing to pay the bill.
   4. Ask the client why he chose to come to this hospital.

9. The matriarch of a family has died on a busy medical unit. The family tells the nurse that the daughter is coming to the hospital from a nearby city to see the body. Which intervention should the nurse implement?
   1. Plan to allow the daughter to see the client in the room.
   2. Take the client to the morgue for the daughter to view.
   3. Request the family to call the daughter and tell her not to come.
   4. Explain that the unit is too busy for family visitation.

10. The unit manager is planning a change in the way postmortem care is provided. Which is the first step in the change process?
    1. Collect data.
    2. Identify the problem.
    3. Select an alternative.
    4. Implement a plan.

11. The female nurse manager is discussing the yearly performance evaluation with a male nurse. Which information regarding communication styles should the nurse manager utilize when talking with the employee?
    1. Men tend to see the work from a global perspective centering on feelings.
    2. Men often see the work environment from a logical, focused perspective.
    3. Men ask many more questions than women and require specific answers.
    4. Men and women communicate similarly in a nursing environment.

12. The newly hired nurse manager has identified that whenever a particular UAP is unhappy with an assignment, the entire unit has a bad day. Which action should the unit manager take to correct his problem?
    1. Meet with the UAP to see why the UAP is unhappy.
    2. Discuss the UAP's attitude and the way it affects the unit.
    3. Place the UAP on a counseling record for the behavior.
    4. Suspend the UAP until the behavior improves.

13. The health-care facility where the nurse works uses e-mail to notify the staff of in-services and mandatory requirements. Which is important information for the nurse manager to remember when utilizing e-mail to disseminate information?
    1. Give as much information as possible in each e-mail.
    2. Use e-mail for all communications with the staff.
    3. Use capital letters to get a point across with emphasis.
    4. Make the e-mail notices quick and easy to read.

14. At 1700, the HCP is yelling at the nursing staff because the early morning lab work is not available for a client's chart. Which action should the charge nurse implement first?
    1. Call the lab and have the lab supervisor talk with the HCP.
    2. Discuss the HCP's complaints with the nursing supervisor.
    3. Form a committee of lab and nursing personnel to fix the problem.
    4. Tell the HCP to stop yelling and calm down.

15. Which nursing action is an example of evidenced-based practice (EBP)?
    1. Turn on the tap water to help a client urinate.
    2. Use two identifiers to identify a client before a procedure.
    3. Educate a client based on current published information.
    4. Read nursing journals about the latest procedures.

16. The charge nurse notices a nurse recapping a needle in a client's room. Which action should the charge nurse take first?
    1. Tell the nurse not to recap the needle.
    2. Quietly ask the nurse to step into the hall.
    3. Reprimand the nurse for not following procedure.
    4. Notify the house supervisor of the nurse's behavior.

17. The UAP is preparing to provide postmortem care to a client with a questionable diagnosis of anthrax. Which instructions is priority for the nurse to provide to the UAP?
    1. The UAP is not at risk for contracting an illness.
    2. The UAP should wear a mask, gown, and gloves.
    3. The UAP may skip performing postmortem care.
    4. Ask whether the UAP is pregnant before she enters the client's room.

18. The client on a medical unit died of a communicable disease. Which information should the nurse provide to the mortuary workers?
    1. No information can be released to the mortuary service.
    2. The nurse should tell the funeral home the client's diagnosis.
    3. Ask the family for permission to talk with the mortician.
    4. Refer the funeral home to the HCP for information.

19. The nurse and UAP are caring for a minimally responsive client who weighs more than 500 pounds. Which action is priority when moving the client in the bed?
    1. Obtain a lifting device made for lifting heavy objects.
    2. Do not attempt to move the client because of the weight.
    3. Get another UAP to help move the client in the bed.
    4. Tell the family that the client must assist in moving in the bed.

20. The terminally ill client has a DNR order in place and is currently complaining of "pain all over." The nurse performs an assessment and notes the client has shallow breathing. The vital signs are P 67, R 8, BP 104/62. Which intervention should the nurse implement?
    1. Administer the narcotic pain medication IVP.
    2. Turn and reposition the client for comfort.
    3. Refuse to administer pain medication.
    4. Notify the HCP of the client's vital signs.

1. 1. Telling the family over the telephone could cause the client's significant other to have an accident while driving to the hospital. The nurse should avoid disclosing this type of information over the telephone.
   2. **This response allows the family/ significant other to know that there has been some incident, but it does not disclose the death. This is the best statement for the nurse at this time.**
   3. Telling the family over the telephone could cause the client to have an accident while driving to the hospital. The nurse should avoid disclosing this type of information over the telephone.
   4. This is a backward way of telling the family that the client died and should be avoided.

2. 1. **The nurse from a medical unit should be capable of caring for a client with a chest tube. This is the best assignment for the nurse.**
   2. Nurses must be certified in administration of antineoplastic agents before they care for clients receiving these agents.
   3. An experienced oncology nurse should care for this client. This client will require teaching and someone who can provide answers to questions.
   4. The staff on the oncology unit may like a break, but client care is the issue, and staff members that have learned how to care for the client should be assigned to this client.

3. 1. Leaving the facility will make client care even more strained.
   2. **The nurse should notify the supervisor that the nurse is concerned that the assignment will not allow the nurse to provide adequate care to any of the three clients. This is the first step the nurse should implement.**
   3. This is the second step. The nurse should put his or her concerns in writing and present the documentation to the supervisor. In states that have a "safe harbor" clause in the nursing practice act, this will prevent the nurse from losing his or her license should a poor outcome result from the assignment.
   4. If the staffing continues to be unsafe, the nurse may choose to resign, but the resignation should follow accepted business practices.

4. 1. **If the family is not causing a disruption in the code, then the supervisor should remain near the family member and explain what the interventions being implemented mean to the family member. The supervisor should be ready to escort the family member out of the code if the family member becomes disruptive.**
   2. This will cause ill will on the part of the family and could result in filing of a needless lawsuit.
   3. The HCP is busy with the care of the client. This is not the time to ask an HCP a question the supervisor can handle.
   4. Ignoring the family member could cause a problem; the supervisor should be proactive in managing the situation.

5. 1. Morphine is a potent narcotic analgesic. A 4 on the 1-to-10 pain scale is considered moderate pain and should be treated with a less potent pain medication.
   2. Promethazine is administered for nausea.
   3. **Hydrocodone is a narcotic analgesic that is less potent than morphine. It has been 5 hours since the hydrocodone was last administered, and no other pain medication has been required by the client. This is the best medication for moderate pain.**
   4. Ibuprofen may be effective for moderate pain, but the client is allergic to ibuprofen. The nurse should tag the MAR and chart to notify the HCP to discontinue this medication.

6. 1. The mother may want to see her infant before the body is removed from the room.
   2. The infant's body will be sent to a funeral home. The parents will not be allowed to take the body home.
   3. The body should be treated with the dignity accorded to any human remains.
   4. **The nurse can present the parents with a lock of the infant's hair and a set of footprints. Giving the parents something of the infant helps with the grieving process.**

7. 1. The infection control nurse should evaluate the problem fully before deciding on a course of action.
   2. The infection control nurse should assess the staff member's delivery of care and use standard nursing practice before deciding on a course of action with the unit manager.

3. This is an action that will allow the infection control nurse to observe compliance with standard nursing practices such as handwashing. Once the nurse has attempted to determine a cause, then a corrective action can be implemented.
4. The entire hospital has not shown an increased infection rate; only one unit has shown an increase.

8. 1. Federal law requires that clients presenting to an emergency department must be assessed and treated without regard to payment. The nurse should initiate steps to assess the client.
2. The nurse must assess the client. If a transfer is made, it will be after the client has been stabilized and the receiving hospital has accepted the transfer.
3. Federal law requires that clients presenting to an emergency department must be assessed and treated without regard to payment. The hospital will attempt to recover the costs after the client has been treated,
4. This is irrelevant information.

9. 1. The daughter lives in a "nearby" city. The client should not be moved anywhere until the daughter arrives.
2. A morgue is a difficult place to view a body. This could be appropriate if the daughter was going to take hours to days to get to the hospital.
3. Many people feel it is necessary to view the body. Not allowing the daughter time to view the body before transfer to a funeral home or the morgue could cause hurt feelings and impede the grieving process.
4. Many people feel it is necessary to view the body. Not allowing the daughter time to view the body before transfer to a funeral home or the morgue could cause hurt feelings and impede the grieving process.

10. 1. The change process can be compared to the nursing process. The first step of each process is to assess the problem. Assessment involves collecting the pertinent data that supports the need for a change.
2. The second step is to identify the problem or, in the nursing process, identify possible nursing diagnoses.
3. The third step is to select an alternative to implement to fix the problem. This is similar to choosing a specific nursing diagnosis.
5. The fourth step is to implement a plan of action. This is similar to implementing the nursing care plan.

11. 1. Women tend to see the big picture and seek solutions based on what makes people feel comfortable rather than on logic.
2. Men often see the world from a logical perspective and focus on a specific intervention.
3. Men tend to ask fewer questions than women, especially if the man perceives that asking the question will make him look foolish or ignorant.
4. Men and women communicate very differently. The female manager of a male employee should recognize the difference when attempting to arrive at a common goal.

12. 1. The attitude of the UAP changes from one day to the next. The "why" is not important for the manager to know. The important thing for the manager to know is whether the UAP can control the attitude.
2. The first step is an informal meeting with the UAP to discuss the UAP's attitude and how it affects the staff. The manager should document the conversation informally with the date and time (the UAP does not need to see this documentation) for future reference. If the situation is not resolved, more formal counseling must take place.
3. This step would follow the informal discussion if the attitude did not improve.
4. This is a step sometimes used to get the attention of the staff member when formal counseling has not been effective. This step occurs just before termination.

13. 1. E-mails should be easy to read and concise. Individuals may not take the time to read and understand poorly worded, lengthy e-mails.
2. Some communication is appropriate by e-mail, but when discussing a problem with an individual, it is best to use face-to-face communication in which both parties can give and receive feedback.
3. Capital letters in e-mails may be interpreted as shouting or yelling to the receiver.
4. E-mail communication should be concise and easy to read. If the e-mail

requires a lot of information, then the writer should use bullets to separate information.

14. 1. The problem is not a nursing problem. The HCP should be discussing the problem with an individual from the department that "owns" the problem.
    2. This is not a nursing problem.
    3. This is not a nursing problem.
    4. This will only make the HCP angrier. The HCP should be directed to discuss the problem with the department that can fix the problem.

15. 1. Many nurses follow this practice, but no research has been completed to support this practice.
    2. This is part of the Joint Commission's Patient Safety Goals, not evidence-based practice.
    3. **Evidence-based practice is the conscientious use of current best evidence in making decisions about nursing care. Using the "evidence" or research to teach a client is evidence-based practice.**
    4. Reading the journal is a step in EBP, but EBP requires using the information in practice.

16. 1. The charge nurse should stop the nurse from recapping the needle, but not in front of the client.
    2. **The charge should not reprimand the nurse in front of the client or family. The charge nurse should ask the nurse to step into the hall where the client cannot hear.**
    3. Reprimanding the nurse is not the first action.
    4. Notifying the house supervisor is not the first action.

17. 1. The UAP may be at risk of contacting the illness.
    2. **The UAP should wear appropriate personal proactive equipment when providing any type of care.**
    3. The UAP should not be told to skip performing assigned tasks.
    4. Pregnancy is not affected by anthrax.

18. 1. The mortuary service is considered part of the health-care team in this case. The personnel in the funeral home should be made aware of the client's diagnosis.
    2. **The mortuary service is considered part of the health-care team. In this case, the personnel in the funeral home should be made aware of the client's diagnosis.**
    3. The nurse does not need to ask the family for permission to protect the funeral home workers.
    4. The nurse, not the HCP, releases the body to the funeral home.

19. 1. **The nurse and the UAP should protect themselves from injury. A lifting device should be used before attempting to move the client.**
    2. The nurse and the UAP should provide the best care that is possible, including turning the client every 2 hours.
    3. One other person may not be enough to turn or move the client adequately without injuring the staff.
    4. The client is not responsive enough to assist in movement.

20. 1. **The nurse should administer the IVP narcotic pain medication even if the client has shallow breathing, with respirations of 8. The American Nurses Association's Code of Ethics states the client has the right to die in comfort and dignity. A nurse should never administer a medication with the intent of hastening the client's death, but medicating a dying client to achieving a peaceful death is an appropriate intervention. If the client is splinting to protect himself or herself from pain, then pain relief can actually improve respiratory function.**
    2. Repositioning the client would not be effective for "all over pain."
    3. This is cruel to do to a client who is dying and has made himself or herself a DNR.
    4. The HCP has all the orders needed in place. There is no reason to notify the HCP.

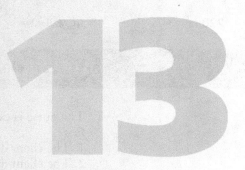

Comprehensive Examination

"Be nice to people on your way up because you meet them on your way down."

—Jimmy Durante

ABBREVIATION LIST

ABG	Arterial Blood Gas	**ICP**	Intracranial Pressure
ACE	Angiotensin-Converting Enzyme	**ID**	Identification
AIDS	Acquired Immunodeficiency Syndrome	**INR**	International Normalized Ratio
AMA	Against Medical Advice	**IV**	Intravenous
ARDS	Acute Respiratory Distress Syndrome	**IVP**	Intravenous Push
		IVPB	Intravenous Piggy Back
BID	Twice a Day	**LPM**	Liters per Minute
BP	Blood Pressure	**LPN**	Licensed Practical Nurse
BSC	Bedside Commode	**MAR**	Medical Administration Record
BUN	Blood Urea Nitrogen	**MHW**	Mental Health Worker (Mental Health UAP)
CABG	Coronary Artery Bypass Graft	**MI**	Myocardial Infarction
CBC	Complete Blood Count	**NPO**	Nothing Per (by) Os (Mouth)
CF	Cystic Fibrosis	**PCA**	Patient-Controlled Analgesia
CHF	Congestive Heart Failure	**PD**	Parkinson's Disease
CPR	Cardiopulmonary Resuscitation	**PO**	Per Os (by Mouth)
COPD	Chronic Obstructive Pulmonary Disease	**PRBCs**	Packed Red Blood Cells
DKA	Diabetic Ketoacidosis	**prn**	As Needed
DVT	Deep Vein Thrombosis	**PT**	Prothrombin Time
ESRD	End-Stage Renal Disease	**PTT**	Partial Thromboplastin Time
GERD	Gastroesophageal Reflux Disease	**RN**	Registered Nurse
		R/O	Rule Out
HCP	Health-Care Provider	**RRT**	Rapid Response Team
HH	Home Health	**TKO**	To Keep Open
HIPAA	Health Insurance Portability and Accountability Act	**UAP**	Unlicensed Assistive Personnel
hs	At Bedtime		
ICU	Intensive Care Unit		

QUESTIONS

1. The nurse is caring for clients on a medical unit. Which client should the nurse assess first?
   1. The client diagnosed with COPD who has a pulse oximeter reading of 93%.
   2. The client diagnosed with CHF who has bilateral 4+ peripheral edema.
   3. The client diagnosed with pneumonia who has a temperature of 100°F.
   4. The client diagnosed with Guillain-Barré syndrome who is unable to feel the hips.

2. Which medication should the nurse administer first after receiving the morning shift report?
   1. The IVPB antibiotic to the client admitted at 0530 this morning.
   2. The sliding scale short-acting insulin to the client with diabetes.
   3. The non-narcotic pain medication to a client with a headache.
   4. The proton-pump inhibitor to the client with a peptic ulcer.

3. The nurse in a critical care unit is administering medications to a client. Which intervention should the nurse implement first?
   1. Check the radial pulse before administering digoxin, a cardiac glycoside.
   2. Monitor the oxygen (O_2) saturation before administering the bronchodilator.
   3. Obtain the latest PTT results on the client with a heparin drip.
   4. Administer the mucosal barrier agent to the client who is NPO.

4. The surgical nurse is admitting a client to the operating room. Which information would require the nurse to call a time-out?
   1. The client is drowsy from the preoperative medication and drifts off to sleep.
   2. The consent form lists a left knee, but the client tells the nurse it is the right knee.
   3. The surgical technician cannot find the surgeon's preferred surgical tray.
   4. The client states his or her name and birth date as it appears on the chart.

5. The nurse is administering medications at 1800 to a client and uses the following medication administration record (MAR). Which intervention should the nurse implement first?

Client's Name: CC	Account Number: 45678-98		Allergies: NKDA	
Diagnosis: Heart Failure	Weight: 178 pounds		Height: 68 inches	
Medication	**0701–1500**	**1501–2300**		**2301–0700**
Digoxin (Lanoxin) 0.125 mg PO daily	0900 DN			
Furosemide (Lasix) 40 mg IVP daily	0900 DN			
Cephalosporin (Keflex) 500 mg PO every 6 hours	1200 DN	1800		
Warfarin (Coumadin) 5 mg PO daily		1800		
Nurse Name/Initials	**Day Nurse RN/ DN**	**Evening Nurse RN/EN**		

    1. Assess the client's potassium and digoxin levels.
    2. Monitor the client's partial thromboplastin level.
    3. Check the client's international normalized ratio (INR).
    4. Verify the client's name and identification (ID) number with the MAR.

6. The nurse is administering medications to clients on a medical unit. Which medication should the nurse question administering?
    1. The steroid, prednisone, to the client diagnosed with COPD.
    2. The anticoagulant, enoxaparin (Lovenox), to a client who had knee surgery.
    3. The antiplatelet, ticlopidine (Ticlid), to a client being prepared for surgery.
    4. The ACE inhibitor, captopril (Capoten), to a client who has a blood pressure (BP) of 100/68.

7. The nurse is caring for a client who has a chest tube. Which interventions should the nurse implement? Rank the interventions in order of performance.
    1. Assess the client's lung sounds.
    2. Note the amount of suction being used.
    3. Check the chest tube dressing for drainage.
    4. Make sure that the chest tube is securely taped.
    5. Place a bottle of sterile saline at the bedside.

8. The nurse is preparing to administer the third unit of packed red blood cells (PRBCs) to a client with a bleeding gastric ulcer. Which interventions should the nurse implement? Select all that apply.
    1. Hang a bag of D_5NS to keep open (TKO).
    2. Change the blood administration set.
    3. Check the client's current vital signs.
    4. Assess for allergies to blood products.
    5. Obtain a blood warmer for the blood.

9. The nurse is assessing clients on a pediatric unit. Which assessment data is priority?
   1. The 6-year-old client diagnosed with leukemia who is sucking his thumb.
   2. The 9-year-old client diagnosed with ulcerative colitis who has bloody diarrhea.
   3. The 13-year-old client diagnosed with cystic fibrosis (CF) who has a pulse oximeter reading of 91%.
   4. The 15-year-old client diagnosed with syphilis who is allergic to penicillin.

10. The home health nurse is caring for a client diagnosed with COPD. Which client problem is priority?
    1. Activity intolerance.
    2. Altered coping.
    3. Impaired gas exchange.
    4. Self-care deficit.

11. The nurse in a rehabilitation facility is evaluating the progress of a female client who sustained a C-6–C-7 spinal cord injury. Which outcome indicates the client is improving?
    1. The client can maneuver the automatic wheelchair into the hallway.
    2. The client states she will be able to return to work in a few weeks.
    3. The client uses eye blinks to communicate yes and no responses.
    4. The client's husband built a wheelchair ramp onto their house.

12. The 46-year-old client in a women's health clinic tells the nurse "I wake up at night sweating." Which statement is the nurse's best response?
    1. "You might want to drink soy milk every day."
    2. "Take calcium pills to prevent osteoporosis."
    3. "Are you having trouble with vaginal dryness?"
    4. "It will help if you sleep under a fan at night."

13. The newborn nursery nurse has received report. Which client should the nurse assess first?
    1. The 2-hour-old infant who has nasal flaring and is grunting.
    2. The 6-hour-old infant who has not passed meconium stool.
    3. The 12-hour-old infant who refuses to latch onto the breast.
    4. The 24-hour-old infant who has a positive startle reflex.

14. The nurse and unlicensed assistive personnel (UAP) are caring for a group of clients on a medical unit. Which action by the UAP requires immediate intervention by the nurse?
    1. The UAP dons unsterile gloves before emptying a urinary catheter bag.
    2. The UAP places clean linen in all of the clients' rooms for the day.
    3. The UAP uses a different plastic bag for every client when getting ice.
    4. The UAP massages the client's trochanter when turing the client.

15. The charge nurse is making assignments on a surgical unit. Which client should be assigned to the least experienced nurse?
    1. The client who had a vaginal hysterectomy and still has an indwelling catheter.
    2. The client who had an open cholecystectomy and has gray drainage in the tube.
    3. The client who had a hip replacement and states something popped while walking.
    4. The client who had a Whipple procedure and reports being thirsty all the time.

16. The unit manager on an oncology unit receives a complaint about the care a client received from the female night shift nurse. Which action should the unit manager implement first?
    1. Ask the night charge nurse to make sure the nurse does the work.
    2. Request the nurse come in to discuss the care provided.
    3. Discuss the situation with the client making the complaint.
    4. Document this occurrence and place in the nurse's employee file.

17. The intensive care unit nurse and a UAP are caring for a client who has had a coronary artery bypass graft (CABG). Which nursing task should the nurse assign to the UAP?
    1. Monitor the client's arterial blood gases.
    2. Re-infuse the client's blood using the cell saver.
    3. Assist the client to take a sponge bath.
    4. Change the client's saturated leg dressing.

18. The nurse and the UAP are caring for clients on a pediatric unit. Which task should the nurse delegate to the UAP?
    1. Sit with the 6-year-old client while the parent goes outside to smoke.
    2. Stay with the 4-year-old client during scheduled play therapy sessions.
    3. Position the 2-year-old client for the postural drainage therapy.
    4. Weigh the diaper of the 6-month-old client who is on intake and output.

19. The charge nurse of a postsurgical unit observes a new graduate telling the elderly client's visitor not to push the client's patient-controlled analgesia (PCA) pump button. Which action should the charge nurse implement?
    1. Encourage the visitor to push the button for the client.
    2. Ask the nurse to step into the hallway to discuss the situation.
    3. Discuss the hospital protocol for the use of PCA pumps.
    4. Continue to perform the charge nurse's other duties.

20. The male home health nurse is planning his rounds for the day. Which client should the nurse plan to see first?
    1. The 56-year-old client diagnosed with multiple sclerosis who is complaining of a cough.
    2. The 78-year-old client diagnosed with congestive heart failure who reports losing 3 pounds.
    3. The 42-year-old client diagnosed with an L-5 spinal cord injury who has developed a stage 4 pressure ulcer.
    4. The 80-year-old client diagnosed with a cerebrovascular accident (CVA) who has right-sided paralysis.

21. The quality control nurse in a long-term care facility observes a licensed practical nurse (LPN) telling a newly hired medication aide to crush nifedipine (Procardia XL) before administering the medication to a client who has difficulty swallowing pills. Which action should the quality control nurse take first?
    1. Tell the medication aide to take the client's blood pressure.
    2. Notify the director of nurses of the charge nurse's instructions.
    3. Show the medication aide where to find pudding for the client.
    4. Ask the charge nurse to speak privately with the nurse.

22. The psychiatric clinic nurse is returning telephone calls. Which telephone call should the nurse return first?
    1. The female client who reports being slapped by her husband when he got drunk last night.
    2. The male client who reports he is tired of living because his wife just left him because he lost his job.
    3. The female client diagnosed with anorexia who reports she does not think she can stand to eat today.
    4. The male client diagnosed with Parkinson's disease who reports his hands are shaking more than yesterday.

23. The psychiatric nurse and mental health worker (MHW) on a psychiatric unit are caring for a group of clients. Which nursing task should the nurse delegate to the MHW?
    1. Take the school-aged children to the on campus classroom.
    2. Lead a group therapy session on behavior control.
    3. Explain the purpose of recreation therapy to the client.
    4. Give a bipolar client a bed bath and shampoo the hair.

24. The administrative supervisor is staffing the hospital's medical surgical units during an ice storm and has received many calls from staff members who are unable to get to the hospital. Which intervention should the supervisor implement first?
    1. Inform the chief nursing officer.
    2. Notify the on-duty staff to stay.
    3. Call staff members who live close to the facility.
    4. Implement the emergency disaster protocol.

25. The nurse is working in a community health clinic. Which nursing task should the nurse delegate to the UAP?
    1. Instruct the UAP to take the client's history.
    2. Request the UAP to document the client's complaints.
    3. Ask the UAP to obtain client's weight and height.
    4. Tell the UAP to complete the client's follow-up care.

26. The staff nurse is working with a colleague who begins to act erratically and is loud and argumentative. Which action should the nurse implement?
    1. Ask the supervisor to come to the unit.
    2. Determine what is bothering the nurse.
    3. Suggest the nurse go home.
    4. Smell the nurse's breath for alcohol.

27. The nurse is taking a history on a client in a women's clinic when the client tells the nurse "I have been trying to get pregnant for 3 years." Which question is the nurse's best response?
    1. "How many attempts have you made to get pregnant?"
    2. "What have you tried to help you get pregnant?"
    3. "Does your insurance cover infertility treatments?"
    4. "Have you considered adoption as an option?"

28. The nurse working at the county hospital is admitting a client who is Rh-negative to the labor and delivery unit. The client is gravida 2, para 0. Which assessment data is the most important for the nurse to assess?
    1. Why the client did not have a viable baby with the first pregnancy.
    2. If the mother received a RhoGAM injection after the last pregnancy.
    3. The period of time between the client's pregnancies.
    4. When the mother terminated the previous pregnancy.

29. The UAP notifies the charge nurse that the male client is angry with the care he is receiving and is packing to leave the hospital. Which action should the charge nurse implement first?
    1. Ask the client's nurse why the client is upset.
    2. Discuss the problem with the client.
    3. Notify the health-care provider (HCP).
    4. Have the client sign the against medical advice (AMA) form.

30. The nurse is preparing to administer 2 units of PRBCs to a client diagnosed with CHF. Which HCP order should the nurse question?
    1. Administer each unit over 2 hours.
    2. Administer the loop diuretic, furosemide (Lasix), intravenous push (IVP) once.
    3. Restrict the client's fluids to 1000 mL per 24 hours.
    4. Have a complete blood count (CBC) done the following morning.

31. The nurse is assessing a client with a spontaneous pneumothorax who has a left-sided chest tube. Which data indicate the treatment is effective?
    1. The chest x-ray indicates consolidation.
    2. The client has bilateral breath sounds.
    3. The suction chamber has vigorous bubbling.
    4. The client has crepitus around the insertion site.

32. The nurse is planning care for the client diagnosed with Parkinson's disease (PD). Which client problem is priority?
    1. Altered nutrition.
    2. Altered mobility.
    3. Altered elimination.
    4. Altered body image.

33. The HCP ordered the loop diuretic, bumetanide (Bumex), to be administered stat to a client diagnosed with pulmonary edema. Which assessment data 4 hours later indicates the client may be experiencing a complication of the medication?
    1. The client develops jugular vein distention.
    2. The client has bilateral rales and rhonchi.
    3. The client complains of painful leg cramps.
    4. The client's output is greater than the intake.

34. The UAP accidentally pulled the client's chest tube out while assisting the client to the bedside commode (BSC). Which intervention should the nurse implement first?
    1. Securely tape petroleum gauze over the insertion site.
    2. Instruct the UAP how to move a client with a chest tube.
    3. Assess the client's respirations and lung sounds.
    4. Obtain a chest tube and a chest tube insertion tray.

35. The 24-year-old client diagnosed with a traumatic brain injury is being transferred to a rehabilitation unit. Which HCP order should the nurse question?
    1. Physical therapy to work on lower extremity strength daily.
    2. Occupational therapy to work on cognitive functioning BID.
    3. A soft diet with mechanical ground meats and thickening agent in fluids.
    4. Methylprednisolone (Solu-Medrol), a steroid, IVP q 6 hours.

36. The 36-year-old client in the women's health clinic is being prescribed birth control pills. Which information is important for the nurse to teach the client? Select all that apply.
    1. Do not smoke while taking birth control pills.
    2. Take one pill at the same time every day.
    3. If a birth control pill is missed, do not double up.
    4. Stop taking the pill if breakthrough bleeding occurs.
    5. There are no interactions with other medications.

37. The nurse on the medical unit is preparing to administer 0900 medications. Which medication should the nurse administer first?
    1. The mucosal barrier agent, sucralfate (Carafate), to a client who has GERD.
    2. The proton-pump inhibitor, pantoprazole (Protonix), to a client with an ulcer.
    3. The Humulin N insulin to a client who is no longer NPO for an x-ray.
    4. The steroid, prednisone, to a client with asthmatic bronchitis.

38. The nurse and UAP are caring for clients on an orthopedic unit. Which task can be delegated to the UAP?
    1. Ambulate the client who had a knee replacement and is weak.
    2. Place a client who had a spinal fusion on a regular bed pan.
    3. Turn, cough, and deep breathe a client who is 2 days post-op.
    4. Feed the client for the first time after a partial laryngectomy.

39. The unit manager of a medical unit is over budget for the year and must transfer one staff member to another unit. Which option is the best action for the unit manager to take before deciding on which staff member to transfer?
    1. Assess each staff member's abilities.
    2. Choose the last staff member hired.
    3. Ask for input from the staff members.
    4. Request the transfer documentation form.

40. The female client was admitted to the orthopedic unit for injuries received during a domestic argument. The client tells the nurse, "I am afraid my husband will kill me if I leave him. It was my fault anyway." Which statement is the nurse's best response?
    1. "What did you do to set him off like that?"
    2. "Do you have a plan for safety if you go back?"
    3. "Why do you think it was your fault?"
    4. "You should leave him before it is too late."

41. The husband of a client on the surgical unit comes to the desk and asks the nurse, "What is my wife's biopsy report?" Which intervention is the nurse's best action?
    1. Check the chart to see whether the client has allowed the spouse to have information.
    2. Obtain the pathology report and tell the husband the results of the biopsy.
    3. Call the HCP and arrange a time for the husband to meet with the HCP.
    4. Inform the client and husband of the biopsy results at the same time.

42. The new graduate nurse is assigned to work with a UAP to provide care for a group of clients. Which action by the nurse is the best method to evaluate that delegated care is being provided?
    1. Check with the clients to see whether they are satisfied.
    2. Ask the charge nurse whether the UAP is qualified.
    3. Make rounds to see that the clients are being turned.
    4. Watch the UAP perform all the delegated tasks.

43. The charge nurse is making assignments on a pediatric unit. Which client should be assigned to the LPN?
    1. The 6-year-old client diagnosed with sickle cell crisis.
    2. The 8-year-old client diagnosed with biliary atresia.
    3. The 10-year-old client diagnosed with anaphylaxis.
    4. The 11-year-old client diagnosed with pneumonia.

44. The client involved in a motor vehicle accident is being prepped for surgery when the client asks the emergency department nurse, "What happened to my child?" The nurse knows the child is dead. Which statement is an example of the ethical principle of nonmalfeasance?
    1. "I will find out for you and let you know after surgery."
    2. "I am sorry but your child died at the scene of the accident."
    3. "You should concentrate on your surgery right now."
    4. "You are concerned about your child. Would you like to talk?"

45. The new graduate has accepted a position at a facility that is accredited by the Joint Commission. Which statement describes the purpose of this organization?
    1. The Commission reviews facilities for compliance with standards of care.
    2. Accreditation by the Commission guarantees the facility will be reimbursed for care provided.
    3. Accreditation by the Commission reduces liability in a legal action against the facility.
    4. The Commission eliminates the need for Medicare to survey a hospital.

46. The client in a critical care unit died. Which intervention is priority for the nurse to implement?
    1. Stay with the significant other.
    2. Gather the client's belongings.
    3. Perform postmortem care.
    4. Ask about organ donation.

47. The nurse caring for client BC is preparing to administer medications. Based on the laboratory data given in this table, which intervention should the nurse implement?

Client's Name: BC	Account Number: 55678-78	Allergies: Sulfa
Diagnosis: Deep Vein Thrombosis	Height: 70 inches	Weight: 150 pounds
LABORATORY REPORT		
Lab Test	Client Value	Normal Value
PT	19.3	10–13 seconds
INR	1.7	2.0–3.0 (therapeutic)
PTT	53	34 seconds

    1. Administer warfarin (Coumadin) IVP.
    2. Continue the heparin drip.
    3. Hold the next dose of warfarin.
    4. Administer the daily aspirin.

48. In the intensive care unit (ICU), the critical care nurse assesses a client diagnosed with an asthma attack who has a respiration rate of 10 and an oxygen saturation of 88%. Which intervention should the nurse implement first?
    1. Call a Rapid Response Team (RRT).
    2. Increase the oxygen to 10 LPM.
    3. Check the client's ABG results.
    4. Administer the fast-acting inhaler.

49. The client in the ICU has been on a ventilator for 2 weeks with an endotracheal tube in place. Which intervention should the nurse expect to prepare the client for next?
    1. Transfer to a long-term care facility.
    2. Daily arterial blood gases.
    3. Removal of life support.
    4. Placement of a tracheostomy.

50. A 90-year-old male client was recently widowed after more than 60 years of marriage. The client was admitted to a long-term care facility and is refusing to eat. Which intervention is an example of the ethical principle of autonomy?
    1. Place a nasogastric feeding tube and feed the client.
    2. Discuss why the client does not want to eat anymore.
    3. Arrange for the family to bring food for the client.
    4. Allow the client to refuse to eat if he wants to.

51. The nurse is admitting a client who professes to be a member of the Jesus Christ Church of Latter Day Saints (Mormons). Which action by the nurse indicates cultural sensitivity to the client?
    1. The nurse does not insist on administering a blood transfusion.
    2. The nurse pins the client's amulet to the client's pillow.
    3. The nurse keeps the client's undershirt on during the bath.
    4. The nurse notifies the client's curandero of the admit.

52. The home health (HH) nurse is teaching the parents of a child diagnosed with cystic fibrosis. Which information is priority to teach the parents?
    1. Explain that the child's skin tastes salty.
    2. Observe the consistency of the stools daily.
    3. Give pancreatic enzymes with every meal.
    4. Increase the intake of salt in the child's diet.

53. The UAP enters the elderly female client's room to give the bath, but the client is watching her favorite soap opera. Which instructions should the nurse give to the UAP?
    1. Tell the UAP to complete the bath at this time.
    2. Have the UAP skip the client's bath for the day.
    3. Instruct the UAP to give the bath after the program.
    4. Document the attempt to give the bath as refused.

54. The nurse has been made the chairperson of a quality improvement committee. Which statement is an example of effective group process?
    1. The nurse involves all committee members in the discussion.
    2. The nurse makes sure all the group agrees with the decisions.
    3. The nurse asks two of the committee members to do the work.
    4. The nurse does not allow deviation from the agenda to occur.

55. While the nurse is caring for a client on a ventilator the ventilator alarm sounds. Which intervention should the nurse implement first?
    1. Check the client's ventilator.
    2. Notify the respiratory therapist.
    3. Assess the client's respiratory status.
    4. Ventilate the client using an Ambu bag.

56. The rehabilitation nurse is planning the discharge of a 68-year-old client whose status post subarachnoid hemorrhage includes residual speech and balance deficits. Which referral should the nurse initiate at this time?
    1. Referral to a hospice organization.
    2. Referral to the speech therapist.
    3. Referral to the physical therapist.
    4. Referral to a home health agency.

57. The psychiatric nurse has received morning report. Which client should the nurse assess first?
    1. The 23-year-old male client who is blocking the other clients' view of the television.
    2. The 31-year-old client who is sitting in the day room, rocking back and forth, and humming.
    3. The 46-year-old female client who is eating multiple candy bars in her room.
    4. The 50-year-old client who refuses to change out of night clothes.

58. The clinic nurse is caring for a 10-year-old client diagnosed with diabetes mellitus type 2. Which client problem is priority?
    1. Altered nutrition, excessive intake.
    2. Risk for low self-esteem.
    3. Hypoglycemia.
    4. Risk for loss of body part.

59. The overhead page has just announced a Code Red on a unit two floors below the unit where the nurse is working. Which action should the nurse implement?
    1. Turn off the oxygen supply to the rooms.
    2. Evacuate the clients to a lower floor.
    3. Close all of the doors to the clients' rooms.
    4. Make a list of clients to discharge.

60. The nurse administered erythropoietin alpha (Epogen), a biologic response modifier, to a client diagnosed with anemia. Which data indicates the client may be experiencing an adverse reaction?
    1. BP 200/124.
    2. Apical pulse 54.
    3. Hematocrit 38%.
    4. Long bone pain.

61. The female client diagnosed with end-stage renal disease (ESRD) who has a left forearm graft is assigned to the nurse and UAP. Which action by the UAP requires immediate intervention by the nurse?
    1. The UAP avoids using soap while bathing the client.
    2. The UAP takes the BP on the client's left arm while the client is lying down.
    3. The UAP tells the client that she should not eat chips.
    4. The UAP measures a scant amount of urine in the BSC.

62. The client diagnosed with sickle cell disease complains of joint pain rated "10" on a 1-to-10 pain scale. Which intervention should the nurse implement first?
    1. Administer a narcotic analgesic to the client.
    2. Check the ID prior to administering the medication.
    3. Assess the client to rule out (R/O) complications.
    4. Obtain the medication for the narcotics box.

63. The elderly client was found on the floor by the bed. Which information should the nurse document in the client's chart?
    1. Fell. No injuries noted. Incident report completed. HCP notified.
    2. Found on floor. No complaints of pain. Able to move all extremities.
    3. States no one answered call light, so attempted to get up without help.
    4. Got out of bed without assistance and fell by the bedside.

64. The HH nurse is caring for an elderly client. Which nursing task should the nurse delegate to the home health aide?
    1. Cook and freeze meals for the client.
    2. Assist the client to sit on the front porch.
    3. Take the client for outings to the store.
    4. Monitor the client's mental status.

65. The client admitted to R/O a myocardial infarction is complaining of substernal chest pain radiating to the left arm and jaw. Which intervention should the nurse implement first?
    1. Take the client's pulse, respirations, and blood pressure.
    2. Call for a stat electrocardiogram and a troponin level.
    3. Place sublingual nitroglycerin 1/150 gr under the tongue.
    4. Notify the HCP that the client has pain.

66. The client diagnosed with acute respiratory distress syndrome (ARDS) is having increased difficulty breathing. The arterial blood gas indicates an arterial oxygen level of 54% on O_2 at 10 LPM. Which intervention should the intensive care unit nurse implement first?
    1. Prepare the client for intubation.
    2. Bag the client with a bag/mask device.
    3. Call a Code Blue and initiate cardiopulmonary resuscitation (CPR).
    4. Start an IV with an 18-gauge catheter.

67. The nurse is caring for a 14-year-old female client diagnosed with bulimia. Which intervention should the nurse delegate to the UAP?
    1. Talk with the parents about setting goals for the client.
    2. Stay with the client for 15 to 20 minutes after each meal.
    3. Encourage the client to verbalize low self-esteem.
    4. List for the dietitian the amount of food the client consumed.

68. The client tells the nurse in the bariatric clinic, "I have tried to lose weight on just about every diet out there but nothing works." Which statement is the nurse's best response?
    1. "Which diets and modifications have you tried?"
    2. "How much weight are you trying to lose?"
    3. "This must be difficult. Would you like to talk?"
    4. "You may need to get used to being overweight."

69. The nurse is preparing to administer medications for clients on a medical unit. The client diagnosed with hypothyroidism is complaining of being hot all the time, feeling palpations, and being jittery. Which intervention should the nurse implement first?
    1. Check the client's serum thyroid levels.
    2. Assess the client for diarrhea.
    3. Document the finding in the chart.
    4. Hold the client's thyroid medication.

70. The nurse is caring for a client diagnosed with acquired immunodeficiency syndrome (AIDS). Which client problem is priority?
    1. Body image disturbance.
    2. Impaired coping.
    3. Risk for infection.
    4. Self-care deficit.

71. The client's arterial blood gas (ABG) results are pH 7.34, $PaCO_2$ 50, HCO_3 24, PaO_2 87. Which intervention should the nurse implement first?
    1. Have the client turn, cough, and deep breathe.
    2. Place the client on oxygen via nasal cannula.
    3. Check the client's pulse oximeter reading.
    4. Notify the HCP of the ABGs.

72. The client is admitted to the emergency department with an apical pulse 134, respirations 28, and BP 92/56, and the skin is pale and clammy. Which intervention should the nurse implement first?
    1. Type and crossmatch the client for PRBCs.
    2. Start two IVs with large-bore catheters.
    3. Obtain the client's history and physical.
    4. Check the client's allergies to medications.

73. The nurse and LPN are caring for clients on an oncology unit. Which client should be assigned to the LPN?
    1. The client diagnosed with acute leukemia who is on a continuous infusion of antineoplastic medications.
    2. The client newly diagnosed with cancer of the lung who is being admitted for placement of an implanted port.
    3. The client diagnosed with an ovarian tumor weighing 22 pounds who is being prepared for surgery in the morning.
    4. The client diagnosed with pancreatic cancer who complains of frequent, unrelenting abdominal pain.

74. Which client should the nurse on a pulmonary unit assess first after receiving the shift report?
    1. The client diagnosed with pneumonia whose ABG results are pH 7.44, PaO_2 89, $PaCO_2$ 37, HCO_3 25.
    2. The client diagnosed with ARDS with a pulse oximeter reading of 91%.
    3. The client diagnosed with respiratory failure who is complaining of shortness of breath when ambulating to the bathroom.
    4. The client diagnosed with a pulmonary embolism whose intravenous heparin infusion was discontinued.

75. The charge nurse of a long-term care facility is making assignments. Which client should be assigned to the most experienced UAP?
    1. The client who is unable to perform personal hygiene.
    2. The client who is angry about the family's not visiting.
    3. The client who needs a full body lift to get in the wheelchair.
    4. The client who is particular about the way things are done.

76. The client 2 days after a laparoscopic cholecystectomy tells the office nurse, "My right shoulder hurts so bad I can't stand it." Which statement is the nurse's best response?
    1. "This is a result of the carbon dioxide gas used in surgery."
    2. "Call 911 and go to the emergency department immediately."
    3. "Increase the pain medication the surgeon ordered."
    4. "You need to ambulate in the hall to walk off the gas pains."

77. The client in a long-term care facility complains of chest pain on deep inspiration. Which intervention should the nurse implement first?
    1. Place the client on oxygen.
    2. Assess the client's lungs.
    3. Notify the HCP.
    4. Arrange for an ambulance transfer.

78. The nurse is caring for a female client 3 days post knee replacement surgery when the client complains of vaginal itching. The MAR indicates the client has been receiving the antacid, calcium carbonate (Maalox), the antibiotic, ceftriaxone (Rocephin), and the anticoagulant, enoxaparin (Lovenox). Which priority intervention should the nurse implement?
    1. Request the dietary department to send yogurt on each tray.
    2. Explain to the client this is the result of the antibiotic therapy.
    3. Notify the HCP on rounds of the client's vaginal itching.
    4. Ask the client whether she is having unprotected sexual activity.

79. The nurse manager of the maternal/child department is developing the budget for the next fiscal year. Which statement best explains the first step of the budgetary process?
    1. Ask the staff for input about needed equipment.
    2. Assess any new department project for costs.
    3. Review the department's current year budget.
    4. Explain the new budget requirements to the staff.

80. The nurse on the psychiatric unit observes one client shove another client. Which intervention should the nurse implement first?
    1. Discuss the aggressive behavior with the client.
    2. Document the occurrence in the client's chart.
    3. Approach the client with another staff member.
    4. Instruct the client to go to the unit's quiet room.

81. The client in the operating room states, "I don't think I will have this surgery after all." Which intervention should the nurse implement first?
    1. Have the surgeon speak with the client.
    2. Ask the client to discuss the concerns.
    3. Continue to prep the client for surgery.
    4. Immediately stop the surgical procedure.

82. Which data indicates therapy has been effective for the client diagnosed with bipolar disorder?
    1. The client only has four episodes of mania in 6 months.
    2. The client goes to work every day for 9 months.
    3. The client wears a nightgown to the day room for therapy.
    4. The client has had three motor vehicle accidents.

83. The nurse is caring for a client newly diagnosed with multiple sclerosis. Which referral is appropriate at this time?
    1. To a social worker to apply for disability.
    2. To a dietitian for a nutritional consult.
    3. To a psychological counselor for therapy.
    4. To a chaplain to discuss spiritual issues.

84. The nurse and LPN have been assigned to care for clients on a pediatric unit. Which nursing task should be assigned to the LPN?
    1. Administer PO medications to a client diagnosed with gastroenteritis.
    2. Take the routine vital signs for all the clients on the pediatric unit.
    3. Transcribe the HCP's orders into the computer.
    4. Assess the urinary output of a client diagnosed with nephrotic syndrome.

85. The nurse is administering medications on a rehabilitation unit. Which medication should the nurse administer first?
    1. The digoxin to a client with a comorbid condition of CHF.
    2. The morning medications to the client scheduled for therapy.
    3. The narcotic pain medication to a client with increased intracranial pressure.
    4. The thyroid medication to a client with hypothyroidism.

86. The charge nurse observes the new graduate nurse delegating tasks to the UAP and the UAP seeming to ignore the new nurse. Which action should the charge nurse implement first?
    1. Wait and observe how the new nurse handles the situation.
    2. Tell the UAP to get busy and complete the assigned tasks.
    3. Discuss learning to assert authority with the new graduate.
    4. Informally counsel the UAP about the response to the nurse.

87. The nurse has received the morning shift report on an oncology unit. Which client should the nurse assess first?
    1. The client diagnosed with leukemia that has a white blood cell (WBC) count of 1.2 (10^3).
    2. The client diagnosed with a brain tumor who has a headache rated as a "2" on the 1-to-10 pain scale.
    3. The client diagnosed with breast cancer who is upset and crying.
    4. The client diagnosed with lung cancer who is dyspneic on exertion.

88. The client on the medical unit has a cardiac arrest. Which is the administrative supervisor nurse's first intervention during the code?
    1. Begin to take notes to document the code.
    2. Make sure all the jobs are being done.
    3. Arrange for an intensive care unit bed.
    4. Administer the emergency medications.

89. Which client should the evening nurse assess first after receiving the P.M. shift report?
    1. The client who is completing the second unit of PRBCs.
    2. The client who was informed of a terminal diagnosis this morning.
    3. The client who refused to eat the dietary tray but got food from home.
    4. The client who became short of breath ambulating in the hallway.

90. The hospital has declared a major disaster. Which action should the charge nurse of the medical unit implement first?
    1. Make rounds with the discharge officer.
    2. Instruct the staff in the disaster plan.
    3. Send one nurse to the disaster command post.
    4. Maintain the functioning of the unit.

91. Which of the staff nurse's personal attributes is an important consideration for the unit manager when discussing making an experienced nurse a preceptor for new graduates? Select all that apply.
    1. The nurse's need for the monetary stipend.
    2. The nurse's ability to organize the work.
    3. The ability of the nurse to interact with others.
    4. The quality of the care the nurse provides.
    5. The nurse's willingness to be a preceptor.

92. The new nurse has accepted a position on a unit that is run using the shared governance model. Which statement is an important precept of this system?
    1. The nurse must cover a shift if the manager asks.
    2. The nurses are responsible for the care they provide.
    3. The nurses schedule themselves to cover the unit.
    4. Nurses are never asked to go to another unit to work.

93. The new graduate on a surgical unit does not take breaks or go to lunch and still cannot complete the work in a timely manner. Which statement is the preceptor's best recommendation to the new graduate?
    1. Suggest the new graduate look for a different position.
    2. Start administering medications 2 hours early.
    3. Clock out at the end of the shift and then finish the charting.
    4. Do not skip the allowed breaks except during an emergency.

94. Which medication should the nurse question administering?
    1. The ACE inhibitor to the client diagnosed with a myocardial infarction (MI) who is on a ventilator and has a BP of 88/62.
    2. The calcium channel blocker to a client diagnosed with hypertension who has a headache and a BP of 220/98.
    3. The beta blocker to a client diagnosed with migraine headaches who has an apical pulse of 52.
    4. The cardiac glycoside to a client diagnosed with heart failure who denies being nauseated.

95. The hospice nurse caring for a client diagnosed with diabetes mellitus type 2 observes the client eating a bowl of ice cream. Which intervention should the nurse implement first?
    1. Allow the client to enjoy the ice cream.
    2. Check the client's blood glucose.
    3. Remind the client not to eat ice cream.
    4. Suggest the client eat low-fat sweets.

96. Which information is most important for the primary nurse to determine prior to referring a terminally ill client to a hospice agency?
    1. Determine exactly how long the client will live.
    2. Check the ability of the client to pay for hospice.
    3. Assess the client's need for supportive care.
    4. Ask whether the client wants palliative care only.

97. The charge nurse of a surgical unit has been notified of an external disaster with multiple casualties. Which client should the charge nurse request to be discharged from the hospital?
    1. The client scheduled for a repair of an abdominal aortic aneurysm (AAA) in the morning and whose preoperative teaching has not been started.
    2. The client who had an abdominal hysterectomy 2 days ago and whose catheter has been removed.
    3. The client who has a bleeding peptic ulcer and now has a hemoglobin of 7 mg/dL and a hematocrit of 22.1%.
    4. The client who was in a motor vehicle accident and has a 6 on the Glasgow coma scale and decorticate posturing.

98. Which laboratory data should the charge nurse notify the HCP?
    1. The potassium level of 3.6 mEq/L in a client diagnosed with heart failure who is taking the loop diuretic furosemide (Lasix).
    2. The PTT level of 78 in the client diagnosed with pulmonary embolism who is receiving IV heparin.
    3. The blood urea nitrogen (BUN) of 84 mg/dL in a client diagnosed with end-stage renal disease and peripheral edema.
    4. The blood glucose level of 543 mg/dL in a client diagnosed with uncontrolled diabetes mellitus type 1.

99. Which nursing intervention is priority for the intensive care nurse to implement when caring for a client diagnosed with diabetic ketoacidosis?
    1. Assess for a fruity breath odor.
    2. Check blood glucose levels ac and hs.
    3. Monitor the client's pulse oximeter readings.
    4. Maintain the IV rate on an infusion pump.

100. The client diagnosed with diabetes mellitus type 2 has a hemoglobin A_{1C} of 11 mg/dL. Which intervention should the nurse implement first?
    1. Check the client's current blood glucose level.
    2. Assess the client for neuropathy and retinopathy.
    3. Teach the client about the effects of hyperglycemia.
    4. Monitor the client's BUN and creatinine levels.

1. 1. A pulse oximeter reading of 93% is considered to be within normal limits; this would be an excellent reading for a client diagnosed with COPD. The nurse would not need to assess this client first.
   2. In a client diagnosed with CHF, 4+ edema is expected. The nurse would not need to assess this client first.
   3. The client diagnosed with pneumonia is expected to have a fever. The nurse would not need to assess this client first.
   4. **Guillain-Barré syndrome is a condition that involves ascending paralysis that can lead to respiratory failure. The client complains of being unable to feel the hips. The nurse should assess this client first to determine the level of impairment.**

2. 1. **First-dose intravenous antibiotic medications are priority medications and should be administered within 1 to 2 hours of when the order was written. This should be the first medication administered.**
   2. This is an important medication and should be administered before the breakfast meal, but it is not priority over initiating the intravenous antibiotic treatment.
   3. The client should be medicated but not before initiating the intravenous antibiotic.
   4. This medication can be administered within the allowable 30 minutes before and after the scheduled administration time.

3. 1. The nurse checks an apical pulse, not a radial pulse, prior to administering digoxin.
   2. The bronchodilator will not be held based on the pulse oximeter reading. The nurse does not need to check the oxygen saturation level.
   3. **Intravenous heparin increases the client's partial thromboplastin time and causes an anticoagulant effect. The nurse should always be aware of the client's most current PTT levels when therapeutic heparin is being administered.**
   4. Mucosal barrier agents are given to coat the stomach prior to eating. Oral medications are held when the client is NPO.

4. 1. The client would be expected to be drowsy after a narcotic preoperative medication. The nurse would not need to call a time-out for this client.

   2. Any time that there is a discrepancy on the chart or with what the client says, the nurse should call an immediate time-out until the situation has been resolved.
   3. This may cause an upsetting situation in the operating room, but it is not a reason to stop the client's surgery.
   4. Because this is what is supposed to happen, the nurse would not need to call a time-out.

5. 1. The day shift nurse should check the client's potassium and digoxin levels prior to administering the digoxin. The digoxin has been administered for the day.
   2. A partial thromboplastin time is monitored for IV heparin, not Coumadin.
   3. **The nurse should monitor the INR prior to administering warfarin (Coumadin). The therapeutic level for warfarin is 2 to 3.**
   4. This should be done immediately prior to administering the medication at the bedside.

6. 1. Steroid medications are frequently prescribed for clients diagnosed with COPD. The nurse would not question administering this medication.
   2. Lovenox is prescribed to prevent deep vein thromboses (DVT) in clients who are immobile.
   3. **The nurse should not administer an antiplatelet medication to a client going to surgery. The nurse should hold this medication and discuss this with the surgeon.**
   4. The client's blood pressure is within an acceptable range. The nurse should administer this medication.

7. 1, 4, 3, 2, and 5.
   1. The nurse should begin the care by assessing the client. Remember the nursing process.
   4. The nurse should have the client's chest and dressing exposed and should check to make sure the chest tube is securely taped at this time.
   3. The nurse then follows the chest tube to the drainage system and assesses the system.
   2. The last part of the chest tube drainage system to assess is the suction system.
   5. The nurse should make sure that emergency supplies are at the bedside last.

8. 2 and 3 are correct.
   1. The only solution compatible with blood is normal saline. Dextrose causes the blood to coagulate.
   2. The blood administration set is changed after every 2 units.
   3. The nurse must assess the client's vital signs before every unit of blood is administered.
   4. The nurse should assess for allergies prior to administering medications. Before administering blood products, the nurse should assess to determine compatibility with the client's blood type. The client may have an incompatible blood type, but this is not an allergy.
   5. A blood warmer is used when the client has identified cold agglutinins. This is not in the stem.

9. 1. A 6-year-old client would be expected to regress in the hospital. The nurse would not need to assess this client first.
   2. A client diagnosed with ulcerative colitis is expected to have bloody diarrhea. The nurse would not need to assess this client first.
   3. A pulse oximeter reading of 91% equates to approximately a 60% arterial saturation. Cystic fibrosis involves thick, tenacious secretions in the lungs and gastrointestinal tract. The nurse should assess this client first.
   4. There are other antibiotics that can be prescribed for the client. The nurse would not need to assess this client first.

10. 1. Activity intolerance is not priority over gas exchange. If gas exchange does not occur, the client will die.
    2. Coping is a psychosocial problem, and physiologic problems are priority.
    3. Impaired gas exchange is the priority problem for this client. If the client does not have adequate gas exchange, the client will die. Remember Maslow's Hierarchy of Needs.
    4. Self-care deficit is not priority over gas exchange.

11. 1. The client's being able to maneuver a wheelchair indicates that the client has progressed in therapy.
    2. This statement indicates the client is in denial about the prognosis of the injury.
    3. Eye blinks may be used for communication in a client with a higher-level injury.
    4. The building of a wheelchair ramp indicates the husband is preparing for the client's return home, not that the client is progressing in therapy.

12. 1. Soy products have been shown to improve the symptoms of menopause, and many women use them because estrogen therapy has proven to increase the risk of cardiovascular problems.
    2. Calcium replacement will help to prevent osteoporosis, but the client is complaining of symptoms related to menopause, not osteoporosis.
    3. This is another symptom of menopause, but the nurse should help the client deal with the symptom she is complaining about.
    4. This may be true, but the client does not need the nurse to suggest an intervention that the client can determine by herself.

13. 1. Nasal flaring and grunting indicate the infant is in respiratory distress. The nurse should assess this infant first.
    2. The nurse would not worry about the infant not passing meconium until 20 to 24 hours after birth. The nurse would not assess this infant first.
    3. This situation requires teaching the mother and patience, but the infant is not in distress. The nurse would not assess this infant first.
    4. This is normal for a newborn. The nurse would not assess this infant first.

14. 1. This is the correct procedure when coming into contact with blood and body fluids. The nurse does not need to intervene.
    2. This may be wasteful if the linens are not used because the client is discharged, but it does not warrant immediate intervention by the nurse until the unit has a problem with linen over usage. This action saves the UAP time.
    3. This is the correct procedure for getting ice. The nurse does not need to intervene.
    4. Massaging pressure points increases tissue damage and increases the risk of skin breakdown. The nurse should intervene and stop this action by the UAP.

15. 1. This client has had a common surgical procedure and is not experiencing a complication. The least experienced nurse could care for this client.
    2. Green bile in a T-tube is expected, but a gray tint to the drainage indicates an infection. An experienced nurse should be assigned to this client.

3. A popping feeling when ambulating indicates the hip joint may have dislocated. An experienced nurse should be assigned to this client.
4. A Whipple procedure involves removing most of the pancreas. The symptoms indicate the client is not metabolizing glucose (symptom of diabetes mellitus). An experienced nurse should be assigned to this client.

16. 1. The unit manager should talk to the client first, not ask the night charge nurse to watch the nurse. This step may be needed if a doubt does surface about the nurse's actually performing the appropriate nursing tasks.
2. This is the second step in this process if the manager determines the complaint is valid.
3. **The first step is to discuss the complaint with the client. This step lets the client know that the client is being heard, and the manager is able to ask any questions to clarify the complaint.**
4. The occurrence may need to be documented and placed in the employee's file, but this is not the unit manager's first intervention.

17. 1. The nurse and respiratory therapist, not the UAP, are responsible for monitoring the ABGs.
2. Infusion of blood and blood products, even the client's own, cannot be delegated to a UAP.
3. **The UAP can assist with hygiene needs; this is one of the main tasks that may be delegated to UAPs.**
4. The nurse must assess the surgical site for bleeding, infection, and healing. The UAP cannot perform assessments.

18. 1. This is not an appropriate delegation. Taking the UAP from the floor to stay with a child so the parent can smoke is supporting a bad health habit.
2. The play therapist will stay with the client during the therapy.
3. The respiratory therapist will position the client for postural therapy.
4. **The UAP is capable of completing intake and outputs on clients. Weighing a diaper is the method of obtaining the output in an infant.**

19. 1. Only the client should activate the PCA pump. Allowing family or significant others to push the button places the client at risk for an overdose.

2. The nurse is acting appropriately; there is no reason to discuss the instructions further.
3. The nurse is acting appropriately; there is no reason to discuss the instructions further.
4. **The nurse is acting appropriately, and there is no reason to discuss the instructions further. The charge nurse should continue with other duties.**

20. 1. **This client may be developing a complication of immobility, one of which is pneumonia. The nurse should assess this client first.**
2. Loss of weight in a client with CHF indicates the client is responding to therapy. This client does not need to be assessed first.
3. Pressure ulcers are a chronic problem, which frequently occur in clients who are paralyzed. This client does not need to be assessed first.
4. Paralysis is expected for a CVA. This client does not need to be assessed first.

21. 1. The medication aide should not administer the medication if the client's BP is less than 90/50, but this is not the first action the nurse should do.
2. The director of nurses may need to be informed that the charge nurse does not know basic medication administration procedures, but this is not the first action for the quality control nurse to implement.
3. The medication aide should be shown where to find pudding or applesauce to mix in crushed medications, but this medication should not be crushed.
4. **The XL in the name of the medication indicates that this medication is a sustained-released formulation and should not be crushed. The quality control nurse should speak privately with the charge nurse and not correct the charge nurse in front of the medication aide. This should be done immediately so that the client does not receive a crushed sustained-release medication.**

22. 1. Because this client is reporting an incident that occurred hours ago and she is not in imminent danger, this client is not the first client the nurse should call.
2. **The nurse should return this call first because the nurse must determine whether the client has a plan for suicide.**

3. Not wanting to eat is part of the anorexia disease process. The nurse does not need to return this call first.
4. Hand trembling is part of the Parkinson's disease process. Control of the symptoms of Parkinson's disease is affected by several factors, including the amount of sleep the client had, fatigue, and the development of tolerance to the medications. Because this client is not at risk for suicide, he is not the first client for the nurse to see.

23. 1. **Pediatric clients in a psychiatric facility must keep up with school work. Clients must be escorted from one building to another. The MHW should be assigned to this task.**
2. The MHW is not qualified for this task to lead a group therapy session.
3. Explaining the purpose of recreation therapy is teaching, and teaching cannot be delegated to an MHW.
4. Clients in a psychiatric facility are expected to meet their own hygiene needs as part of assuming responsibility for themselves. This is not the best task to assign to the MHW.

24. 1. The chief nursing officer should be informed, but this is not the first action.
2. **The first action for the administrative supervisor is to make sure the clients receive care. The supervisor cannot allow the on-duty staff to leave until replacement staff members have been arranged.**
3. The supervisor should call any staff that can get to the hospital in an attempt to staff the hospital, but this is not the first action to implement.
4. An emergency disaster protocol may be implemented, but the first intervention is to ensure the clients have a nurse on duty.

25. 1. The nurse cannot delegate any task that requires nursing judgment. History taking requires knowing which questions need to be asked to assess the client's problems.
2. Documenting the client's complaints is a nursing responsibility that the nurse must perform. It cannot be delegated to UAP.
3. **This UAP can obtain the heights and weights on clients. This is the task the nurse should delegate.**
4. The follow-up care may require teaching, judgment, or further assessment; therefore, the nurse should not delegate this action to a UAP. When delegating to a

UAP, the nurse must provide clear concise and specific instructions. The nurse cannot delegate teaching.

26. 1. **The actions of the colleague indicate possible drug or alcohol impairment. The staff nurse is not in a position of authority to require the potentially impaired nurse to submit to a drug test. The administrative supervisor should assess the situation and initiate the appropriate follow up. The nurse must make sure an impaired nurse is not allowed to care for clients.**
2. The nurse is not a counselor, and a staff nurse should not attempt to confront an impaired colleague.
3. The administrative supervisor and the charge nurse are the only staff members who have the authority to send a nurse home.
4. The nurse should not attempt to determine the cause of the behavior. This is outside the nurse's authority.

27. 1. The nurse could ask this question, but the client has already told the nurse that 3 years have passed, so the client has tried approximately 36 times.
2. **This is the best question to assess the client. The nurse would not want to suggest an intervention that has been futile.**
3. Infertility treatments are very expensive, but the nurse should assess the client's attempts.
4. This question is not helpful for assessing the client or addressing the client's statement.

28. 1. The reason that the first pregnancy did not yield a viable infant is not relevant at this time. The relevant information is whether the mother received the RhoGAM injection.
2. **The important information to assess is whether the client received the RhoGAM injection within 72 hours of the loss of the first pregnancy. If the client did not receive the injection, the fetus is at risk for erythroblastosis fetalis (blue baby).**
3. This is not important information at this time.
4. This is not important information at this time.

29. 1. The charge nurse should discuss the client's anger with the client immediately because the client is preparing to leave the

hospital. The charge nurse can talk with the primary nurse after talking with the client.

2. **This is the first action for the charge nurse. The client is preparing to leave, and a delay in going to the client's room could result in the client's leaving before the situation can be resolved.**

3. The HCP should be notified, but the charge nurse should assess the situation first.

4. The client will be asked to sign the against medical advice form if he insists on leaving, but the charge nurse should attempt to resolve the situation successfully first.

30. 1. **The nurse should administer a unit of blood over the greatest length of time possible (4 hours) to a client diagnosed with congestive heart failure to prevent fluid volume overload. The nurse should question this order.**

2. Administering a diuretic to a client diagnosed with CHF who is receiving blood is an appropriate order. The nurse would not question this HCP order.

3. Restricting fluids to a client diagnosed with CHF is an appropriate order depending on the severity of the client's condition. The nurse would not question this order, especially when administering IV fluids to the client.

4. The HCP should evaluate the effects of the 2 units of blood. The nurse would not question this HCP order.

31. 1. Consolidation indicates fluid or exudates in the lung—pneumonia. This would not indicate the client is improving.

2. **Bilateral breath sounds indicate the left lung has re-expanded and the treatment is effective.**

3. Vigorous bubbling in the suction chamber indicates that there is a leak in the system, but this does not indicate the treatment is effective.

4. Crepitus (subcutaneous emphysema) indicates that oxygen is escaping into the subcutaneous layer of the skin, but this does not indicate the lung has re-expanded, which is the goal of the treatment.

32. 1. Altered nutrition is a physiologic problem but is not priority over safety.

2. **Altered mobility is a problem experienced by clients diagnosed with Parkinson's disease. It leads to many**

other concerns, including the risk for falls resulting from the client's shuffling gait. This is the priority problem.

3. Altered elimination is a problem that the client's altered mobility can cause. This is not, however, the priority problem.

4. Altered body image is a psychological problem and is not priority.

33. 1. Jugular vein distention would indicate the client has CHF. This is not a complication of a loop diuretic.

2. Rales and rhonchi are symptoms of pulmonary edema, not a complication of a loop diuretic.

3. **Leg cramps may indicate a low serum potassium level, which can occur as a result of the administration of a diuretic.**

4. This would indicate the medication is effective and is not a complication of the medication.

34. 1. **Taping petroleum gauze over the chest tube insertion site will prevent air from entering the pleural space. This is the first intervention.**

2. The nurse should make sure the UAP knows the correct method to assist a client with a chest tube, but the safety of the client is the first priority.

3. This is the second intervention the nurse should implement. Remember, if the client is in distress and the nurse can do something to relieve that distress, then the nurse should not assess first. The nurse should take action to take care of the client.

4. The nurse should obtain the necessary equipment for the HCP to reinsert the chest tube, but the priority intervention is to prevent air from entering the pleural space.

35. 1. The client admitted to a rehabilitation unit is expected to participate in therapy for at least 3 hours each day. The nurse would not question this order.

2. The client admitted to a rehabilitation unit is expected to participate in therapy for at least 3 hours each day. The nurse would not question this order.

3. Clients with neurological deficits may have trouble swallowing. The nurse would not question this order.

4. **A client in a rehabilitation unit for a brain injury should not require IV medications. The nurse should question this order.**

239

36. 1, 2, and 5 are correct.
    1. Smoking while taking birth control pills increases the risk of adverse reactions such as formation of blood clots.
    2. The client should take the pill at approximately the same time each day to maintain a blood level of the hormone.
    3. The client should be instructed to take a missed pill as soon as the client realizes she missed the dose during the intervening 24 hours. However, if the client doesn't realize she missed the pill until the next day, she should not take two pills at that time.
    4. Breakthrough bleeding may indicate a change in dose is needed, but the client should not stop taking the pill.
    5. There may be interactions with other medications. Many antibiotics interfere with the action of the birth control pill, and the client should use other contraceptive methods when on an antibiotic.

37. 1. A mucosal barrier agent must be administered on an empty stomach for the best results. The nurse would question administering this medication 1 to 1½ hours after breakfast.
    2. The proton-pump inhibitor can be administered within the 30-minute leeway before and after the scheduled administration time.
    3. The client who is no longer NPO should receive the long-acting insulin as soon as possible. This medication should be administered first.
    4. The steroid medication can be administered within the 30-minute leeway before and after the scheduled administration time.

38. 1. This client is weak, and the UAP could dislocate the joint. The physical therapist should ambulate this client.
    2. A regular bed pan would be too large for the client with a spinal fusion. The client needs a fracture pan.
    3. The client is 2 days post-op, and the nurse could instruct the UAP to turn the client and encourage the client to deep breathe and cough.
    4. A partial laryngectomy can cause the client to have difficulty swallowing. The nurse should assess the client's swallowing the first time the client is allowed to eat.

39. 1. The manager should assess the abilities of each staff member for the needs of the unit before deciding on which staff member to transfer.

2. This may be the method used by many managers, but the best action is to evaluate the needs of the unit and the abilities of the staff.
3. In many instances, the unit manager must make hard decisions without consulting the staff members. Asking for the staff members' input could cause tension among the staff; therefore, this is not an appropriate intervention.
4. This will be completed after the decision has been made and the staff member notified.

40. 1. This is blaming the client. No one has the right to abuse the client.
    2. The nurse must assess the client's safety and provide a referral to a women's center. This is the nurse's best response.
    3. The client does not owe the nurse an explanation of her feelings. This is not a good response to the client.
    4. The nurse is advising. The decision whether to leave the abuser or not must be the client's decision.

41. 1. Even though the spouse of the client is making the request, the nurse should still check to make sure that the client has listed the husband as allowed to receive information. The Health Information Privacy and Portability Act (HIPAA) regulations do not allow for release of information to anyone not specifically designated by the client.
    2. The nurse cannot do this unless the client has designated the husband as allowed to receive information.
    3. The HCP as well as the nurse must abide by HIPAA.
    4. The HCP is responsible for divulging biopsy results. If the spouse is present when the HCP enters the room and the client allows the spouse to stay, then consent for receiving information is implied.

42. 1. The clients would not understand the importance of the specific tasks. Clients will tell the nurse whether the UAP is pleasant when in the room but not whether the delegated tasks have been completed.
    2. The nurse retains responsibility for the delegated tasks. The charge nurse may be able to tell the nurse that the UAP has been checked off as being competent to perform the care but would not know whether the care was actually provided.

3. The nurse retains responsibility for the care. Making rounds to see that the care has been provided is the best method to evaluate the care.
4. The nurse would not have time to complete his or her own work if the nurse watched the UAP perform all of the UAP's work.

43. 1. A client in a crisis should be assigned to the registered nurse (RN).
2. Biliary atresia involves liver failure, involving multiple body systems. This client should be assigned to the RN.
3. Anaphylaxis is an emergency situation. The client should be assigned to the RN.
4. **The LPN can administer routine medications and care for clients who have no life-threatening conditions.**

44. 1. **Nonmalfeasance means to do no harm. This statement is letting the client know that the concern has been heard but does not give the client bad news before surgery. The nurse is aware that someone having surgery should be of sound mind, and finding out your child is dead would be horrific.**
2. This is an example of veracity.
3. This is an example of paternalism, telling the client what he or she should do.
4. This is a therapeutic response, not an example of nonmalfeasance.

45. 1. **The Joint Commission is an organization that monitors health-care facilities for compliance with standards of care. Accreditation is voluntary, but most third-party payers will not reimburse a facility that is not accredited by some outside organization.**
2. Accreditation does not guarantee reimbursement, although most third-party payers require some accreditation by an outside organization.
3. Accreditation does not reduce the hospital's liability.
4. Medicare/Medicaid will not review a facility routinely if the Joint Commission has accredited the facility, but a representative will review the facility in cases of reported problems.

46. 1. The nurse should "offer self" to the significant other. Ignoring the needs of the significant other at this time makes the significant other feel that the nurse does not care, and if the nurse does not care for "me," then did the nurse provide adequate care to my loved one? This action is very important to assist in the grieving process.
2. The UAP can gather the deceased client's belongings.
3. The UAP can perform postmortem care.
4. **The representative of the organ donation team will make this request. Organ banks think it is best for specially trained individuals to discuss organ donation with the significant others.**

47. 1. Coumadin is an oral, not intravenous, medication.
2. **The therapeutic PTT results should be 1½ to 2 times the control, or 51 to 68 seconds. The client's value of 53 is within the therapeutic range. The nurse should continue the heparin drip as is.**
3. The INR is not up to therapeutic range yet, so warfarin (Coumadin) should be administered.
4. These lab values do not provide any information about aspirin administration, but the nurse should ask the HCP whether aspirin (an antiplatelet) should be discontinued because the client is receiving two anticoagulants-heparin and warfarin.

48. 1. A rapid response team (RRT) is called when the nurse assesses a client whose condition is deteriorating. The purpose of an RRT is to intervene to prevent a code. In the scenario described, the situation has not progressed to an arrest. The nurse should call an RRT, but administering oxygen is the first intervention.
2. **The first action is to increase the client's oxygen to 100%.**
3. The nurse could check the ABG results, but the client is in distress and the nurse should implement an intervention to relieve the distress.
4. A fast-acting inhaler should be used, but not until after the oxygen has been increased and an RRT called.

49. 1. The client may eventually need to be transferred to a facility that accepts long-term ventilator-dependent clients, but the nurse would not anticipate this at this time.
2. The client on a ventilator will have blood gases ordered more often than daily.
3. The stem does not indicate that the client is ready to be removed from the ventilator.
4. **A client who has been intubated for 10 to 14 days and still requires mechanical ventilation should have surgically placed tracheostomy to prevent permanent vocal cord damage.**

50. 1. This is an example of paternalism or beneficence.
    2. This is an example of beneficence.
    3. This is an example of nonmalfeasance or beneficence.
    4. **This is an example of autonomy.**

51. 1. This would be culturally sensitive to a client who is a Jehovah's Witness.
    2. Mormons do not wear amulets.
    3. **The devout Mormon client wears a religious undershirt that should not be removed; this action indicates cultural sensitivity on the part of the nurse.**
    4. Mormons do not consult curanderos. Some Hispanic cultures consult curanderos.

52. 1. The child's skin will normally taste salty, but this is not the priority intervention to teach.
    2. The parents should be asked about the client's stools during an assessment because the effectiveness of the pancreatic enzymes is evaluated by the consistency of the stool. This is not the priority intervention because the child must take the enzymes before monitoring the consistency of the stool.
    3. **Cystic fibrosis is a genetic condition that results in blockage of the pancreatic ducts. The child needs pancreatic enzymes to be administered with every meal and snack so the enzymes will be available when the food gets to the small intestine.**
    4. Cystic fibrosis is one of the few diseases that require salt replacement, but salt replacement is not more important than taking the pancreatic enzymes.

53. 1. The UAP should be sensitive to the client's preferences and not insist that the client miss the program.
    2. The UAP should arrange an acceptable time for the client, and the UAP can return to complete the task at the agreed-on time.
    3. **This is the best instruction for the nurse to give to the UAP.**
    4. The bath has not been refused. The client does not want the program interrupted.

54. 1. **Effective group process involves all members of the group.**
    2. Unanimous decisions may indicate group think, which can be a problem in a group process.
    3. Effective group process involves all members of the group, not just two.

4. Not allowing deviation from the agenda is an autocratic style and limits the creativity and involvement of the group.

55. 1. **The ventilator should be checked to determine which alarm is sounding. This is the first step in assessing the client's problem.**
    2. The nurse should assess the ventilator and the client and then notify the respiratory therapist, if needed.
    3. The client should be assessed, but the ventilator may require only a simple adjustment to fix the problem and turn off the alarm. This is one instance in which the nurse should assess the machine prior to assessing the client because the machine is breathing for the client.
    4. The client should be manually ventilated if the nurse cannot determine the cause of the ventilator alarm.

56. 1. A hospice organization is designed for terminally ill clients. The client is not terminally ill.
    2. The speech therapist helps clients regain speech and swallowing abilities. This therapy should have been occurring while the client was in the rehab facility.
    3. The physical therapist assists the client with gait and muscle strengthening. This therapy should have been occurring while the client was in the rehab facility.
    4. **The client is being discharged. The nurse should plan for continuity of care by arranging for a home health agency to follow the client at home.**

57. 1. **This client is creating a disturbance with the other clients and could be at risk for harm from the other clients. The nurse should assess this client first.**
    2. This behavior does not place the client or others at risk. This client does not need to be assessed first.
    3. This behavior does not place the client or others at risk. This client does not need to be assessed first.
    4. This behavior does not place the client or others at risk. This client does not need to be assessed first.

58. 1. **Children are being diagnosed with type 2 diabetes mellitus because of excessive intake of calories and lack of exercise. This is the priority problem.**
    2. The client has a risk of low self-esteem because of the excess weight, but if the

client and parents adhere to the recommended treatment regimen for weight control, diet, and exercise, the client's self-esteem should improve.

3. The client's problem is hyperglycemia, not hypoglycemia.

4. Amputation is a chronic problem associated with diabetes and occurs after years of uncontrolled blood glucose levels. This is not the priority problem at this time.

59. 1. On a floor not directly affected by the fire, the oxygen is turned off only at the instruction of the administrative supervisor or plant operations director.

2. The clients are safer on the floor where they are, not in an area closer to the fire.

3. **The first action in a Code Red (actual fire) is to Rescue (R) the clients in immediate danger, followed by confine (C), closing the doors. Doors in a hospital must be fire rated to confine a blaze for an hour and a half.**

4. This could be done, but it is a charge nurse responsibility that is not called for at this time.

60. 1. **Erythropoietin stimulates the bone marrow to produce red blood cells. An adverse reaction to Epogen is hypertension, which this client whose BP is 200/124 has. Hypertension can cause the dose of erythropoietin to be decreased or discontinued.**

2. Epogen does not affect the pulse.

3. A hematocrit of 38% would indicate the medication is effective.

4. A side effect of the medication is long bone pain. This can be treated with a non-narcotic analgesic. This is not an adverse reaction.

61. 1. The UAP should not use soap when bathing a client diagnosed with ESRD. Soap is drying, and the client diagnosed with ESRD has poor skin integrity.

2. **The nurse should stop the UAP from using the arm with the graft. Pressure on the graft could occlude the graft.**

3. The UAP can tell the client not to eat contraband food. This is not teaching.

4. This is an appropriate action for the UAP; the nurse would not need to intervene.

62. 1. **The nurse should assess the client for complications before administering the medication.**

2. This should occur but not before assessing the client for complications.

3. **The first step in administering a prn pain medication is to assess the client for a complication that may require the nurse to notify the HCP or implement an independent nursing intervention.**

4. This is not the first intervention.

63. 1. The nurse should not document that the client fell unless the nurse observed the client fall. The nurse should never write "incident report" in a chart. This becomes a red flag to a lawyer.

2. **The nurse should document exactly what was observed. This statement is the correct documentation.**

3. This statement is not substantiated and should not be placed in the chart.

4. This statement is documenting something the nurse did not observe, a fall.

64. 1. Cooking and cleaning are jobs that can be arranged through some home health agencies, but these jobs would be done by a housekeeper, not by the UAP.

2. **The home health aide is responsible for assisting the client with activities of daily living and transferring from the bed to the chair. Sitting outside is good for the client and is a task that can be delegated to the home health aide.**

3. This is boundary crossing by the UAP and could create legal difficulties if the UAP had an accident.

4. This is assessment and cannot be delegated to a UAP.

65. 1. If the client is in distress, assessment is not the first intervention if there is an action the nurse can take to relieve the distress. The nurse should administer the nitroglycerin first.

2. Calling for an electrocardiogram and troponin level should be implemented but not before administering the nitroglycerin.

3. **Placing nitroglycerin under the client's tongue may relieve the client's chest pain and provide oxygen to the heart muscle. This is the nurse's first intervention.**

4. Notification of the HCP can be done after the nurse has stabilized the client.

66. 1. **Acute respiratory distress syndrome is diagnosed when the client has an arterial blood gas of less than 50% while receiving oxygen at 10 LPM. The nurse should prepare for the client to be intubated.**

2. The nurse should intervene while the client is breathing by calling the HCP and assisting in the intubation and setup of the mechanical ventilator. If the client has an arrest before this can be arranged, the client would be ventilated with a bag/mask device.
3. If the nurse does not intervene immediately, an arrest situation will occur, at which time a Code Blue would be called and CPR started.
4. If the client does not have a patent IV, the nurse should start one, but not before preparing for intubation.

67. 1. Planning the care of the client cannot be delegated to a UAP, and, the client, not the parents, should set the goals.
2. The UAP should stay with the client for an hour after a meal. Leaving the client after 20 minutes would allow the client time to induce vomiting.
3. This requires the nurse to utilize therapeutic conversation and nursing judgment. The nurse cannot delegate this intervention to a UAP.
4. **The UAP can document the amount of food consumed on a calorie count form for the dietitian to evaluate.**

68. 1. **This is an assessment question that should be asked to determine what the client has attempted that has been unsuccessful.**
2. The amount of weight loss desired is not as important as assessment of previous unsuccessful strategies.
3. This is a therapeutic statement, but the nurse should assess the client.
4. This statement is not helpful, and the nurse working in a bariatric clinic should know that there are many options for weight loss, including surgery.

69. 1. The nurse should check the laboratory tests to determine the thyroid levels, but this is not the first intervention.
2. Assessing the client for diarrhea could be done, but it is more important not to worsen the problem, and therefore, the nurse should hold the thyroid medication first.
3. Documentation of client complaints is always important, but it is not the first intervention.
4. **The client is describing symptoms of hyperthyroidism. Because the client is diagnosed with hypothyroidism and has been prescribed thyroid hormone**

replacement and now has symptoms of hyperthyroidism, it can be assumed that the client now has an excess of thyroid hormone. Therefore, the nurse should hold the thyroid medication and check the client's thyroid profile.

70. 1. Clients diagnosed with acquired immunodeficiency syndrome (AIDS) may have body image disturbance issues related to weight loss and Kaposi's sarcoma lesions, but these are psychological problems, and physiologic problems have priority.
2. Impaired coping is a psychological problem, and physiologic problems are priority.
3. **The basic problem with a client diagnosed with AIDS is that the immune system is not functioning normally. This increases the risk for infection. This is the priority client problem.**
4. Self-care deficit is a psychosocial problem, not a physiologic problem.

71. 1. **These blood gases indicate respiratory acidosis that could be caused by ineffective cough, with resulting air trapping. The nurse should encourage the client to turn, cough, and deep breathe.**
2. The PaO_2 level is within normal limits, 80 to 100. Administering oxygen is not the first intervention.
3. The nurse knows the arterial blood gas oxygen level, which is an accurate test. The pulse oximeter only provides an approximate level.
4. This is not the first intervention. The nurse can intervene to treat the client before notifying the HCP.

72. 1. The nurse should first prevent circulatory collapse by starting two IVs and initiating normal saline or Ringer's lactate. The crossmatch may be needed if the shock condition is caused by hemorrhage.
2. **The client is exhibiting symptoms of shock. The nurse should start IV lines to prevent the client from progressing to circulatory collapse.**
3. All clients have a history taken and physical examination performed as part of the admission process to the emergency department, but this is not the first intervention.
4. Checking the client's allergies to medications is important, but it is not the first intervention in a client exhibiting signs of shock.

73. 1. The infusion of antineoplastic medications is limited to chemotherapy- and biotherapy-competent registered nurses. A qualified registered nurse should be assigned to this client.
    2. This client should be assigned to a registered nurse who can answer the client's questions about the cancer and cancer treatments.
    3. **This client is pre-op, and the LPN can prepare a client for surgery. A 22-pound tumor indicates a benign ovarian cyst.**
    4. An experienced registered nurse should be assigned to this client because the client is unstable, with unrelenting pain.

74. 1. These are normal blood gases. This client does not need to be assessed first.
    2. **A pulse oximeter reading of 91% is approximately a 60% arterial oxygenation level. The nurse should assess this client first.**
    3. The client diagnosed with respiratory distress would be expected to be short of breath on exertion. This client does not need to be assessed first.
    4. This client is improving or the heparin would not have been discontinued. This client does not need to be assessed first.

75. 1. The inexperienced UAP can assist the client with a bath and brushing the teeth and hair. This client does not need to be assigned to the most experienced UAP.
    2. The nurse should be assigned to care for this client who is angry about the family's not visiting because the client requires assessment, nursing judgment, and therapeutic communication and intervention, which are not within the UAP's scope of practice.
    3. **This client requires an experienced UAP who is skilled in client lifts so that the client is lifted safely and the UAP is not injured in the process.**
    4. The experienced UAP could care for this client, but then other UAPs would not learn to care for the client. This client should be rotated through the UAPs so that all the UAPs can learn to care for the client.

76. 1. **During a laparoscopic cholecystectomy, carbon dioxide is instilled into the client's abdomen. Postoperatively, the gas migrates to the shoulder by gravity and causes shoulder pain.**

2. This is not an emergency situation, and the nurse should explain this to the client.
    3. The nurse should not tell the client to increase the pain medication. This is prescribing.
    4. These pains are "gas" pains, but they are not intestinal gas pains that can be relieved by ambulation.

77. 1. **Chest pain on deep inspiration is a symptom of pulmonary embolism. The nurse should first place the client on oxygen.**
    2. The first intervention is to provide the client with oxygen. The test taker should not assess when the client is in distress.
    3. The HCP should be notified, but oxygen is the priority intervention.
    4. The client needs interventions not available in a long-term care facility. The nurse should arrange for a transfer, but the client should be placed on oxygen first.

78. 1. Vaginal itching while receiving antibiotics indicates that the good bacterial flora in the vagina is being destroyed. Yogurt contains these bacteria and can replace the needed bacteria. However, requesting the dietary department to send yogurt each day is not the priority intervention.
    2. **The nurse should first explain to the client that this is a side effect of the antibiotic medication. Then, the nurse should notify the dietitian and HCP. The antibiotic therapy cannot be discontinued because of the need for antibiotic therapy after knee replacement surgery.**
    3. The HCP should be notified of the vaginal itching, but it is not an emergency and can wait until the HCP makes rounds.
    4. The client's sexual history is not a concern because the vaginal infection is secondary to the antibiotic therapy.

79. 1. The manager should ask for input into the budgetary needs from the staff, but an assessment of the current year's budget is the first step.
    2. An assessment of the costs of any new department projects should be done, but the first step is to assess the present budget.
    3. **The first step in a budgetary process is to assess the current budget.**
    4. Explaining the new budget to the staff is the last step in the process.

80. 1. The nurse should confront the client with the behavior, but this is not the first intervention.
   2. The nurse should document the behavior in the client's chart, but this is not the first intervention.
   3. **The nurse should intervene to stop the behavior first before one of the clients is injured. Approaching the client with another staff member shows strength and provides the nurse with the ability to perform a safe "take down."**
   4. The client should be told to return to the room, but stopping the behavior is the first intervention.

81. 1. This surgeon should speak with the client, but the first intervention is to stop the procedure.
   2. Asking the client to discuss concerns should be done, but the first intervention is to stop the procedure.
   3. Continuing to prep the client for the surgery can be done, but is inappropriate when the client no longer is giving consent.
   4. **Stopping the surgical procedure is the first intervention for the nurse to implement.**

82. 1. Four episodes of mania in 6 months do not indicate therapy has been effective.
   2. **The ability to hold a job for 9 months indicates the client is responding to therapy.**
   3. Wearing a nightgown to the day room does not indicate the client is responding to treatment.
   4. Three motor vehicle accidents do not indicate the client is responding to treatment.

83. 1. The client may be able to maintain the ability to work for several years before needing to apply for disability. The stem does not suggest the client is disabled.
   2. The client is newly diagnosed; nutrition would not be a problem at this time.
   3. **The client should be referred to a psychological counselor to develop skills for coping with the long-term chronic illness.**
   4. The chaplain may need to see the client, but the stem did not indicate the client was having a problem with spiritual distress.

84. 1. **The LPN can administer routine medications.**

2. The UAP, not the LPN, should be assigned to take the routine vital signs.
   3. The unit secretary, not an LPN, should be assigned to transcribe the HCP orders.
   4. The RN, not the LPN, should assess the urinary output of the client. The RN should not delegate assessment.

85. 1. Digoxin can be administered within the 30-minute leeway before and after the scheduled administration time.
   2. **The nurse should administer the medications to the client who will be off the unit first.**
   3. Before administering a narcotic, the nurse must first assess the client to make sure that administering the medication is not going to mask symptoms.
   4. Thyroid medication can be administered within the 30-minute leeway before and after the scheduled administration time.

86. 1. **The charge nurse will not always be available to intercede for the new graduate. The charge nurse should wait and see whether the new graduate is capable of handling the situation before intervening.**
   2. The charge nurse should wait to allow the new graduate to deal with the UAP.
   3. The charge nurse should wait to allow the new graduate to deal with the UAP.
   4. The charge nurse should wait to allow the new graduate to deal with the UAP.

87. 1. A low WBC count is expected in a client diagnosed with leukemia. This client does not need to be assessed first.
   2. A client diagnosed with a brain tumor would be expected to have a mild headache. This client does not need to be assessed first.
   3. **The client is upset and crying. When all the information in the options is expected and not life threatening, then psychological issues have priority. This client should be seen first.**
   4. Dyspnea on exertion is expected in a client diagnosed with lung cancer. This client does not need to be assessed first.

88. 1. The supervisor can take notes documenting the code until relieved, but the supervisor needs to be free to supervise the code and coordinate room assignments and staffing.
   2. **The first intervention for the supervisor is to ensure that all the jobs in the code are being filled.**

3. This is the responsibility of the supervisor, but it is not the first intervention.
4. The supervisor can administer medications, but the supervisor needs to be flexible to complete the duties of the supervisor.

89. 1. This client is being treated, and if the blood is almost finished, then it can be assumed that the client is tolerating the blood without incident.
2. **The client has been given devastating news. When all the information in the options is expected and not life threatening, then psychological issues have priority. This client should be seen first.**
3. The client has eaten. The nurse could arrange for the dietitian to consult with the client about food preferences, but this client does not need to be assessed first.
4. Dyspnea on exertion is not priority if the client is exerting himself or herself.

90. 1. Rounds with the discharge officer will be completed when the discharge officer gets to the charge nurse's unit. Before this happens, the charge nurse must make a list of possible discharges.
2. The staff may need to be reminded of the specific duties during the disaster, but this is not the first intervention.
3. **The charge nurse must send a qualified nurse to the command post to assume duties during the disaster. This is the first intervention.**
4. The charge nurse is responsible to see that all clients on the unit are receiving care. This is not the first responsibility, but it is an ongoing one.

91. 2, 3, 4, and 5 are correct.
1. Monetary need is not a good reason to select a nurse to become a preceptor.
2. **The nurse should be able to organize his or her own workload before becoming a role model for a new nurse. If the nurse is not organized, taking on new responsibilities will be very frustrating for the preceptor and for the preceptee.**
3. **The nurse who acts as a preceptor should have good people skills and be approachable.**
4. **The nurse should consistently provide quality care that others should emulate.**
5. **The nurse should be willing to take on this responsibility or the preceptor will resent the new nurse.**

92. 1. A nurse cannot be responsible for covering any shift that he or she is requested to cover.
2. The nurse is responsible for the care he or she provides regardless of the staffing model.
3. **Under the shared governance system, the staff is given the opportunity to self-schedule. This provides the nurses with flexibility and autonomy.**
4. The nurse may be asked to float to another unit.

93. 1. The preceptor is not being supportive by suggesting the nurse go elsewhere to work.
2. Starting medication administration 2 hours early is not in the acceptable guidelines for medication administration.
3. Finishing charting after clocking out at the end of a shift is not in accordance with wage and hour laws.
4. **This is an appropriate suggestion to give to a new nurse. The nurse is having difficulty staying up with the tasks, and this can be overwhelming. If the nurse takes a break from the tasks, his or her mind will have a chance to rethink the tasks and set priorities.**

94. 1. This BP is low, but the client is on a ventilator and not ambulating, and the client is receiving an ACE inhibitor for its cardiac protective properties. The ACE inhibitor can prevent the client who has had an MI from experiencing heart failure as a result of the increased workload placed on the cardiac muscle. The nurse would not question administering this medication.
2. A calcium channel blocker is administered for hypertension, which this client has. The nurse would not question administering this medication.
3. **The client diagnosed with a migraine headache may be prescribed a beta blocker to prevent migraine headaches, but beta blockers reduce the heart rate. The nurse would question administering this medication because the client's apical pulse is low, at 52.**
4. The nurse would not question administering a medication based on the client's having no nausea.

95. 1. A terminally ill client should be allowed comfort measures even when the activity would normally not be encouraged or allowed. The client can receive sliding scale insulin, if needed, to cover the ice cream.

2. The nurse could do this after the ice cream has been metabolized to determine whether an insulin injection is needed.
3. The nurse should tell the client that food such as ice cream may be consumed in moderation and with the appropriate coverage.
4. Low-fat sweets may be a good substitute for some of the foods the client may want to eat.

96. 1. No one knows exactly how long the client will live. The HCP must think that the client has 6 months or less to live for the client to be placed on a hospice service, but some clients on hospice service have lived for several years.
2. Some hospice agencies have charitable funds. The client's inability to pay would not exclude the nurse from making the referral.
3. The client's need for supportive care is not the most important information. The client must desire comfort measures only.
4. Clients placed on hospice service cannot desire to continue curative treatments. The philosophy of hospice is to provide comfort measures to ensure a peaceful dignified death.

97. 1. A client's aneurysm is at least 5 to 6 cm before being scheduled for an AAA. This client's aneurysm is at risk for rupture. This client should have the surgery as scheduled.
2. This client is stable and could be discharged.
3. This client is not stable and should not be discharged.
4. This client is critically ill and should not be discharged.

98. 1. This is a normal potassium level, and the HCP does not need to be notified.
2. This data is within therapeutic range. and the HCP does not need to be notified.
3. A BUN of 84 mg/dL is an abnormal lab value, but it would be expected in a client diagnosed with ESRD. The HCP does not need to be notified.
4. This is a very high blood glucose level, and the client diagnosed with type 1 diabetes will be catabolizing fats at this level and is at risk for diabetic ketoacidosis (DKA) coma.

99. 1. The client with DKA would have fruity breath; therefore, this nursing intervention does not have priority.
2. Glucose levels are monitored at least every hour.
3. The pulse oximeter reading is not priority for a client in DKA.
4. The client will be on a regular insulin drip, which must be maintained at the prescribed rate on an intravenous pump device. Decreasing the client's blood glucose level is the priority nursing intervention.

100. 1. The client's hemoglobin A_{1C} is a test that reveals the average blood glucose for the previous 2 to 3 months. The current blood glucose level may or may not be in the desired range, but the client's diabetes with this level of hemoglobin A_{1C} is not controlled.
2. The nurse should assess for complications of diabetes, but this is not the first intervention. Getting the client to realize the meaning of a high hemoglobin A_{1C} is the priority at this time.
3. The client must be taught the long-term effects of hyperglycemia. A hemoglobin A_{1C} of 11 indicates an average blood glucose of 310 mg/dL. Over time, a level higher than 120 to 140 mg/dL can lead to damage to many body systems.
4. Monitoring blood work is not priority over teaching the client about complications of diabetes when having such a high A_{1C}.

Appendix

Normal Laboratory Values

These values are obtained from *Davis's Comprehensive Handbook of Laboratory and Diagnostic Tests with Nursing Implications*. Laboratory results may differ slightly depending on the resource manual or the laboratory normal values.

Test	Adult
pH	7.35 to 7.45
Pco_2	35 to 45 mm Hg
Hco_3	22 to 26 mEq/L
Pao_2	80 to 100 mm Hg
O_2 saturation	93% to 100%

Test	Adult
Cholesterol HDL LDL	Less than 200 mg/dL 40 to 65 mg/dL Less than 185 mg/dL
Creatinine	0.6 to 1.2 mg/dL
Glucose	60 to 110 mg/dL
Potassium	3.5 to 5.5 mEq/L
Sodium	135 to 145 mEq/L
Triglycerides	Less than 150 mg/dL
Blood urea nitrogen	10 to 31 mg/dL

Test	Adult
Hematocrit (Hct)	Male: 43% to 49% Female: 38% to 44%
Hemoglobin (Hgb)	Male: 13.2 to 17.3 g/dL Female: 11.7 to 15.5 g/dL
Activated partial thromboplastin time (APTT)	25 to 35 seconds
Prothrombin time (PT)	10 to 13 seconds
Red blood cell count (RBC)	Male: 4.7 to 5.1 10^6 cells/mm³ Female: 4.2 to 4.8 10^6 cells/mm³
White blood cell count (WBC)	4.5 to 11.0 1000/mm³
Platelets	150 to 450 10^3/ul/mm³
Erythocyte sedimentation rate (ESR)	Male: 0 to 20 mm/hr Female: 0 to 30 mm/hr

Test	Adult
Digoxin (Lanoxin)	0.8 to 2.0 ng/mL
International normalized ratio (INR)	2 to 3 2.5 to 3.5 if the client has a mechanical heart valve
Lithium mEq/L	0.6 to 1.2 mEq/L
Phenytoin (Dilantin)	10 to 20 mcg/mL
Theophylline (Aminophyllin)	10 to 20 mcg/mL
Valproic acid (Depakote)	50 to 100 mcg/mL
Vancomycin trough level	10 to 20 mcg/mL
Vancomycin peak level	30 to 40 mcg/mL

Bibliography

Catalano, J. (2006). *Nursing now: Today's issues, tomorrows trends* (4th ed.). Philadelphia: F.A. Davis.

Grossman, S., & Valiga, T. (2005). *The new leadership challenge: Creating the future of nursing* (2nd ed.). Philadelphia: F.A. Davis.

Harkreader, H., & Hogan, M. (2004). *Fundamentals of nursing: Caring and clinical judgment.* Philadelphia: W. B. Saunders.

James, S., Ashwill, J., & Droske, S. (2002). *Nursing care of children: Principles and practice.* Philadelphia: W. B. Saunders.

McKinney, E., Ashwill, J., & Murry, S. (2000). *Maternal-child nursing.* Philadelphia: W. B. Saunders.

Schnell, Z., Leeuwen, A., & Kranpitz, T. (2003). *Davis's comprehensive handbook of laboratory and diagnostic tests with nursing implications.* Philadelphia: F.A. Davis.

Smeltzer, S., Bare, B., Hinkle, J., & Cheever, K. (2008). *Brunner & Sudderath textbook of medical-surgical nursing* (11th ed.). Philadelphia: Lippincott Williams & Wilkins.

Tappen, R., Weiss, S., & Whitehead, D. (1998). *Essentials of nursing leadership and management.* Philadelphia: F.A. Davis.

Venes, Donald (Ed.). (2005). *Taber's cyclopedic medical dictionary.* Philadelphia: F.A. Davis.

Videbeck, S. (2001). *Psychiatric mental health nursing.* Philadelphia: Lippincott.

Zerwekh, J., & Claborn, J. (2005). *Nursing today: Transition and trends* (5th ed.). Philadelphia: W. B. Saunders.

Index